RIGHT TO DIE VERSUS SACREDNESS OF LIFE

Edited by
Kalman J. Kaplan

T0144653

Baywood Publishing Company, Inc.
AMITYVILLE, NEW YORK

RIGHT TO DIE VERSUS SACREDNESS OF LIFE

ISBN: 0-89503-218-X (Paper)

Right to Die versus Sacredness of Life
Edited by Kalman J. Kaplan

This book has been printed simultaneously as a special issue of *OMEGA: Journal of Death and Dying*, Volume 40 Number 1, 1999-2000.

Cover Art: Jack Kevorkian at trial in March 1999, in Oakland County, Michigan

Detroit News photograph by Charles V. Tines. Used with permission.

TABLE OF CONTENTS

RIGHT TO DIE VERSUS SACREDNESS OF LIFE

INTRODUCTION

KALMAN J. KAPLAN, PH.D.*
Wayne State University and
Michael Reese Hospital and Medical Center

RIGHT TO DIE VERSUS SACREDNESS OF LIFE

We are all aware of the controversy in the United States concerning legalized abortion emerging from the *Roe v. Wade* decision of 1973. Abortion rights supporters advocated "freedom of choice" while those opposing abortion promoted "right to life." A similar debate is now occurring for doctor assisted suicide, where "right to die" advocates have been spurred on by the continuing physician-aided deaths of Dr. Jack Kevorkian in Michigan. Although the Supreme Court ruled unanimously in 1997 against a constitutional right to physician-assisted suicide, it left the matter up to individual states to decide. The results have been mixed. The voters in Oregon voted to pass the Death With Dignity Act of 1994 and reaffirmed this vote in 1998. The voters in Michigan, in contrast, voted 3 to 1 against a 1997 proposal to legalize physician-assisted suicide. The right to euthanasia (coming from the Greek "a good death") and assisted suicide have been advocated by the Hemlock Society in terms of a philosophical freedom to die. This position is not neutral, but reflects patterns of Greek thinking, especially those of the Greek and Roman Stoics. Most Biblical religions, in contrast, have strongly opposed the Hemlock Society's position, stressing the sacredness of life and the idea that only a Creator has the power to give life or to take it away. Clearly the very language in which the issue is couched, i.e., either as a

---

*The author would like to thank Flint Lachemeier, Ph.D. for his help in editing this introduction.

1

civil liberty or as a protection from totalitarianism has much to say on how it is resolved.

THE GRAECO-ROMAN WORLD

Historically, the issue underpinning the belief in the right to life and the right to death is the perception of life ownership—does God, the state or the individual own a life (Ross & Kaplan, 1993). The Graeco-Roman world was quite divided on this question. Socrates, for example was ambivalent about suicide. On the one hand, he condemns suicide on the grounds that humans are the property of the gods and have no right to do away with that which does not belong to them (Plato, *Phaedo,* 1955, p. 62b-c). At the same time, however, he describes philosophy as a "preparation for death" (p. 64a) and goes on to argue that death frees the soul from the prison of the body (Plato, *Phaedo,* 1955).

Aristotle, in contrast, opposed suicide on the grounds that the human being is obligated to the state.

> But the man who cuts his throat in a fit of temper is voluntarily doing an injury which the law does not allow. It follows that the suicide commits an injustice. But against whom? Is it not the State rather than himself? . . . It is for this reason that the State attaches a penalty (Aristotle, *The Poetics,* 1936, pp. 11-13).

Durkheim maintains that Aristotle's view underlies Greek and Roman laws on suicide (Durkheim, 1951, pp. 329-332). Suicide is illegal and prohibited when it is not authorized by the state and legal and assisted when it is so authorized. In Athens, Cyprus, and Thebes, a suicide was denied regular burial and, perhaps because of some primitive superstition, the hand of the deceased was cut off and buried separately. The punishment was even more severe in Sparta (Aeschines, 1919). On the other hand suicide was tolerated and even assisted when it had received prior state approval. In Athens, as well as in Massilia and Ceos, the suicide was actually supplied with hemlock (Maximus, 1823). According to Libanius (quoted by Durkheim, 1951, p. 330), the law in Athens read as follows: "Whosoever no longer wishes to live shall state his reasons to the Senate, and after having received permission shall abandon life."

Finally, the Roman Stoic, Seneca, an actual suicide, gave an eloquent defense of suicide as a means of control over the kind of life one should accept. "For mere living is not a good, but living well." He also stresses the quality and not the quantity of life. "Dying well means escape from the danger of living ill" (Seneca, 1979, Epistle LXX). Further, suicide is equated with liberty. "You see that yawning precipice? It leads to liberty. You see that flood, that river, that well? Liberty houses within them . . . Do you inquire the road to freedom? You shall find it in every vein of your body" (De Ira III, 15:3-4). It is clear that Seneca sees an individual as the owner of his/her own life, life as determined and fated, and suicide as freedom.

THE BIBLICAL WORLD

The attitude toward suicide in the Biblical world is much more uniform. God gives and takes life and humans must not intervene in this process in ordinary circumstances. God clearly instructs humans to choose life rather than death "so that you and your children may live" (Deut. 30;19). The first rule of criminal law which God gave Noah and his sons (i.e., all humankind) after the Flood, namely, "whoever sheds the blood of man, by man shall his blood be shed" (Gen. 9:6) was proceeded by this solemn warning: "For your lifeblood, too I will require a reckoning" (Gen. 9:5). The Rabbinic view puts it this way. "Against your will you are born, against your will you live, against your will you die. Against your will you shall in the future give account before the King of Kings" (Avot. 4:9).

Post-Biblical Talmudic opinions stress that while suicide is abominable, it is preferable to committing idolatry, adultery, or murder (Babylonian Talmud, 1975, Sanhedrin 74A). However, this refers to letting oneself be killed rather than actively killing oneself. Further, while actively assisting suicide is prohibited, removing unnatural life support systems is acceptable (Babylonian Talmud, 1975, Avodah Zarah, 18A).

THE CONTEMPORARY LEGAL CONTEXT OF PAS

The issue of doctor-assisted suicide has been a major legal consideration in recent years. In 1996, two important decisions were made separately by the Second and Ninth Circuit Courts of Appeal. The Second Circuit Court overturned the New York State law against Physician-Assisted Suicide (PAS) citing the equal protection clause of the Fourteenth Amendment of the Constitution and denying the distinction between the doctor's withholding of life-support and PAS (*Quill v. Vacco,* 1996). The Ninth Circuit Court overturned the Washington State law banning PAS citing a compelling liberty interest contained within the Fourteenth Amendment (*Washington v. Glucksberg,* 1997).

In June 1997, the U.S. Supreme Court overturned both their courts, denying that there is a constitutional right for PAS (*Washington v. Glucksberg,* 1997). More recently, however, the Supreme Court refused to hear the appeal of Oregon's "Death With Dignity" act, which was reaffirmed by the voters of Oregon in 1997. The upshot of the court position is then to deny that PAS represents a constitutional issue. However, it does not preclude individual states from enacting laws to either allow or forbid PAS.

THE OREGON SITUATION

The situation in Oregon is quite complex as the law permitting doctor-assisted suicide is paralleled by a law rationing health care. Although part of an initiative to universalize health care, the effect of the Oregon waiver to the federal

Medicaid law allows reducing medical coverage for conditions deemed too expensive or not providing sufficient benefits to a large enough number of people. The Oregon Health Services Commission ranked all medical procedures by cost and benefits. This produced a list on which a "budget line" may be drawn—providing coverage for only those procedures above the line. The height of this limbo bar (i.e., the number of procedures covered) is subject to the whim of the budget process—or in a frightening turn, may be lowered to save money for pork-barrel spending.

At least one HMO in Oregon has offered a $75 physician reimbursement for prescribing drugs to assist in a suicide. It is hard to imagine a lower reimbursement amount for any other "medical" procedure. Perhaps a severe enough budget shortfall for Medicaid could result in PAS being the *only* reimbursed medical treatment available. This is a question for the reader to keep in mind throughout the reading of the articles in this volume.

REFERENCES

Aeschines (1919). *The speeches of Aeschines (including against Ctesiphon)* (C. B. Adams Trans.). London, UK: W. Heinemann.

Aristotle (1936). *The Poetics* (S. H. Butcher Ed. and Trans.). London, UK: Macmillan.

Babylonian Talmud (1975). *Vilna Edition.* Jerusalem, Israel.

Durkheim, E. (1951). *Suicide* (J. A. Spaulding & G. Simpson Trans.). Glencoe, IL: The Free Press.

The Holy Scriptures. Philadelphia, PA: The Jewish Publication Society of America.

Maximus, V. (1823). *Valeri Maximi Factorum Dictorumque Memorabilium Liborinovem.* Londini: A. J. Valpy.

Plato (1955). *Phaedo.* (R. W. Bluck Trans.). London, UK: Routledge and Paul.

Roe vs. Wade (1973).

Ross, L. T., & Kaplan, K. J. (1993). Life ownership orientation and attitudes toward abortion, suicide, doctor-assisted suicide, and capital punishment. *Omega, 28* (1), 17-30.

Seneca, The Younger, L. A. (1979). *Seneca.* Cambridge, MA: Harvard University Press.

Quill v. Vacco (1996).

Washington v. Glucksberg, Vol U.S. (1997) see p. 228 APA Style.

WHO DECIDES? THE CONNECTING THREAD OF EUTHANASIA, EUGENICS, AND DOCTOR-ASSISTED SUICIDE*

KIRK CHEYFITZ
New York, New York

ABSTRACT

Throughout recorded history, a series of seemingly unrelated ideas have been consistently intertwined: suicide, euthanasia, infanticide, eugenics, genocide and, most recently, the practice termed physician-assisted suicide. From Plato and Hippocrates to a pair of twentieth-century American physicians named Haiselden and Kevorkian, an examination of history shows these disparate notions always involve two troublesome questions: Which lives are not worth living? And who will decide? The same examination of history teaches that separating the worthy from the not worthy is a very dangerous proposition, especially for those whose lives are deemed marginal.

When the patient died, it was exactly what the doctor intended. In fact, the physician was so morally certain the patient *ought* to die that he had called in reporters to join the deathwatch. Compliantly, his young patient expired the next night at 10 p.m. (Kuepper, 1981)

Alive, the patient was a "burden to society" and himself, the doctor told the press. Faced with a life of pain, misery, and diminished mental capacity—a life not worth living—the patient was better off dead. With those words, the physician lit a blaze of publicity that made medically sanctioned killing front-page news around the country (The Chicago Daily Tribune, Nov. 17 and 18, 1915).

The story sounds very modern and familiar. But this tall, thin, death-dispensing doctor was not Jack Kevorkian, the place was not Michigan, and the date was not yesterday or tomorrow. This was 1915, in Chicago's German-American

*Research assistance was provided by Cathy McKeown. Much of this material originally appeared in *The Detroit Free Press.*

Hospital, and the physician was the chief surgeon and hospital president, Harry J. Haiselden.

Haiselden's story is part of the history of the uses and misuses of euthanasia in America, a history which teaches important lessons: Evil things can be done for supposedly good reasons, even by doctors and even here in the United States. The way a society understands good and evil can change dramatically in a relatively short time. And America finds it relatively easy to forget its past.

The warnings of history are needed now as this country and the entire Western world once again grapple with the age-old issues of providing death to the suffering (or apparently suffering), the terminally ill (or those who appear to be terminal), and the severely impaired. Today, the central moral questions raised by euthanasia are the same as those raised by Harry Haiselden's crusade and by the entire history of this debate over some 3,000 years: Which lives are not worth living? And who will decide?

Perhaps even more importantly, understanding the past may help clarify the more immediate dilemma underlying the current euthanasia debate—American medicine's continuing, abject failure to provide comfort and care for dying people.

This medical failure comes as an historic shift toward an older population is dramatically transforming our culture. The exponential aging of the population and modern medical advances are multiplying the rate of lingering deaths. Against this backdrop, the failure to give the dying the care they want has created a practical and moral crisis for medicine, the law, and society as a whole.

This is the dying crisis. It is, without a doubt, one of the most complex and difficult issues facing the human race, and the numbers alone tell us it's going to get a lot worse before it gets better.

"I think the issue of assisted suicide is a distraction," says Dr. John W. Finn, who has sat at the bedsides, literally and figuratively, of tens of thousands of dying men, women, and children. Finn is the medical director of Hospice of Michigan, a highly praised institution which cares exclusively for the terminally ill. Without rancor, he dismisses the media "circus" surrounding Jack Kevorkian. "The issue's not about physicians and suicide. It's about how we die in this country. It's about what needs to be available and what is society doing and what do we want to offer to people. It's not about the circus" (Finn, March 1997, personal interview).

The underlying social issues were different eighty years ago, but the euthanasia debate was much the same when Dr. Harry Haiselden called a highly unusual press conference on Nov. 16, 1915. Haiselden told the world he would refuse steadfastly to perform a simple operation that could save the life of a badly deformed boy born five days earlier to Allen and Anna Bollinger, a working-class Chicago couple. "Over the next three years, he withheld treatment from, or actively speeded the deaths of, at least five more abnormal babies," writes Martin S. Pernick, a University of Michigan history professor whose book, "The Black Stork," rediscovers Haiselden's forgotten story (Pernick, 1996, pp. 3-4).

Following the death of Baby Bollinger, Haiselden pursued his euthanasia crusade very publicly, aggressively selling his ideas to a mass audience through newsreels and newspaper stories, some of which he wrote himself. He even co-wrote and starred in a feature-length silent movie, *The Black Stork*, which played in theaters for more than a quarter-century. Released in 1916, the movie fictionalized the planned death of the Bollinger baby in order to preach Haiselden's gospel that it was good for society, as well as merciful, for "defectives" to die at birth (Pernick, 1996, p. 16).

Many prominent doctors, social workers, lawyers, and judges strongly condemned Haiselden, some calling him a murderer. Illinois's attorney general demanded his prosecution. But the local prosecutor refused to seek an indictment and, at various times, Haiselden's crusade won editorial support from major newspapers in Chicago, New York, Philadelphia, Detroit, and Baltimore, and "a surprising number of prominent Americans," Pernick's history relates (Pernick, 1996, p. 7).

Haiselden, like many prominent turn-of-the-century Americans, was a believer in eugenics, a powerful movement to rid the world of certain human traits which were thought to be bad and certain diseases believed to be hereditary. Most eugenics promoters wanted to achieve their goals by not allowing the "unfit" to have children, so they pressed for, and ultimately won, state laws to allow the forced sexual sterilization of criminals, the insane, and the retarded. In 1927, the U.S. Supreme Court ruled such laws were constitutional, reasoning that they protected America from plagues of mental defects in much the same way as required immunizations protected society against smallpox (*Buck v. Bell*, 274 U.S. 200, 1927.)

Like Haiselden, however, many also saw a need to marry eugenics with euthanasia and "humanely" kill "unfit" people. Dr. Haiselden was the first to publicly turn eugenic theory to lethal action, and he soon escalated from withholding potentially life-saving treatment to actively hastening the death of deformed babies, while advocating mercy killings for a wide variety of adults.

A 1917 ad for Haiselden's movie quoted him as urging Americans, "Kill defectives, save the nations, and see *The Black Stork*," Pernick recounts in his book (Pernick, 1996, p. 88). In the summer of 1917, Haiselden took the first part of his own advice. Removing the stitches which tied off the umbilical cord of another severely malformed newborn, he let the baby bleed to death, producing more headlines around the world. Later that same year, he "prescribed potentially lethal doses of opiates" for a severely malformed infant "who was taking longer than expected to die," Pernick reports (Pernick, 1996, p. 87).

Using reasoning that will sound very familiar today, Haiselden defended actively causing death by explaining that his intent was simply to relieve the babies' suffering. Their deaths, he said, were incidental to his granting them relief. As Pernick says, however, "this doctrine could become a rationalization for almost any action." And, in fact, it soon did.

The joining of eugenics and euthanasia found its most horrifying expression in Germany, where some 100,000 mentally disturbed, retarded, and disabled Germans were given, in Adolph Hitler's words, a "mercy death" between 1939 and 1941 as part of the Nazis' now infamous T4 program. The techniques used in these "mercy killings," flooding fake shower rooms with carbon monoxide gas, soon were turned on other groups. The resulting holocaust killed millions. "Haiselden's anticipation of themes central to Nazi ideology does not make him the . . . moral equivalent of a Nazi," writes historian Pernick. "But if Haiselden's ideas did not cause the holocaust, both grew in similar soil" (Pernick, 1996, p. 167).

As Pernick and other scholars see it, the "soil" that grows such evil is the very notion upon which the entire concept of euthanasia depends—that it is possible to decide which lives are and are not worth living, which human differences are "good" and which are "bad," when life should be ended and when extended.

Inevitably, Pernick notes, such decisions are value judgments, even though the people making the judgments may claim "scientific objectivity." Haiselden and his supporters advocated using euthanasia to eliminate human traits and diseases as disparate as insanity, retardation, criminality, poverty, crippling disability, and dark skin color. Some of these traits, of course, are no longer seen as bad and most are not viewed as hereditary (Pernick, 1996, p. 15).

By the 1970s, however, when euthanasia and permitting abnormal newborns to die began being debated anew, and these same questions came forward again, America had voluntarily contracted a case of almost total amnesia regarding Harry Haiselden and the public use of euthanasia by physicians in America, Pernick points out.

Pernick, a leading expert in the history of medicine, medical ethics and mass culture, is intrigued and concerned by our collective forgetfulness. "It's pretty clear that physicians have been practicing euthanasia for centuries," he said in an interview. "But public awareness—the amount of publicity about it—is very cyclical. Each time the issue is rediscovered, the previous history has been forgotten" (Pernick, April 1997, personal interview).

Now, euthanasia is back in the news. Once again, it has been propelled to the front pages by a publicity-seeking doctor using shock tactics to get the mass media's attention. This time the form of euthanasia being promoted is called physician-assisted suicide. Once again, the practice is being widely advocated as humanitarian and passionately denounced as murder. Once again, euthanasia is being publicly performed in the United States despite laws forbidding it.

This generation's Harry Haiselden is one-time pathologist Jack Kevorkian, who has used lethal drugs and carbon monoxide to help (by his report) more than 130 people kill themselves in Michigan over the last decade. (Where local prosecutors refused to charge Haiselden with murder, Kevorkian has not been treated similarly. In April 1999, Kevorkian was sentenced in Michigan's Oakland County Circuit Court to ten to twenty-five years in prison for second-degree murder and three to seven years for illegally delivering a controlled drug. Both charges stem from the killing of a seriously ill man whose videotaped death at Kevorkian's hands was broadcast on CBS's "Sixty Minutes." Kevorkian is appealing both verdicts from his Michigan prison cell and seeking to be released on bail pending his appeals. But most legal experts are predicting Kevorkian will be in jail for years to come. Meanwhile, Kevorkian, who often threatened to starve himself to death if jailed, is reportedly eating well and permitting himself to be treated for high blood pressure. Unlike Haiselden, Kevorkian limited his practice to adults requesting to die. But like Haiselden, Kevorkian performed euthanasia to spread a set of theories. Once again, just as in Haiselden's day, it is a gospel of "planned death" which is justified because "the benefit for society is incalculable," as Kevorkian once told an Oakland County, Michigan, judge. This time the broad social benefits being claimed include more organ harvesting for transplants and more human medical experimentation, Kevorkian has said and written (Kevorkian, 1991; pp. 23, 33, 43, 74-78, 82-83, 95-98, 125-129, 133, 201).

The publicity seeking by both Haiselden and Kevorkian is "not simply self-seeking," Pernick believes. The goal is to break through the informal censorship that society and the media impose on certain ideas. In Haiselden's time, he was frequently criticized as harshly for publicizing euthanasia as for practicing it, and the same is true of Kevorkian today. "I think individuals like Dr. Kevorkian do have a great deal of ability to reshape the public agenda if they are willing to put themselves completely on the line," says Pernick, adding, "It's a tactical decision—a strategic decision. It's a way of bringing out otherwise quiet supporters and shifting the spectrum of debate" (M. Pernick, April, 1997, personal interview).

As Kevorkian has successfully shifted the focus of the public debate to physician-assisted suicide, social changes are dramatically shifting the context. When the baby boom generation begins reaching the prime dying ages in roughly thirty years, the pressures for a different way of dying in America will be at their most intense. The dying crisis will be in full howl.

The extent of the population shift is evident in the latest U.S. Census Bureau projections. "We're going to move into an era when a quarter of the population will be in the elderly age groups," says Peter Morrison, a demographer with the RAND Corporation, the well known California think-tank. This is roughly double the current percentage. By the middle of the year 2025, the oldest of the baby boomers will be in their late 70s and average life expectancy will be in the 80s, says Morrison. By then, the total U.S. population will be up 26 percent to 335 million. But the elderly population will have increased many times faster. The number of people sixty-five years old and over in America will have risen 83 percent to sixty-two million, and the population over ninety-five will have more than doubled to 1.1 million. Annual deaths will have gone from 2.3 million to more than 3 million in the same period, up nearly one-third. (U.S. Department of Commerce, Economics and Statistics Administration, Bureau of the Census, February 1996. Population Projections of the United States by Age, Sex, Race, and Hispanic Origin: 1995 to 2050. P25-1130).

Within roughly another decade, by the year 2037, the death rate will have taken an historic up-tick from less than nine deaths per 1,000 population to more than ten. And the number of Americans dying each year will be up to 3.6 million—another 20 percent jump.

"We go . . . to a plateau with a significantly higher death rate," points out morrison. "And it never goes back" (Morrison, April 1997, personal interview).

So if the dying crisis were bad weather, it would be a hurricane poised to engulf the entire country in the 2030s. Which means the present debate over the American way of death may feel like a storm, but it's really just a faint, offshore breeze.

One thing seems certain about the coming rough weather: Medicine in particular and society in general are completely unprepared for the dying crisis. Most people still fear a technological death in a modern hospital. Most doctors still do not pay attention to their dying patients' wishes. Similarly, the state of public policy and the law is completely confused. (The SUPPORT principal investigators, A controlled trial to improve care for seriously ill hospitalized patients, The Study to Understand Prognoses and Preferences for Outcomes and Risks of Treatments (SUPPORT), JAMA, November 22/29, 1995—Vol. 274, No. 20, pp. 1591-1598.)

The polls tell us that the public, by varying margins depending on the wording of the questions, approves of physician-assisted suicide under certain circumstances. In large part, of course, the public's uneasy embrace of physician-assisted suicide is merely a symptom of medicine's failure to make peace with the very modern, very popular and only partly defined notion of informed consent—the revolutionary idea that doctors must share information and decision-making power with their patients. Ordinary people tend to agree that they should play a role in making decisions about their treatment and their dying; physicians still are trained to believe that such decisions are best made by physicians.

The medical establishment certainly appears chagrined at the results of studies like SUPPORT, which demonstrate that medical decision-making is largely unburdened by considerations of the patients' wishes or desires. But rather than entertain any fundamental reforms of medical education and practice to empower patients as actors in their own care, the reaction of organized medicine has been to create a new specialty out of treating the dying, as if the dying and the "non-dying" should be clinically separated and accorded differing levels of candor and participation in their own treatment. Creating specialties and sub-specialties is how medicine traditionally has distanced itself from the patient's reality as a person, choosing to treat discrete symptoms and physical systems rather than whole people. So far the distancing act has worked and even has produced more successful medicine by producing experts in particular procedures, treatments, and disease processes. But this process of specialization has worsened the fundamental lack of honest communication between doctor and patient and so it seems that further specialization will only exacerbate the current crisis in medicine, not cure it. (For a discussion of this fundamental issue, see Katz, 1984.)

How did we get into this mess? It's a long story—at least three-millennia long. Euthanasia was extremely common in ancient times. Its practice included all the present forms, from physician-assisted suicide to causing the death of malformed newborns to simply refusing treatment to patients with serious illnesses. The reasoning behind all these ancient practices was not much different from Harry Haiselden's ideas.

The Hebrew Bible documents the ritual killing of infants in pagan societies and forbids it (2 Kings 16:2-3; 2 Kings 3: 26-27; 2 Kings 23:10; Jeremiah 7:31; Ezekiel 16:20). The book of Genesis specifically condemns the behavior of Hagar who abandons her son Ishmael because she cannot bear to watch him die from thirst in the desert (Genesis 21:15).

Some 400 years before Christ, Plato, the most influential of the ancient Greek philosophers, argued that physicians should refuse to treat chronically ill people who couldn't work. Anyone so afflicted, Plato wrote in his renowned treatise "The Republic," had a "life not worth living" (Plato, *The Republic,* III. 1. 406). Plato praised an early physician who always withheld treatment from such patients, noting "he would not try . . . to prolong a miserable existence and let his patient beget children who would likely be as sickly as himself." Thus the doctor's refusal to treat the patient not only helped end the patient's "useless" life, it also stopped the spread of "bad" human traits (Plato, *The Republic,* III. 1. 407).

Hippocrates, known as the father of modern medicine and medical ethics, seemingly originated at least part of Plato's doctrine. Born some thirty to forty years before Plato, Hippocrates once wrote that physicians should not "treat those who are overmastered by their diseases, realizing that in such cases medicine is powerless." Thus began a long tradition calling for physicians to turn their backs on the dying (Hippocratic Writings, Galv~ao~Sobrinho C.R. October 1996 journal article; History of Allied Science).

But early physicians also provided deadly drugs to their suffering, untreatable patients. This practice was common enough that the Hippocratic Oath, the original code of medical ethics, contained this pledge forbidding euthanasia: "I will neither give a deadly drug to anyone if asked for it, nor will I make a suggestion to this effect" (Hippocratic Writings, Degnin F.D. April 1997, Journal of Medical Philosophy).

In the Middle Ages in Europe, scholars find a general swing away from the Greeks' warning to leave the very ill alone. Physicians moved toward "a commitment to alleviate pain and suffering," according to Dutch philosopher and physician Gerrit Kimsma, a prominent proponent of the brand of physician-assisted suicide now practiced openly in The Netherlands. Kimsma, who teaches at the Free University in Amsterdam, describes the development of the "sleeping sponge, as they called it . . . in which various kinds of drugs were used to sedate a dying person" (Kimsma, March 1997, personal interview).

It is revealing that the modern history of euthanasia, particularly in America, is not so well documented. In fact, the only reliable, general history of euthanasia in this country is found in the unpublished doctoral dissertation of a Rutgers University student in 1981 entitled "Euthanasia in America, 1890-1960: The Controversy, the Movement, and the Law" (Kuepper, 1981).

It was August, 1891, when the first credible call was issued for laws to permit physicians to prescribe lethal drugs to suffering, terminally ill patients. The call came from Felix Adler, a prominent educator and scholar. Adler proposed a six-member commission of judges and doctors "to prevent abuses." Their job, recounts Kuepper, would be to grant death only if they could "unanimously agree on the hopeless condition of any patient requesting to die" (Kuepper, 1981, p. 32).

Two changes in American society set the stage for Adler's proposal, Kuepper maintains. One was the dwindling of religion and the rise of science. Death was becoming less a matter of God's will and more an example of nature at work. Second was the conviction, based on possibly flawed statistics, that suicide and cancer were reaching "crisis proportions." Thus, the public was simultaneously considering both suicide and painful, degenerative illnesses.

In 1906, the Ohio legislature considered the first law to permit physicians to end the lives of terminally ill or mortally injured people who were requesting death. The bill never made it out of committee, but its introduction generated more publicity for the idea.

The broad public debate in America seemingly was dominated by similar calls for voluntary euthanasia—proposals to allow rational adults, suffering and near death, to request medical help to end their lives. But, simultaneously, arguments were being advanced for involuntary euthanasia—the sorts of arguments that soon would lead to Harry Haiselden's mercy killings.

In 1900, a New York physician and author emerged as "the most noteworthy propagandist for involuntary euthanasia," writes Kuepper, proposing a "gentle, painless death" for people with severe inherited defects. W. Duncan McKim, author of "Heredity and Human Progress," suggested that candidates for death by carbonic gas would include the retarded, most epileptics, some habitual drunks, and numerous criminals (McKim, 1900, pp. 208, 209).

The euthanasia debate peaked in the late 1910s as Harry Haiselden took the stage. Then public attention waned during the 1920s. The issue was reborn in the thirties with the formation of England's Voluntary Euthanasia Legalization Society. By 1936, New York clergyman and author Charles Francis Potter had advocated that certain mentally impaired people be "mercifully executed." Soon afterwards he added the call to allow the terminally ill to request death. In 1938, Potter founded the Euthanasia Society of America (ESA), which has survived, although in much altered form, to this day (Potter, 1951, autobiography).

World War II and news of the Nazi atrocities effectively silenced the euthanasia movement in America, making any discussion of forced mercy killing politically impossible. Even when the ESA quietly began to revive after the war, its official policy was to advocate euthanasia only for terminally ill patients who asked for death. And so the debate disappeared again from public view, carried on only by a few scholars.

"The whole debate about care at the end of life really began taking off in the late '60s and early '70s," says Daniel Callahan, a Harvard-trained philosopher and one of the country's leading scholars of ethical issues in medicine. The reappearance of the issue coincided with huge advances in medical technology, giving rise to fears that dying in America had become cold, technical, ugly, isolating, painful, and needlessly extended (Callahan, March 1997, personal interview).

All these fears seem embodied in the case of Karen Ann Quinlan, the twenty-one-year-old New Jersey woman who stopped breathing and lapsed into a coma for no apparent reason at a party on the night of April 14, 1975. In the hospital, she remained comatose and on a respirator for three-and-a-half months. With no improvement in sight, her parents consulted with their priest and Karen's doctors and asked that the respirator be turned off so Karen could die peacefully. The doctors and the hospital refused. After a series of legal battles lasting six months, the Quinlans finally received court authority to remove their daughter from the respirator. With the doctors still resisting, Karen was slowly weaned from the breathing machine. Surprisingly, she could breathe on her own. She remained alive in a come for nine years, maintained by tube feedings and antibiotics, until her death on June 11, 1985, at the age of thirty-one (Healey, 1985).

The Quinlan case brought the "right to die" movement to center stage in America. Numerous similar cases were marched into court, all involving adults and infants who were being kept alive "artificially" by medical technology. "Most of the cases had one feature in common," says Callahan. "Usually, some hospital and/or some doctors didn't want to stop treating and families or patients were asking them to please stop" (Callahan, March 1997, personal interview).

Callahan, president of The Hastings Center, a bioethics think-tank in upstate New York, concludes, "I think that began to convey to the public one simple message. Namely, 'they don't let you die easily in this country, particularly if you are in a hospital.'" By 1977, Callahan says, the Gallup Poll for the first time showed more than half of Americans to be pro-euthanasia (Callahan, March 1997, personal interview).

The trend of the court decisions at the time firmly established the right to refuse medical treatment, even if such refusal clearly would lead to death. Even the Catholic Church agreed with these decisions, reasoning that no one was morally obliged to extend their life through "extraordinary" medical treatment.

This era sparked three strong movements to reform medical care for the dying, Callahan notes, all of them intended to reduce the knee-jerk use of medical technology, better relieve pain, and give the terminally ill more choice and more control over their own dying.

The first great effort was the founding of the hospice movement, which began in England in the 1960s and crossed the ocean to America in the 1970s. Hospice is a method of caring for the terminally ill. Attempts at cures are stopped so care can focus on relieving pain and providing spiritual support. Callahan explains, "The aim was, 'Let's get people in the hands of those who are particularly trained to care for the dying and let's also get them out of high-tech hospitals" (Callahan, March 1997, personal interview).

The second reform wave was the "advance directive" movement to allow people to state in advance their desire to refuse the use of aggressive medical technology. And the third major reform consisted of efforts to get physicians to communicate better with seriously ill patients, so the patients would understand their real condition and doctors would know exactly how the patients wished to be treated as the end of life approached.

"The thing that's striking is that those reform movements really did not have the effect that people expected," Callahan now says. "I think the assumption was: Put those reforms in place and it would pretty well result in proper care for the dying."

But it simply did not work. More than twenty years after the reforms were initiated, nothing much has changed.

Though hospice is widely considered a great success, too few physicians still are willing to refer their terminally ill patients to hospice programs. As a result, hospice reaches only about 325,000 people a year—less than 15 percent of the annual deaths in America. And many of these people are referred to hospice too late in their dying process to receive much benefit (National Home and Hospice Care Survey, 1993).

Advance directives haven't worked because very few people take the trouble to execute legally proper advance directives. More importantly, studies have proven, most doctors ignore advance directives.

Writing in the "Hastings Center Report," the journal of Callahan's institute, one expert gave this summation of the most important modern research study on medical care of the dying: "The findings do not depict gentle, peaceful death, but high technology run amok with poor communication, inadequate relief of symptoms, and little respect for patient preferences" (Lo, Bernard, End of life care after termination of SUPPORT, from Dying Well in the Hospital, The Lessons of SUPPORT, a special supplement to the Hastings Center Report, Nov-Dec 1995, p. 6).

The study, completed in late 1995 and known by the acronym SUPPORT, took four years, looked at over 9,000 seriously ill patients in five major teaching hospitals, and cost nearly $30 million. For the first two years, in the words of one expert commentator, SUPPORT studied "just what is to be feared about the experience of dying in American hospitals" (Dying Well in the Hospital, The Lessons of SUPPORT, a special supplement to the Hastings Center Report, Nov-Dec 1995).

It found plenty for patients to fear, including having specific instructions regarding treatment ignored by doctors, suffering through considerable pointless treatment, and dying in pain. (The SUPPORT principal investigators, A controlled trial to improve care for seriously ill hospitalized patients. The Study to Understand Prognoses and Preferences for Outcomes and Risks of Treatments (SUPPORT), JAMA, November 22/29, 1995—Vol. 274, No. 20, pp. 1591-1598.)

For the next two years, SUPPORT tried to change this dismal picture by putting a plan into action—an "intervention," in medical terms—to make dying better in the hospitals. But nothing worked. "Bluntly put," stated an independent analysis of SUPPORT in the "Hastings Center Report", "the intervention failed" (Moskowitz, E. H. and Nelson, J. L., The Best Laid Plans, from Dying Well in the Hospital, The Lessons of SUPPORT, a special supplement to the Hastings Center Report, Nov-Dec 1995, p. 5).

Perhaps the single most alarming finding of SUPPORT was that doctors routinely ignore terminal patients' requests to be left alone to die peacefully. While 31 percent of the patients expressed a desire not to be resuscitated if their hearts or breathing stopped, less than half of the doctors even knew that such requests had been made. The study also documented excessive time spent in intensive care prior to death and excessive pain for half the patients in the last three days of life, a time when there is usually little or no reason to hold back on pain-relieving drugs.

Dr. Finn, Hospice of Michigan's chief physician, cares for some 7,000 dying people each year. He is passionate about death and dying and, when the small, rumpled physician ticks off the SUPPORT study's major findings, his voice slows and the rising inflection turns statements of fact into incredulous questions. "It essentially gave medicine an F-minus in regards to care of the dying, pain management, autonomy, choices, the physician's communication with patients' families," he says. And he believes the failing grade was earned and fully deserved. "The SUPPORT study shows you can spend $30 million and get nowhere."

"You know, the real issue is that we need a different kind of physician," says Finn. "One that isn't so technically based. One that can share the patient's humanity." Finn adds that this unimaginably complex public debate is really about what the dying want. But he adds, sadly, "Reporters never ask the dying what *they* want" (Finn, March 1997, personal interview).

REFERENCES

Buck v. Bell, 274 U.S. 200, (1927).

Callahan, D. (1995). *The Hastings Center Report,* Briarcliff Manor, New York: The Hastings Center.

Chicago Daily Tribune, (November 17, 1915) page 7, *Doctor to let defective baby expire unaided.*"

Chicago Daily Tribune, (November 18, 1915) page 1, *Baby dies; Physician upheld.*

Degnin, F. D. (1997). Levinas and the Hippocratic Oath: A discussion of physician-assisted suicide, *Journal of Medical Philosophy.*

Galv~ao~Sobrinho, C. R. (1996). Hippocratic ideals, medical ethics, and the practice of medicine in the early middle ages: The legacy of the Hippocratic Oath. *Journal of History of Medical Allied Science.*

The Hastings Center (1995). *The lessons of support: Dying well in the hospital,* A Special Supplement to the Hastings Center Report, Nov-Dec 1995. Moskowitz, Ellen H.; Nelson, James Lindemann; Lo, Bernard; Marshall, Patricia A.; Annas, George J.; Emanuel, Linda L.; Brody, Howard; Berwick, Donald M.; Hardwig, John; Schneider, Carl E.; Solomon, Mildred Z.; Dresser, Rebecca; Callahan, Daniel. Briarcliff, New York: The Hastings Center.

Healey, J. M. (1985), Decisions at the end of life: The legacy of Karen Ann Quinlan, *Conn. Med.*

Holy Scriptures, The. (1995). Philadelphia: The Jewish Publication Society of America.

Katz, J. (1984). *The silent world of doctor and patient.* New York: Free Press.

Kevorkian, J. (1991). *Medicide,* Amherst, N.Y.: Prometheus Books.

Kimsma, G. (1990). *The growth of medical knowledge,* Boston: Dordrecht.

Kuepper, S. L. (1981). *Euthanasia in America, 1890-1960: The controversy, The movement, and the law.* Rutgers University, unpublished doctoral thesis.

McKim, W. D. (1900). *Heredity and human progress.* New York: Free Press.

National Home and Hospice Care Survey (1993). [Raw Data File].

Pernick, M. S. (1996). *The black stork,* New York: Oxford University Press.

Plato, *The collected dialogues.* Edited by Hamilton & Cairns. Princeton: Bollingen Foundation: Princeton University Press.

Potter, C. F. (1951). *The preacher and I,* an autobiography. New YorK.

Quill, T. E. (1993). *Death and dignity: Making choices and taking charge,* New York: Norton.

SUPPORT principal investigators (1995). A controlled trial to improve care for seriously ill hospitalized patients: The Study to Understand Prognoses and Preferences for Outcomes and Risks of Treatments (SUPPORT). *JAMA, 274* (20), 1591-1598.

Personal Interviews Conducted by the Author

Callahan, Daniel. President of the Hastings Center. March, 1997.

Finn, John W., M.D. Medical Director. Hospice of Michigan. March 1997.

Kimsma, Gerrit, M.D. March 1997. Telephone interview from his home in The Netherlands.

Morrison, Peter, Demographer. RAND Corporation. April, 1997.

Pernick, Martin, Ph.D., Professor of the History of Medicine. University of Michigan. Ann Arbor, Michigan. April 1997.

HIPPOCRATES, MAIMONIDES AND THE DOCTOR'S RESPONSIBILITY*

KALMAN J. KAPLAN, PH.D.
Wayne State University and
Michael Reese Hospital and Medical Center

MATTHEW B. SCHWARTZ, PH.D.
Wayne State University

ABSTRACT

Jack Kevorkian criticizes the Hippocratic tradition in Greek medicine, which bans the physician from giving his patient a lethal medication. He sees this prohibition as potentially bringing harm to a suffering patient and not reflective of the larger Greek society which was tolerant and even approving of suicide. However, Kevorkian's advocacy of doctor-assisted suicide can be seen as the polarity of doctor abandonment of the suffering patient rather than as an antidote to it. Both positions involve an outcome of physician removal from the suffering patient, which can be contrasted with Maimonides' command to the physician to watch over the life and death of his patients.

The right to die debate is raging across America spurred on by the assisted suicides conducted by Dr. Jack Kevorkian. The present article explores Dr. Kevorkian's philosophic base and his effort to find support in Greek philosophy, culture, and medicine. We offer in contrast a Biblical view of helping a dying patient as expressed in the physician's prayer that is attributed to Moses Maimonides. Dr. Kevorkian specifically rejects the Biblical views of life, death, and healing and remains trapped instead inside the views of the ancient Greeks of which one expression is the Hippocratic Oath. Kevorkian states his basic case as follows:

---

*An earlier draft of this article appeared in *Ethics and Medicine* (1998), *14* (2), 49-53.

17

As medical services, euthanasia and assisted suicide were always ethical, widely practiced by physicians and endorsed by almost all segments of society in Hippocratic Greece. The only opposition came from the tiny pagan religious sect called Pythagoreanism (which is said to have concocted the oath erroneously ascribed to Hippocrates). Despite their opposition, the Pythagoreans acknowledged that their contrary tenets could not be imposed on all of Greek society without seriously impairing its functional integrity. Later on there was none of that blunt honesty and respect for mores when the Western Judeo-Christian principles, which coincided almost exactly with those of extremely puritanical Pythagoreanism, dictated harshly punitive laws against euthanasia for all of society. Such laws cannot change but can only abuse and subvert ethics by paralyzing humans through brutal intimidation and fear. Eventually, in spite of all the fearful acquiescence and repressive atrocities borne of such transgression, the mores will prevail and ethics will be disabused (Kevorkian, 1992, p. 9).

In this passage Dr. Kevorkian offers several arguments. 1) Euthanasia and assisted suicide were widely practiced in Ancient Greece. Classical sources clearly support this view; 2) The Hippocratic Oath, which opposed doctor assisted suicide, has been construed to be the generally accepted Greek position when in fact it reflected the view of the small Pythagorean school. Ludwig Edelstein (1943) has argued this point convincingly; 3) Kevorkian equates Judeo-Christian principles with abuse, paralysis, and brutal intimidation on the one hand, and with what he calls Pythagorean Puritanism on the other. Here Dr. Kevorkian is seriously misled.

ARGUMENT 1: EUTHANASIA AND SUICIDE WERE WIDELY PRACTICED IN ANCIENT GREECE

With regard to the first point, there is no question that suicide was widespread in Ancient Greece and that assistance was often offered. Diogenes Laertius (1972) documents the suicides of many Greek philosophers in his classic description of their lives. The great poet John Donne (1608/1984) provides a similar list of Greek and Roman suicides in his fascinating book *Biathanatos*. The causes were sometimes so seemingly minute as a stubbed toe (Zeno the Stoic) or a gumboil (Cleanthes). The Greeks and Romans saw suicide as freedom (Seneca, *De Ira*, 3. 15. 34) because they saw life as hopeless, fatalistic, and unfree, and many killed themselves on philosophical grounds. Indeed, the early Greeks and Romans followed a number of practices which modern society would find abhorrent. 1) Child exposure, which was so widespread, that it caused a population decline by the third century B.C.E.; 2) The killing or beating of people as part of religious ceremonies; 3) The forced enslavement or massacre of prisoners of war, including women and children; and 4) The restrictions on women, who lived rather sequestered lives with very limited opportunities for self-expression and personal advancement. The Greeks gave much to mankind with their accomplishment in art, theater, government, science, and philosophy, but many of their social and religious practices would hardly be acceptable to us today.

ARGUMENT 2: HIPPOCRATES REFLECTED A MINORITY POSITION IN ANCIENT GREECE

To answer Kevorkian's second argument requires some study of the Hippocratic Oath:

> I swear by Apollo the physician, and Aesculapius, and Health, and All-heal, and all the gods and goddesses, that, according to my ability and judgment, I will keep this Oath and this stipulation- to reckon him who taught me this Art equally dear to me as my parents, to share my substance with him, and relieve his necessities if required; to look upon his offspring in the same footing as my own brothers, and to teach them this art, if they shall wish to learn it, without fee or stipulation; and that by precept, lecture, and every other mode of instruction, I will impart a knowledge of the Art to my own sons, and those of my teachers, and to disciples bound by a stipulation and oath according to the law of medicine, but to none others. I will follow that system of regimen which, according to my ability and judgment, I consider for the benefit of my patients, and abstain from whatever is deleterious and mischievous. I will give no deadly medicine to any one if asked, nor suggest any such counsel; and in like manner I will not give to a woman a pessary to produce abortion. With purity and with holiness I will pass my life and practice my Art. I will not cut persons laboring under the stone, but will leave this to be done by men who are practitioners of this work. Into whatever house I enter, I will go into them for the benefit of the sick, and will abstain from every voluntary act of mischief and corruption; and, further from the seduction of females or males, of freemen and slaves. Whatever, in connection with my professional practice or not, in connection with it, I see or hear, in the life of men, which ought not to be spoken of abroad, I will not divulge, as reckoning that all such should be kept secret. While I continue to keep this Oath unviolated, may it be granted to me to enjoy life and the practice of the art, respected by all men, in all times! But should I trespass and violate this Oath, may the reverse be my lot (p. xiii).

For Kevorkian (1991, Chapter 13), the real source of doctor's enmity toward death as the arch-enemy of medicine lies less in the Hippocratic Oath per se than in Section II of the Second Constitution of Hippocrates' treatise on epidemics, in which physicians are exhorted by the father of their calling "to do good or to do no harm." Section II of the Second Constitution of Hippocrates' treatise on epidemics contains the following passage.

> The physician must be able to tell the antecedents, know the present, and foretell the future-must meditate these things, and have two special objects in view with regard to diseases, namely, to do good or to do no harm. The art consists in three things—the disease, the patient, and the physician. The physician is the servant of the "art" (according to Galen, "nature" was substituted for "art" in many manuscripts), and the patient must combat the disease along with the physician.

Kevorkian attempts to distinguish Hippocrates' call for "the doctor and the patient to work together to combat the disease" from the position that "the doctor must heroically lead the patient off to do battle with death." Kevorkian attempts to buttress his argument through separating the word "disease" into component parts "dis" and "ease." The main, indeed the only enemy for Hippocrates, he says, is disease—that is, the disturber of a person's "ease." In having taken the oath of combating death," Kevorkian argues, "the medical profession want only infringes upon both aspects of its special and genuinely Hippocratic obligation. In quixotically trying to conquer death, doctors all too frequently do no good for their patients' ease; but at the same time they do harm instead by prolonging and even magnifying patients' dis-ease."

Kevorkian's attempt at linguistic analysis are erroneous and crude. "Disease" was not the Greek word "employed" by Hippocrates but a middle English word. Breaking this middle English word into its component parts obviously has no implications for Hippocrates' use of the word, and to assert otherwise is false and misleading.

Hippocrates' position on several important points is revealed in this passage: 1) The physician is the servant of the "art" or "nature," 2) The "art" consists of three parties: the disease, the patient and the physician, 3) The disease is the enemy, something to be combated by the patient along with the physician, 4) With regard to the disease, the physician is exhorted to do good or to do no harm, and 5) In the Hippocratic Oath per se, the physician swears to "give no deadly medicine to any one, if asked, nor suggest any such counsel."

What is notably absent in Hippocrates is any statement of the doctor's responsibility to care for a dying patient. He must not administer deadly medicine, but what shall he do to ward off death or, at least, to ease the patient's discomfort. Or shall he simply leave the patient to his fate, abandon him as the Goddess Artemis abandoned her worshipper, the hero Hippolytus when he was mortally wounded (Euripides, *Hippolytus*).

Dr. Kevorkian is correct in saying that the Hippocratic Oath is opposed to much that occurred in Greek thought. It is very significant, however, that he fails to see that both the Oath and he himself are operating within the structure of a Greek world view which was obsessed with fatalism, suicide, child exposure and death as freedom.

ARGUMENT 3: PYTHAGOREAN AND BIBLICAL PROHIBITIONS AGAINST SUICIDE ARE EQUIVALENT

In his third argument, Dr. Kevorkian incorrectly equates the mathematical Pythagorean position underlying the Hippocratic Oath with Christian anti-suicide dogma and "western Judeo-Christian principles."

In fact, suicide for the Pythagoreans was wrong because it upset an abstract mathematical discipline set by the gods. There is a set number of souls, according to the Pythagoreans, that is available in the world at any one time. Killing oneself creates a gap by upsetting this mathematical equilibrium, and thus must be rejected (Kaplan & Schwartz, 1993, p. 16).

Further, human beings reject suicide because they fear punishment

> . . . that the souls of all men were found in the body, and in the life which is on Earth, for the sake of punishment . . . On which account all men, being afraid of those threatenings of the Gods, fear to depart from life by their own act, but only gladly welcome death when it comes in old age (Athenaeus, *The Deipnosophists,* 2.216).

The punitive, cold and abstract emphasis of the Pythagorean position was not sufficient to prevent Pythagoras himself from letting himself be killed (Diogenes Laertius, 8. 45) and is not to be equated with the passionate Biblical prohibition against suicide. The Hebrew Bible describes the Creator lovingly involved with the world. He created the world solely as an act of kindness and, in the highest expression of love and benevolence toward man, created him in the divine image. To destroy or damage any human being defaces the divine image, insults and diminishes the whole of God's creation, and reduces the divine plan of love in which the world was brought into being (Soloveitchik, 1973). This is not a cold prohibition based on an abstract mathematical principle but a passionate commitment to the divine quality within each human being.

The Hebrew position is expressed in the physician's prayer attributed to Moses Maimonides, the great Jewish thinker and physician of the 12th century C. E.

> Almighty God, Thou hast created the human body with infinite wisdom. Ten thousand times ten thousand organs hast Thou combined in it that act unceasingly and harmoniously to preserve the whole in all its beauty—the body which is the envelope of the immortal soul. They are ever acting in perfect order, agreement and accord. Yet, when the frailty of matter or the unbridling of passions deranges this order or interrupts this accord, then forces clash and the body crumbles in the primal dust from which it came. Thou sendest to man diseases as beneficent messengers to foretell approaching danger and to urge him to avert it.
>
> Thou has blest Thine earth, Thy rivers and Thy mountains with healing substances; they enable thy creatures to alleviate their sufferings and to heal

their illnesses. Thou hast endowed man with the wisdom to relieve the suffering of his brother, to recognize his disorders, to extract the healing substances, to discover their powers and to prepare and to apply them to suit every ill. In Thine Eternal Providence Thou hast chosen me to watch over the life and health of Thy creatures. I am now about to apply myself to the duties of my profession. Support me. Almighty God, in these great labors, that they may benefit mankind, for without thy help not even the least thing will succeed.

Inspire me with love for my art and for Thy creatures. Do not allow thirst for profit, ambition for renown and admiration, to interfere with my profession, for these are the enemies of truth and of love for mankind and they can lead astray in the great task of attending to the welfare of Thy creatures. Preserve the strength of my body and of my soul that they ever be ready to cheerfully help and support rich and poor, good and bad, enemy as well as friend. In the sufferer let me see only the human being. Illumine my mind that it recognize what presents itself and that it may comprehend what is absent or hidden. Let it not fail to see what is visible, but do not permit it to arrogate to itself the power to see what cannot be seen, for delicate and indefinite are the bounds of the great art of caring for the lives and health of Thy creatures. Let me never be absent-minded. May no strange thoughts divert my attention at the bedside of the sick, or disturb my mind in its silent labors, for great and sacred are the thoughtful deliberations required to preserve the lives and health of Thy creatures.

Grant that my patients have confidence in me and my art and follow my directions and my counsel. Remove from their midst all charlatans and the whole host of officious relatives and know-all nurses, cruel people who arrogantly frustrate the wisest purposes of our art and often lead Thy creatures to their death.

Should those who are wiser than I wish to improve and instruct me, let my soul gratefully follow their guidance; for vast is the extent of our art. Should conceited fools, however, censure me, then let love for my profession steel me against them, so that I remain steadfast without regard for age, for reputation, or for honor, because surrender would bring to Thy creatures sickness and death. Imbue my soul with gentleness and calmness when older colleagues, proud of their age, wish to displace me or to scorn me or disdainfully to teach me. May even this be of advantage to me, for they know many things of which I am ignorant, but let not their arrogance give me pain. For they are old and old age is not master of the passions. I also hope to attain old age upon this earth, before Thee, Almighty God!

Let me be contented in everything except in the great science of my profession. Never allow the thought to arise in me that I have attained sufficient knowledge, but vouchsafe to me the strength, the leisure and the ambition ever to extend my knowledge. For art is great, but the mind of man is ever expanding.

Almighty God! Thou hast chosen me in Thy mercy to watch over the life and death of Thy creatures. I now apply myself to my profession. Support me in this great task so that it may benefit mankind, for without Thy help not even the least thing will succeed.

This approach is fundamentally different from that found in Hippocrates: 1) the physician has been chosen by God to watch over the life and health of his creatures, 2) the doctor prays for inspiration from God for love for his art and for God's creatures, the three parties being God, the doctor and God's creatures, 3) the disease is a beneficent messenger sent by God to foretell approaching danger and to urge him to avert it, 4) the physician has been chosen by God in His mercy to watch over the life and death of his creatures, and 5) the physician specifically prays to remove from his patients "all charlatans and the whole host of officious relatives and know-all nurses, cruel people who arrogantly frustrate the wisest purposes of our art and often lead Thy creatures to their death."

Maimonides can thus be contrasted with Hippocrates on at least five dimensions: 1) Whom does the physician serve? 2) Who are the relevant parties? 3) How is disease viewed? 4) What is the role of the physician with regard to good and harm, life and death? 5) What is the role of the physician with regard to inducing death?

For Hippocrates, the physician serves nature and, along with the patient, combats the disease. Maimonides, in contrast, sees the physician as serving God and views the disease as a beneficent messenger sent by God to foretell and avert approaching danger.

Hippocrates, perhaps reacting to the suicidal nature of the Greek culture, specifically forbids the doctor to give the patient any lethal medicine or to make any suggestions to that effect. But this is a cold injunction, not accompanied by a positive instruction to tend to a patient in his last hours. Maimonides gives no specific instruction to the physician not to give lethal medicine. Indeed, he does not need to, as the Biblical civilization does not equate freedom with suicide, as do the Greco-Roman Stoics, but with fulfilling God's commandments in life (*Avot,* 6.2) Maimonides' physician does pray that his patient be shielded from those charlatans, know-it-alls, officious relatives, and cruel people who would lead him to his death. In addition, however, the physician is specifically instructed to watch over the life and death of God's creatures to give them all the help and comfort possible in their last hours.

WHERE DOES KEVORKIAN GO ASTRAY?

Let us grant that Dr. Kevorkian correctly senses the lack of human compassion in the Hippocratic view, and that he sincerely wishes to alleviate the pain of his patients in the most thorough and foolproof manner. On the surface, Dr. Kevorkian does not turn his back on the dying patient like do Artemis and Hippocrates. However, he seeks to answer a Greek problem with the classic

Greek solution—suicide, which ironically also implies turning away from one's patient, of washing one's hands of the patient in distress.

Kevorkian follows in his practice the way of Sophocles' *Antigone*. Antigone's obsession with burying her dead brother leads to her own being buried alive. "Not burying the dead" symbolizes the indifference of a medicine that unfeelingly turns away from the suffering patient in need; "Burying the living" represents the approach of Dr. Kevorkian, who perhaps fearing that the patient will reach a point where he loses the ability to deal with his own pain, kills him prematurely. Dr. Kevorkian is thus a tragic figure trapped in his misguided inability to escape the Greek polarized and fatalistic vision.

It does not occur to Kevorkian to make use of the higher compassion inherent in a Biblical approach to medicine as reflected in Maimonides' prayer. Indeed, Dr. Kevorkian sees "medicine as a purely secular profession, like engineering and many others." "Any religion ought to be irrelevant to the strictly secular doctor-patient relationship." Medicine is part of the empirical world while religion belongs to the "uninvestigatable" world, and the two cannot mix.

This blind spot of Kevorkian is extremely unfortunate for it is the Biblical world that contains the hope necessary to encounter the Greek sense of despair. Physical, spiritual, and social support of the suffering patient is in harmony with the highest Biblical ideal of freedom, emphasizing the preciousness of every moment of life. Who knows how much good can result from a small act or word of goodness by an apparently insignificant person in a seemingly lost moment— even if that person is in great pain. In Maimonides' view, the doctor's caring for his patient is a religious commandment. The patient is offered freedom within that relationship. Kevorkian is too immersed in the tragic Greek vision to see this. Here freedom can only occur through suicide. Indeed suicide becomes the highest expression of freedom and death becomes a right rather than an inevitable fact. Suicide in itself becomes in itself a worthy goal and objective.

The terminality of a patient is stressed because we are afraid to face the fact that as mortals, we are all terminal. We obsess on control because we sense that we really have very little control over the most important things in our lives. Is not Kevorkian as phobic about death as the medical establishment he opposes? Shall the physician's role be to bring death or to apply as best he can the many methods, physical and psychological, of relieving pain? As Maimonides acknowledges, the physician can help bring a patient into the world. He need not abandon the patient when he leaves the world, helping him with a similar application of technical skill and compassion.

Assisting a suffering patient to kill himself is, in a sense, to help collude with the world's abandonment of him. In Maimonides' view God does not abandon the patient even in great suffering or at the moment of death. The physician acts as representative of a God who cares deeply about human life and who does not rejoice in death even of the wicked. Maybe the patient will repent and "seize his world" even in his last moment (Babylonian Talmud, *Avodah Zarah*, 11a).

Hippocrates being wrong does not make Kevorkian right. Rather, they are two sides of the same coin. The Hippocratic posture is too disengaged from the dying patient while Kevorkian becomes overly-enmeshed in the dying process. Maimonides stands as a bright and hopeful alternative to both Hippocrates and Kevorkian, providing a model for the physician to watch over the life and death of his patient who is God's creature.

Dr. Kevorkian strongly opposes religion and feels that it has no place in the doctor-patient relationship. However, a physician's medical skill alone does not in any sense qualify him to make moral decisions about a patient's life and death any more than it qualifies him to serve as a federal judge or to referee a hockey game. It takes many years of devoted study to learn enough about one's religion to serve as a religious teacher, minister, or rabbi. Obviously, scholars of religion are not qualified to perform surgeries, but they are generally far better prepared than physicians to make moral and ethical judgments even on medical issues. Remarkably too, Dr. Kevorkian makes no effort to tell us about what a patient faces after a suicide. Can we presume that suicide means the utter annihilation and termination of the individual? Or shall we follow the doctrines of Kevorkian's much admired Greeks who believed strongly in continuing existence of the soul. Who knows what will happen when we shuffle off this mortal coil. Plato and many others even wrote at length of the transmigration of souls. Homer depicted the dead warriors of the Trojan War amidst the terrible miseries of Hades. What can Dr. Kevorkian promise his patients about their own post-mortem continuance?

REFERENCES

Athenaeus of Naucratis. (1924). *The Deipnosophists*. London: Heinemann.

Babylonian Talmud. (1975). Jerusalem: Vilna Edition.

Donne, J. (1608/1984). *Biathanatos*. Ernest W. Sullivan II. Cranbury, NJ: Associated University Press.

Edelstein, L. (1943). *The Hippocratic Oath, text, translation, and interpretation*. Baltimore: Johns Hopkins Press.

Golden, W. W. (1900). Maimonides' prayer for physicians. *Transactions of the Medical Society of West Virginia, 33*, 414-415.

Hippocratic Writings. (1984). F. Adams (Tr.) In R. M. Hutchins (Ed.), *Great books of the western world, Vol. 10* (p. xiii). Chicago: The University of Chicago Press.

Holy Scriptures, The. (1955). Philadelphia: The Jewish Publication Society of America.

Kaplan, K. J., & Schwartz, M. B. (1993). *A psychology of hope: An antidote to the suicidal pathology of Western civilization*. Westport, CT: Praeger.

Kaplan, K. J., & Schwartz, M. B. (1998). Watching over patient life and death: Kevorkian, Hippocrates and Maimonides. *Ethics and Medicine, 14* (2), 49-53.

Keller, H. (1931). "Comparison between Hippocratic Oath and Maimonides' Prayer in the Ideal practice of Medicine from the Rabbinical Point of View." In *Modern Hebrew Orthopedic Terminology and Jewish Medical Essays* (pp. 142-146). Boston: Stratford Co.

Kevorkian, J. (1991). *Prescription: Medicide, the goodness of planned death.* Buffalo, N.Y.: Prometheus Books.

Kevorkian, J. (1992). A fail-safe model for justifiable medically-assisted suicide ("Medicaid"). *American Journal of Forensic Psychiatry, 13,* 7-41.

Laertius, D. (1972). *Lives of eminent philosophers.* 2 vols. R. D. Hicks (Trans.). Cambridge: MA: Harvard University Press, Loeb Classical Library.

Oates, W. J., & O'Neill, Jr. (Eds.). (1938). *The complete Greek drama,* 2 vols. New York: Random House.

Oath and Prayer of Maimonides, The. (1955). *Journal of American Medical Association, 157,* 1158.

Seneca, L. A., The younger (1979). *Seneca.* Cambridge: Harvard University Press.

Soloveitchik, J. (1973). *Bet Halevi.* New York: n. p.

GENDER, PAIN, AND DOCTOR INVOLVEMENT: HIGH SCHOOL STUDENT ATTITUDES TOWARD DOCTOR-ASSISTED SUICIDE

KALMAN J. KAPLAN, PH.D.

EVE BRATMAN

Michael Reese Hospital and Medical Center,
Wayne State University and Oberlin College

ABSTRACT

The present study concentrates on the attitudes of high school students toward active doctor-assisted suicide as described in hypothetical doctor-patient scenarios, orthogonally manipulating doctor's reaction to patient's wishes to end his/her life (whether discussed, accepted or encouraged), presence of patient's physical pain, presence of patient's emotional pain, and the gender of the hypothetical patient. Doctor-assisted suicides thoroughly discussed with the patient are judged to be more moral, acceptable, and "legal" than assisted suicides that are simply accepted by the doctor or actively encouraged by him. Significantly, this is not a distinction that is relevant in the eyes of the law. Further, the presence of *both* physical and emotional pain on the part of the patient make the patient death more acceptable in the eyes of high school students. This latter effect is striking, given the result of the Wooddell and Kaplan (1999-2000) study showing that patient depression tends to weaken acceptability of death. Finally, respondents, both male and female, tend to view deaths of patients of the opposite gender as more acceptable than patients of the same gender.

The legal controversy regarding doctor involvement in patient end of life decisions has tended to turn on two issues. First, whether the method is *passive* (i.e., withholding of a life maintaining substance or apparatus) or *active* (i.e., the introduction of a life ending substance or apparatus). Second, whether the doctor's response involves euthanasia (carrying out the act himself), assisted-suicide

27

(helping the patient carry out the end of life act), or simply observed suicide (witnessing the patient's end of life act).

With regard to the first issue, the Supreme Court makes a clear distinction (*Washington et al. v. Glucksberg et al.* 1997). The patient has the right to physician aid in passive end of life decisions (i.e., to refuse life sustaining treatment from a physician) but not in active end of life decisions (i.e., to demand a life ending substance from a physician). With regard to the second issue, euthanasia is illegal in all fifty states, while doctor-assisted suicide is illegal by law or tradition in forty-four states. It is currently legal only in one state (Oregon) and has been practiced *de facto* in another (Michigan). Witnessing the patient death is not illegal in any state.

The realities of doctor-patient relations, however, reveal that the legal distinctions do not encompass the entire psycho-social dimensions of the issue. The fear of a slippery slope, where the doctor influences the patient to make an end of life decision that do not reflect the patient's original wishes, is not limited to active euthanasia or assisted suicide. Emanuel and Emanuel (1992), for example, discussed the relationship of the doctor and the patient in regards to paternalistic, and informative models of doctor reactions. In the paternalistic model, the doctor may make decisions for the patient without exploring the patient's options and desires, and convictions. It is not hard to imagine cases where this would occur; for example, ending dialysis treatment of a patient for the good of his/her family. This act would be legally acceptable, but it is morally questionable. One can likewise imagine the situation of a doctor encouraging a patient's death, but remaining a witness to the act, thereby remaining legally secure, but perhaps morally culpable.

The results of Wooddell and Kaplan (1999-2000) reflect the difference of the psycho-social and the legal boundaries of acceptability, especially in regard to the second dimension: doctor response. Their work orthogonally manipulates the active versus passive nature of the life ending act, the degree of doctor involvement in the suicide (observed, assisted, or acted) and the doctor's reaction to the patient's wishes (discussed, accepted, or encouraged). Wooddell and Kaplan found that passive means of bringing about death were perceived as generally more acceptable than active ones. However, their results also revealed that the doctor's reaction to the patient's request to die (whether thoroughly discussed, simply accepted, or actively encouraged) was more important in determining public acceptance than the actual involvement of the doctor in the patient's death (observed, assisted, or acted) even though it is only the latter dimension which is of legal significance (observed is legal while assisted or acted are illegal). Indeed, Wooddell and Kaplan report conditions where doctor assistance or action is less unacceptable than simple doctor observance.

Wooddell and Kaplan also found that physical pain and depression were mitigating factors. Physical pain tended to make the patient's death more acceptable while depression tended to make it less acceptable. Also, the Wooddell and

Kaplan study did not manipulate the gender of the patient. Finally, in contrast to the Detroit Free Press poll (see Lachenmeier, Kaplan, & Caragacianu, 1999-2000) Wooddell and Kaplan surveyed college students rather than adults.

The present study extends that of Wooddell and Kaplan in a number of ways. First, we focus only on active rather than passive end of life acts. Second, we vary only the doctor's reaction to the patient's wishes (discussed, accepted, or encouraged) as opposed to his actual action, which we limit to assisted suicide. Third, we orthogonally manipulate the physical and emotional pain of the patient. Finally, we manipulate the gender of the patient.

Specifically, the present study asks the following six research questions:

1. Does respondent gender affect judgments of morality, legality, and acceptability of the end-of-life action taken in the hypothetical scenario, and the likelihood of the respondent behaving similarly to the patient and/or the doctor?
2. Does patient gender affect judgments of morality, legality, and acceptability of the end-of-life action taken in the hypothetical scenario, and the likelihood of the respondent behaving similarly to the patient and/or the doctor?
3. Does the degree of the patient's emotional pain affect judgments of morality, legality, and acceptability of the end-of-life action taken in the hypothetical scenario, and the likelihood of the respondent behaving similarly to the patient and/or the doctor?
4. Does the degree of the patient's physical pain affect judgments of morality, legality, and acceptability of the end-of-life action taken in the hypothetical scenario, and the likelihood of the respondent behaving similarly to the patient and/or the doctor?
5. Does the degree of doctor involvement in the patient's action affect judgments of morality, legality, and acceptability of the end-of-life action taken in the hypothetical scenario, and the likelihood of the respondent behaving similarly to the patient and/or the doctor?
6. Do any significant interactions emerge?

METHODS

Participants and Procedure

This study attempts to examine teenage perspectives on doctor assisted suicide in regard to the issues of gender, doctor involvement, and the nature of the patient's pain. The sample group contained seventy-five students from a Chicago high school (25 males and 50 females, representing an ethnically diverse group of high school juniors and seniors ages 16 to 18) were presented with twelve hypothetical scenarios describing a doctor-patient relationship involving an end-of-life action. Twelve of the twenty-five male participants were presented with scenarios involving hypothetical male patients, while the remaining thirteen males were presented with scenarios involving hypothetical female patients. Twenty-five of the fifty female respondents received "male" scenarios, while the remaining twenty-five received "female" scenarios.

Independent Variables

The twelve scenarios independently manipulated patient's emotional pain (yes or no), patient's physical pain (yes or no), and the degree of doctor involvement in the patient's suicide (discussed, accepted, or encouraged). In short, the present study manipulated five independent variables. There were two between-factors: respondent gender (male = 1, female = 2) and patient gender (male = 1, female = 2), and three within-factors: patient's emotional pain (yes = 1, no = 2) patient's physical pain (yes = 1, no = 2), and nature of doctor's reaction to patient's decision (discussed patient's decision = 1, accepted patient's decision = 2, encouraged patient's decision = 3).

Two sample scenarios are presented below.

Female—Physical Pain—Encouraged

Ruth is a patient suffering from an incurable medical condition that appears to cause her extreme physical pain without any emotional effects. Ruth approaches her doctor and explains that the physical pain is so overwhelming that she wishes to end her life. The patient requests that the doctor assist this effort by giving her a substance that will painlessly end her life. The doctor actively encourages Ruth to stick to her decision and agrees to go along with the plan by assisting Ruth in her suicide.

Male—Physical and Emotional Pain—Discussed

Duane is a patient suffering from an incurable medical condition that appears to cause him both extreme physical and emotional pain. Duane approaches his doctor and explains that his pain is so overwhelming that he wishes to end his life. The patient requests that the doctor assist this effort by giving him a substance that will painlessly end his life. The doctor has a long discussion with Duane in which they thoroughly review a number of alternative solutions, the negative consequences of his death for other people including his family, and the patient's moral and ethical beliefs regarding suicide. In the end, however, Duane wishes to end his life, and the doctor goes along with the plan by assisting Duane in his suicide.

Dependent Variables

Social attitudes were measured by seven different questions:

1. Overall, do you consider the actions/decisions of the doctor to be morally right or morally wrong? (1 = Right, 6 = Wrong)
2. Do you consider the actions/decisions of the doctor to be legal or illegal (1 = Legal, 6 = Illegal)
3. Should the actions of the doctor, as described above, be regulated by the law in any way? (1 = Yes, 2 = No)
4. In the above situation, rate the acceptability of the patient's death. (1 = Acceptable, 6 = Unacceptable)
5. If alternative treatments exist to make the patient more comfortable, rate the acceptability of the patient's death. (1 = Acceptable, 6 = Unacceptable)
6. If you were in the above patient's situation, rate the similarity of the action you would take. (1 = Completely different, 6 = Exactly the same)
7. If you were in the above doctor's position, rate the similarity of the action you would take. (1 = Completely different, 6 = Exactly the same)

Analysis

Seven five-way ANOVAS were conducted following a $2 \times 2 \times 2 \times 2 \times 3$ factorial design, with the first two variables (respondent gender and patient gender) representing between-factors. The remaining three (physical pain, emotional pain, and nature of doctor reaction) represent within-factors.

RESULTS

ANOVAS were conducted on each of the seven measures of attitudes toward the doctor-assisted suicides. We highlight the significant results below, grouping them according to main effects and interactions of each of these variables.

Respondent and Patient Gender

Table 1 presents the main effects attributable to gender, both of the respondent and the hypothetical patient.

The significant main effects are as follows:

1. Male respondents judged that the doctor's action should be regulated by the law (Mean = 1.05) more than did the female respondents (Mean = 1.16, $F = 23.95, p < .001$).
2. Male respondents rated themselves as more likely to take a similar action to that of the patients in their situation (Mean = 2.87) than did female respondents (Mean = 2.45, $F = 17.34, p < .001$). This is especially true when the patient is described as being in physical pain (Mean for male respondents = 3.59, Mean for female respondents = 2.87). A much smaller difference exists between the male and female respondents if the patients are not described as in physical pain (Male Mean = 2.15, Female Mean = 2.03, $F = 2.03, p < .01$).

Table 1. Mean Difference as a Function of Respondent and Patient Gender

Question	Respondent Gender				Patient Gender			
	Male	Female	$F(1,36)$	p	Male	Female	$F(1,36)$	p
Do you consider the actions/decisions of the doctor to be morally right or morally wrong? (1 = right, 6 = wrong)	4.04	4.03	.00	n.s.	3.93	4.14	4.20	<.05
Do you consider the actions/decisions of the doctor to be legal or illegal? (1 = legal, 6 = illegal)	3.93	3.96	.08	n.s.	3.87	4.03	1.91	n.s.
Should the actions of the doctor be regulated by law in any way? (1 = yes, 2 = no)	1.05	1.16	23.95	<.001	1.14	1.11	.81	n.s.
In the above situation, rate the acceptability of the patient's death. (1 = acceptable, 6 = unacceptable)	3.70	3.86	2.17	n.s.	3.68	3.93	6.53	<.01
If alternate treatments exist to make the patient more comfortable, rate the acceptability of the patient's death. (1 = acceptable, 6 = unacceptable)	4.91	4.88	.13	n.s.	4.83	4.95	2.17	n.s.
If you were in the above patient's situation, rate the similarity of the action you would take. (1 = completely different, 6 = exactly the same)	2.87	2.45	17.34	.001	2.80	2.38	18.81	<.001
If you were in the above doctor's situation, rate the similarity of the action you would take. (1 = completely different, 6 = exactly the same)	2.50	2.42	.64	.42	2.63	2.27	13.59	<.001

3. Respondents judged the deaths of male patients to be less morally wrong (Mean = 3.93) than those of female patients (Mean = 4.14, F = 4.20, $p < .05$).

4. The deaths of male patients were judged as more acceptable (Mean = 3.68) than the deaths of female patients (Mean = 3.93, F = 6.53, $p < .01$).

5. Respondents judged themselves as more likely to take a similar action to that of male patients (Mean = 2.80) than female patients (Mean = 2.38, $F = 18.81, p < .001$), if they were in the patient's situation.

6. Respondents judged themselves as more likely to take a similar action to that of the doctor for male patients (Mean = 2.63) than for female patients (Mean = 2.27, F = 13.59, $p < .001$). In addition, a number of significant interactions emerge between respondent gender and patient gender.

7. Male respondents judged the deaths of female patients as less morally wrong (Mean = 3.96) than the deaths of male patients (Mean = 4.13). In contrast, female respondents judged the deaths of male patients as less morally wrong (Mean = 3.83) than the deaths of female patients (Mean = 4.23, $F = 6.80, p < .01$).

8. Male respondents judged the deaths of female patients as less illegal (Mean = 3.72) than the deaths of male patients (Mean = 4.17). In contrast, female respondents judged the deaths of male patients as less illegal (Mean = 3.73) than the deaths of female patients (Mean = 4.20, $F = 13.40$, $p < .001$).

9. Given alternative treatments to make the patient more comfortable, male respondents judged the deaths of female patients as less unacceptable (Mean = 4.73) than the deaths of male patients (Mean = 5.11). In contrast, female patients judged the deaths of male patients as less unacceptable (Mean = 4.69) than the deaths of female patients (Mean = 5.07, $F = 17.80$, $p < .001$).

10. Male respondents judged themselves as slightly more likely to behave similarly to the doctor in the cases of female patients (Mean = 2.51) than in the cases of male patients (Mean = 2.49), whereas female patients judged themselves as more likely to behave similarly to the doctor with regard to male patients (Mean = 2.70) than with regard to female patients (Mean = 2.15, $F = 7.83, p < .01$).

Patient's Emotional and Physical Pain

Table 2 presents the main effects attributable to patient pain, both emotional and physical.

The significant main effects are as follows:

Table 2. Mean Difference as a Function of Patient's
Emotional and Physical Pain

Question	Emotional Pain				Physical Pain			
	Yes	No	$F(1,36)$	p	Yes	No	$F(1,36)$	p
Do you consider the actions/decisions of the doctor to be morally right or morally wrong? (1 = right, 6 = wrong)	3.74	4.33	32.56	<.001	3.60	4.47	69.99	<.001
Do you consider the actions/decisions of the doctor to be legal or illegal? (1 = legal, 6 = illegal)	3.74	4.17	13.19	<.001	3.60	4.30	35.66	<.001
Should the actions of the doctor be regulated by law in any way? (1 = yes, 2 = no)	1.13	1.11	.81	n.s.	1.13	1.12	.56	n.s.
In the above situation, rate the acceptability of the patient's death. (1 = acceptable, 6 = unacceptable)	3.44	4.18	53.27	<.001	3.19	4.42	145.85	<.001
If alternate treatments exist to make the patient more comfortable, rate the acceptability of the patient's death. (1 = acceptable, 6 = unacceptable)	4.67	5.11	26.81	<.001	4.58	5.20	53.78	<.001
If you were in the above patient's situation, rate the similarity of the action you would take. (1 = completely different, 6 = exactly the same)	2.91	2.27	43.42	<.001	3.11	2.07	111.82	<.001
If you were in the above doctor's situation, rate the similarity of the action you would take. (1 = completely different, 6 = exactly the same)	2.70	2.20	26.53	<.001	2.83	2.07	61.64	<.001

11. Patient's death was judged to be more morally right if the patient was in emotional pain (Mean = 3.74) than if the patient was not (Mean = 4.33, $F = 32.56, p < .001$).

12. Patient's death was judged to be more legal if the patient was in emotional pain (Mean = 3.74) than if the patient was not (Mean = 4.17, $F = 13.19$, $p < .001$).

13. Patient's death was judged to be more acceptable if the patient was in emotional pain (Mean = 3.44) than if the patient was not (Mean = 4.18, $F = 53.27, p < .001$).

14. Given alternative treatments to make the patient more comfortable, his death was considered to be more acceptable if the patient was in emotional pain (Mean = 4.67) than if the patient was not (Mean = 5.11, $F = 26.81, p < .001$).

15. Respondents judged themselves to be more likely to behave similarly to the patient if the patient was in emotional pain (Mean = 2.91) than if the patient was not (Mean = 2.27, $F = 43.42, p < .001$).

16. Respondents judged themselves to be more likely to behave similarly to the doctor if the patient was in emotional pain (Mean = 2.70) than if the patient was not (Mean = 2.20, $F = 26.53, p < .001$).

17. Patient's death was considered to be morally right if the patient was in physical pain (Mean = 3.60) than if the patient was not (Mean = 4.47, $F = 69.99, p < .001$).

18. Patient's death was considered to be more legal if the patient was in physical pain (Mean = 3.60) than if the patient was not (Mean = 4.30, $F = 35.66, p < 001$).

19. Patient's death was considered to be more acceptable if the patient was in physical pain (Mean = 3.19) than if the patient was not (Mean = 4.42, $F = 145.85, p < .001$).

20. Given alternative treatments to make the patient more comfortable, the patient's death was considered to be more acceptable if the patient was in physical pain (Mean = 4.58) than if the patient was not (Mean = 5.20, $F = 53.78, p < .001$).

21. Respondents judged themselves as more likely to behave similarly to the patient if the patient was in physical pain (Mean = 3.11) than if the patient was not (Mean = 2.07, $F = 111.82, p < .001$).

22. Respondents judged themselves as more likely to behave similarly to the doctor if the patient was in physical pain (Mean = 2.83) than if the patient was not (Mean = 2.07, $F = 61.64, p < .001$).

In addition, the following significant interactions emerge between the patient's emotional and physical pain:

23. Patient's death was judged to be least immoral if the patient was in both emotional and physical pain (Mean = 3.49) than if he was in neither

physical nor emotional pain (Mean = 4.95). If the patient was only in physical pain his death was judged as less immoral (Mean = 3.71) than if the patient was only in emotional pain (Mean = 3.98), although both of these conditions were judged to fall between the two extreme conditions discussed above ($F = 13.30, p < .001$).

24. Patient's death was judged to be least illegal if the patient was in both physical and emotional pain (Mean = 3.58) and slightly more illegal if the patient was in only physical pain (Mean = 3.62). The death of a patient only in emotional pain was judged to be somewhat more illegal (Mean = 3.90), while the death of a patient in neither physical nor emotional pain was judged to be moderately illegal (Mean = 4.71, $F = 10.78, p < .001$).

25. Patient's death was judged at least unacceptable if the patient was in both emotional and physical pain (Mean = 3.04) than if the patient was in neither physical nor emotional pain (Mean = 4.83). If the patient was only in physical pain his death was judged as less unacceptable (Mean = 3.34) than if the patient was only in emotional pain (Mean = 5.01, $F = 19.09$, $p < .001$).

26. Respondents judged themselves as more likely to behave similarly to the patient if the patient was in both emotional and physical pain (Mean = 3.34), and least similarly to the patient if the patient was in neither physical nor emotional pain (Mean = 1.65). The respondents judged themselves as more likely to emulate the patient's decision if the patient was only in physical pain (Mean = 2.88) than if the patient was only in emotional pain (Mean = 2.49), although both of these conditions were judged to fall between the two extreme conditions discussed above ($F = 3.70, p < .05$).

27. Respondents judged themselves as more likely to behave similarly to the doctor if the patient was in both emotional and physical pain (Mean = 2.93), and least similarly to the doctor if the patient was in neither physical nor emotional pain (Mean = 1.67). The respondent judged himself as more likely to emulate the doctor's decision if the patient was only in physical pain (Mean = 2.73) than if the patient was only in emotional pain (Mean = 2.47), although both of these conditions were judged to fall between the two extreme conditions discussed above ($F = 9.83, p < .01$).

Finally, Table 3 presents the main effects due to the degree of doctor reaction to the patient's decision.

Doctor Reaction to Patient Decision

The main effects are as follows:

28. The patient's death was considered to be less immoral if the doctor had discussed the patient's decision with him (Mean = 3.23) than if the

Table 3. Mean Difference as a Function of Doctor's Reaction
to Patient Decision

Question	Discussed Decision	Accepted Decision	Encouraged Decision	$F(2,36)$	p
Do you consider the actions/decisions of the doctor to be morally right or morally wrong? (1 = right, 6 = wrong)	3.23	4.37	4.50	61.13	<.001
Do you consider the actions/decisions of the doctor to be legal or illegal? (1 = legal, 6 = illegal)	3.39	4.20	4.27	23.24	<.001
Should the actions of the doctor be regulated by law in any way? (1 = yes, 2 = no)	1.17	1.09	1.11	4.73	<.01
In the above situation, rate the acceptability of the patient's death. (1 = acceptable, 6 = unacceptable)	3.40	4.06	3.96	16.35	<.001
If alternative treatments exist to make the patient more comfortable, rate the acceptability of the patient's death. (1 = acceptable, 6 = unacceptable)	4.70	4.99	4.98	5.06	<.01
If you were in the above patient's situation, rate the similarity of the action you would take. (1 = completely different, 6 = exactly the same)	2.72	2.46	2.59	2.40	n.s.
If you were in the above doctor's situation, rate the similarity of the action you would take. (1 = completely different, 6 = exactly the same)	3.19	2.09	2.07	58.64	<.001

doctor either simply accepted (Mean = 4.37) or actively encouraged (Mean = 4.50) the patient's decision ($F = 61.13, p < .001$).

29. The patient's death was considered to be less illegal if the doctor had discussed the patient's decision (Mean = 3.39) than if the doctor simply accepted (Mean = 4.20) or actively encouraged (Mean = 4.27) the patient's decision ($F = 23.24, p < .001$).

30. Respondents were less inclined to judge that the doctor's actions should be regulated by law if the doctor had discussed the patient's decision (Mean = 1.17) than if the doctor had simply accepted (Mean = 1.09) or actively encouraged (Mean = 1.11) the patient's decision ($F = 4.73$, $p < .01$).

31. The patient's death was considered to be more acceptable if the doctor had discussed the patient's decision (Mean = 3.40) than if the doctor had either accepted (Mean = 4.06) or encouraged (Mean = 3.96) the patient's decision ($F = 16.35, p < .001$). This effect is more pronounced for male than female respondents. Male respondents judged the patient's death as more acceptable if the doctor discussed the decision with the patient (Mean = 3.03) than did female respondents (Mean = 3.59). No such gender difference was found in terms of the acceptability of the patient's death when the doctor simply accepted the patient's decision (Male Mean = 4.09, Female Mean = 4.05) or when the doctor actively encouraged the patient's decision (Male Mean = 3.99, Female Mean = 3.94, $F = 3.46, p < .05$).

32. Given the possibility of alternative treatments to make the patient more comfortable, the patient's death was judged to be more acceptable if the doctor had discussed the patient's decision (Mean = 4.70) than if the doctor either simply accepted (Mean = 4.99) or actively encouraged (Mean = 4.98) the patient's decision ($F = 5.06, p < .01$).

33. Respondents judged themselves as more likely to behave similarly to the doctor if the doctor had discussed the patient's decision (Mean = 3.19) than if he had simply accepted (Mean = 2.09) or actively encouraged the patient's decision (Mean = 2.07, $F = 58.64, p < .001$).

DISCUSSION AND CONCLUSIONS

The results may be summarized as follows:

1. Male respondents are more likely to feel that the doctor's behavior should be legally regulated by law than are female respondents, though no difference exists between the two genders with regard to their judgment of the moral acceptability of the doctor's behavior. Finally, male respondents are more likely to identify with the patient's decision to end his/her life, especially under conditions of physical pain, than are female respondents.

2. The assisted suicides involving male patients were judged to be significantly more moral, more acceptable, and easier to identify with than those involving female patients. No such patient gender difference emerged regarding attitudes toward legal regulation.

3. Respondents of each gender found that doctor-assisted suicide scenarios involving patients of the opposite gender to be more moral, legal, and acceptable than of scenarios involving their own gender. In other words, male respondents found female assisted suicides more acceptable, while female respondents found male assisted suicides more acceptable.

4. The deaths of patients in emotional pain were judged as more moral, acceptable, legal, and easier to identify with than those not in emotional pain. This tendency exists for both male and female respondents.

5. The deaths of patients in physical pain were judged as more moral, legal, acceptable, and easier to identify with than those not in physical pain. This tendency is accentuated for male as compared to female respondents.

6. The effects of emotional and physical pain seem to augment, rather than diminish, each other. That is, the deaths of patients in both physical and emotional pain were judged to be more acceptable, legal, and easier to identify with than the deaths of patients with only one source of pain, which in turn were judged to be more acceptable than the deaths of patients in neither physical nor emotional pain. Physical pain seems to be more important in increasing the acceptability of doctor-assisted suicide than emotional pain. The effects of the patient's physical pain are greatest in this regard in the absence of emotional pain, and the effects of emotional pain are greatest in the absence of physical pain.

7. Patient's deaths are generally judged to be more moral, acceptable, legal, and easier to identify with when the doctor has discussed the patient's decision with the patients than when the doctor either simply accepts or actively encourages the patient's decision. The difference is more pronounced for male as compared to female respondents. Whether the doctor accepted or actively encouraged the patient's decision did not significantly affect the acceptability of the patient's death.

A number of significant implications emerge from the above results.

First, the study highlights the differences in respondent judgment between issues of morality, legality, and acceptability in regard to assisted suicides. While all of the scenarios presented in the survey are illegal, respondents clearly felt that doctor's reaction to the patient's death request not only affects the acceptability and the morality of the act, but also whether it should be regulated legally, based on the doctor's level of discussion, acceptance, or encouragement of the patient's decision.

Second, the study highlights the important and potentially dangerous role of gender in the end of life decision. Each gender felt that the death of the opposite gender was more legal, acceptable, and moral than the death of one's own gender. This finding is highly significant in regard to the Kevorkian patients, where 67 percent of the patients were women, and these women show a lesser degree of terminality and objective signs of pain (Kaplan & deWitt, 1996; Kaplan, Lachenmeier, Harrow et al., 1999-2000; Kaplan, O'Dell, Dragovic et al., 1999-2000). This may indicate that many of these women patients have committed suicide for psychosocial rather than medical reasons. This is particularly plausible in light of national gender differences in regard to suicide: in 1993, four times as many men than women *completed* suicide, whereas three times as many women than men *attempted* suicide. Thus, it is possible that Kevorkian's assisted suicides represent the attempted suicides of the population rather than the completed suicides. His suicide patients often draw attention to the feeling of misery of the patient rather than the patient's certainty in their desire to die; further, Kevorkian has sometimes encouraged a patient in suicidal plans about which they were initially ambivalent. There may also be a correlation between the legality of assisted suicides and the level of female assisted suicides. Before the Michigan law against assisted suicide was signed by the governor, Kevorkian assisted the suicides of eight females and no males. In the time in between the signing of the law against assisted suicide and his acquittal on charges of assisted suicide, Kevorkian killed nine females and eleven males. In the time period following his acquittal, Kevorkian killed two males and nine females. These data suggest that the legalization of assisted suicide may encourage this solution for women. Thus, the correlation between the gender of the patient and the occurrence of the suicide has definite implications not only in terms of the perceived "acceptability" of the death, but also in terms of legality issues.

Third, the study helps to convey the question of emotional pain and its relation to doctor-assisted suicide. This represents an important point of difference from the Wooddell and Kaplan study. Wooddell and Kaplan (1999-2000) specifically described the patient's emotional pain as depression, and found that it *diminished* the acceptability and morality of the doctor-assisted suicide. In the present study, the definition was left more open, not precisely specifying the exact nature of the emotional pain. Here emotional pain further *increased* the acceptability of the doctor-assisted suicide.

The exact nature of the physical pain of the patient is also an important issue. This is true in the present study, in the Wooddell and Kaplan study (1999-2000), and in Dr. Kevorkian's patients. For example, Marjorie Wantz, Dr. Kevorkian's second assisted suicide, claimed that she had intense physical pain in her vagina. Autopsy revealed however, no physical reason for her pain. Indeed, all of her reproductive organs had been removed in surgery several years before her death. Thus, this discrepancy regarding the nature and definition of suffering may be a significant slippery slope in terms of the patient's decision to commit suicide, the doctor's involvement in the patient's decision, the possibility of alternative treatments for the pain, and as the current study reveals, the overall acceptability of the death of the patient. More generally, the autopsies show that Kevorkian's female patients have less anatomical basis for pain than do his male patients, even though the two genders report equal levels of pain. Is some of this pain masked depression, and how does this affect attitudes toward assisted suicide?

Finally, both this study and that of Wooddell and Kaplan (1999-2000) indicate the importance psychologically of the doctor's reaction to the patient's wish rather than to his actual action, which is of more legal consequence. What young people in these samples seem to be worried about is that a doctor will encourage a depressed patient to take his or her own life, not whether his act is assisted suicide or euthanasia. This issue is not currently effectively addressed. Most of the worst doctor abuses in patient deaths may be currently legal and not directly related to the debate regarding doctor-assisted suicide or euthanasia. Encouraging a patient to die, even if it is by the patient's own hands without any physical assistance, is seen as unacceptable, immoral, and illegal. The doctor's tremendous potential influence on the patient makes this issue especially dangerous in the present period of changing conceptions in health care.

REFERENCES

Emanuel, E. J., & Emanuel, L. J. (1992). Four models of the physician-patient relationship. *Journal of the American Medical Association, 267,* 2221-2226.

Kaplan, K. J., & De Witt, J. (1996). "Kevorkian's list:" Gender bias or what? *Newslink, 22,* 1, 14.

Lachenmeier, F., Kaplan, K. J., & Caragacianu, D. (1999-2000). Doctor-assisted suicide: An analysis of public opinion of Michigan adults, *Omega, 40* (1), 61-87 (this issue).

The New York State Task Force on Life and the Law. (1994). *When death is sought: Assisted suicide and euthanasia in the medical context.* New York: New York State Task Force on Death and the Law.

Washington et al. v. Glucksberg et al. U.S. 996-110, 95-1858, 1997.

Wooddell, V., & Kaplan, K. J. (1998). An expanded typology of suicide, assisted suicide and euthanasia, *Omega, 36,* 201-208.

Wooddell, V., & Kaplan, K. J. (1999-2000). Effect of the doctor on college students' attitudes toward physician-assisted suicide. *Omega, 40* (1), 43-60 (this issue).

EFFECT OF THE DOCTOR ON COLLEGE STUDENTS' ATTITUDES TOWARD PHYSICIAN-ASSISTED SUICIDE

VICTOR WOODDELL, PH.D.

KALMAN J. KAPLAN, PH.D.

Wayne State University and
Michael Reese Hospital and Medical Center

ABSTRACT

Ninety-six students were presented with eighteen different vignettes describing different types of active and passive observed suicide, assisted suicide, and euthanasia. Attitudes regarding the morality and desired legality of each situation were measured. Results indicate that the interaction between the doctor and the patient, and, to a lesser extent, the active or passive nature of the agent of death, were more important than the actual actions of the doctor in allowing or causing death to occur.

In a previous article, the authors (Wooddell and Kaplan, 1998) presented a typology graphically depicting different types of suicide according to the actions and reaction of the doctor, as well as the nature of the agent of death. This typology presented twenty-four types of suicide ranging from private unobserved suicide to enforced euthanasia, and included physician assisted, as well as observed, suicide. The emphasis of that typology was on the doctor-patient relationship: whether the doctor discussed, accepted, or encouraged the patient's desire to die, and whether the doctor observed, assisted, or carried out the act of death. In addition, active and passive methods of dying were distinguished. This typology is presented in Figure 1.

Frank Boehm, a physician who has written on a wide variety of medical issues, has made distinctions which are useful in the context of this discussion (Boehm, 1997). One distinction is between treatment which is intended to relieve pain, but which may cause death (i.e., delivering large doses of pain killers), and actions

Doctor's Action:	Patient's Decision is:						
	Solitary/ Private	Disapproved/ Refused	Discussed/ Debated	Accepted/ Allowed	Encouraged/ Pressured	Unconsulted/ Incapable	Ignored/ Over-Ruled
Doctor Unaware	Solitary Suicide	X	X	X	X	X	X
Doctor Uninvolved	X	Disapproved Suicide	X	X	X	X	X
Doctor Observes	X	X	Discussed Observed Suicide	Accepted Observed Suicide	Encouraged Observed Suicide	X	X
Doctor Assists	X	X	Discussed Assisted Suicide	Accepted Assisted Suicide	Encouraged Assisted Suicide	X	X
Doctor Acts	X	X	Discussed Voluntary Euthanasia	Accepted Voluntary Euthanasia	Encouraged Voluntary Euthanasia	X	X
Doctor Decides	X	X	X	X	X	Nonvoluntary Euthanasia	X
Doctor Imposes	X	X	X	X	X	X	Involuntary Euthanasia

In each category, the agent of death can be: Active (adding, increasing, or continuing something life-destroying); Passive (subtracting, decreasing, or withholding something life-preserving).

Figure 1. Death Typology

which are explicitly intended to cause the death of the patient (even if death is seen as a way of relieving suffering). He also makes a distinction between the stopping of treatment which may cause death and the administration of a substance which is certain to cause death. Boehm's conclusion is that doctors cannot resolve these dilemmas themselves, but require guidelines and direction that can only come from social debate and consensus. In terms of our typology, Boehm's second distinction is a contrast between active and passive modes of euthanasia (doctor commits the act). Other authorities also emphasize a moral difference between the two modes, often highlighting the difference between "passive euthanasia" and (active) "assisted suicide" (Glick, 1992).

Searles (1995) has conducted a study of Manitoba physicians regarding their attitudes toward physician assisted suicide and euthanasia. In that study, 88 percent of the 112 physicians who responded agreed that stopping treatment was ethically different from assisting a suicide. Yet 60 percent also agreed that in the case of a patient with an incurable disease and great suffering the law should allow a doctor to help end the patient's life. On the other hand, Hendin (1995) argues that legalizing physician assisted suicide and euthanasia would be a very dangerous and unnecessary solution, given the availability of therapy for suicidal depression. Hendin, who is also a medical doctor, makes no distinction between euthanasia and assisted suicide in either the passive or active modes.

Yet it is apparent that all of these arguments are given from the point of view of the doctor. And as Hendin (1995) points out, it is not enough to simply ask people "Are you in favor of euthanasia?" Boehm's social consensus can only result from a more in-depth analysis of the way people frame this issue. Do educated members of the public make the same distinctions as medical professionals? Do they agree with the concerns voiced by doctors, or do they come to different conclusions?

In his analysis of euthanasia and popular culture, as exemplified by an early twentieth-century movie "The Black Stork," Pernick (1996) points out several important dimensions of the current debate. One of these is a supposedly modern emphasis on individual autonomy and empowerment, although thoughtful advocates recognize that individual preferences need to be regulated in some way. It is not unlikely that members of the public frame their opinions in terms of their own perceived power of choice in such situations, thus leading them to reject a doctor who either refuses categorically to consider carrying out their wishes, or who encourages patients to die.

The goal of this study is to gauge the attitudes of college students by presenting them with a series of vignettes describing hypothetical examples of a doctor interacting with a patient who has requested to die. Various types of observed suicide, assisted suicide, and euthanasia are described, and a number of "mitigating circumstances" are presented, in order to evaluate the "Zone of Acceptance," if there is any, that people may have toward these situations. It is hoped that these results will assist policy makers and concerned citizens in forming a fuller understanding of the dimensions of this issue.

METHOD

Participants

A total of ninety-six students were recruited from several undergraduate psychology courses being offered at a large mid-western university. This sample included fifty-nine white students, twenty-seven African-American students, and ten students of other ethnic backgrounds. Eighteen male and seventy-five female students participated.

Procedure

These students were recruited from courses for which permission had been granted by the course instructor. While not a random selection of courses, a large enough selection of courses were included in the study that it was felt the resulting sample was fairly representative of the student body at large. All students within each course were given the survey to complete during class time. Assignment to the three experimental groups was done randomly, and students in each class were assigned to each of the three groups.

Conditions

Eighteen different vignettes were employed to represent the different experimental conditions. Each participant was given six scenarios to read, with the same questions to answer after reading each scenario. Three different sets of six scenarios each corresponded to each of the experimental groups. One between-groups and two within-subjects variables were included within this study. "Doctor's Actions" was the between-groups variable and consisted of three levels: Doctor Only Observes Death, Doctor Assists the Death, Doctor Commits the Act. The two within-subjects variables included "Type of Death Agent" and "Doctor's Reaction (or response) to Request for Death." Type of Death Agent consisted of two levels: Active (i.e., a toxin) or Passive (i.e., withdrawal of treatment). Doctor's Response to Request for Death consisted of three levels: Doctor Discusses Implications of Request, Doctor Accepts Request Without Comment, and Doctor Encourages Decision to Die. This yielded a $3 \times 2 \times 3$ mixed between/within design, and each combination of factors was represented by a different vignette. These vignettes were constructed by matching together phrases corresponding to each experimental condition. Two sample vignettes are presented in Table 1.

Table 1. Sample Vignettes

(Doctor Discusses, Observes, Passive Agent of Death)

A patient receiving treatment for a serious medical condition approaches his/her doctor and explains that he/she no longer wishes to continue receiving the treatment which is keeping him/her alive. The patient is aware that this will result in his/her own death. However, the patient requests that the doctor remain with the patient until the patient dies. The doctor has a long discussion with this patient in which they review a number of alternative solutions, the negative consequences of the patient's death for other people including the patient's family, and the patient's moral and ethical beliefs regarding suicide. In the end, however, the patient still wishes to end their own life, and the doctor goes along with this decision.

(Doctor Encourages, Commits Act, Active Agent of Death)

A patient suffering from a serious medical condition approaches his/her doctor and explains that he/she wishes the doctor to give them a substance which will end his/her life. The patient requests that the doctor inject the chemical which will kill the patient. The doctor is very supportive of this idea and encourages the patient in this decision by expressing approval and agreeing that the patient's present condition makes life not worth living.

Measures

The same ten questions immediately followed each vignette. The first item asked "Overall, do you consider the actions of the doctor to be morally right or morally wrong?" This was followed by a 6-point scale ranging from 1= right to 6 = wrong. The next item asked "Should the actions of the doctor, described above, be regulated by law in any way?" This was followed by the choices Yes and No. Next, participants were instructed to use a 6-point scale ranging from 1 = legal to 6 = illegal to answer the next seven items.

The next item, item 3, simply asked "Should the actions of the doctor, described above, be legal or illegal?" The next three items, 4 through 6, concerned various mitigating circumstances which were felt might change the attitude of the respondent toward the actions described in the scenario. These first three items concerned circumstances which are often given as reasons for physician-assisted suicide. These included: "What if the patient, described above, is suffering from intense, constant pain?," "Now imagine that the patient described above is not in intense, constant pain, but is terminal, that is, has less than a year to live," and "Now imagine that the patient described above is not in intense, constant pain and is not terminal, but is physically incapable of taking care of himself or herself." In each case, these statements were followed by "Should the actions of the doctor, described above, be legal or illegal?" and the 6-point scale described above.

The next three items, items 7 through 9, concerned mitigating circumstances which were felt might decrease the legality of the doctor's actions. These included "Now imagine that the patient, described above, does not have any physical problems but is afflicted with a loss of mental capacity, for example as a result of Senile Dementia or Alzheimer's Disease," "Now imagine that the patient described above does not have any physical problems, and has not lost mental capacity, but has been diagnosed as experiencing severe clinical depression, a mental condition which can affect judgment (but is often treatable)," and "Now imagine that the patient does not have any physical problems and has not lost mental capacity nor is severely depressed, but that some alternative type of treatment is available to make the life of the patient described above more comfortable (hospice care, pain control, etc.)." Each of these statements were followed by "Should the actions of the doctor, described above, be legal or illegal?" and the 6-point scale. The last item, item 10, asked "If you were the patient described in the story above, would you do the same thing?" This was followed by the options Yes and No.

RESULTS

The mean response to each item, for each experimental condition, is displayed in Table 2. The scale scores correspond to the following: 1 = right and 6 = wrong for item 1, and 1 = legal and 6 – illegal for items 3 through 9 (see Table 2). Two different patterns of results are evident from an examination of Table 2, one regarding the independent variables and one regarding the dependent variables. Table 2 is arranged so that the independent variables (the experimental conditions) are displayed in the columns ranging from left to right. The different dependent variables in the study (the various "Mitigating Circumstances") are displayed in rows from top to bottom. Thus, there are two different patterns of results to discuss, a "right to left" pattern of the effects of the experimental conditions, and a "top to bottom" pattern of the effects of different mitigating circumstances. These will be discussed independently.

EXPERIMENTAL EFFECTS

Mean Differences

To begin with, the effects of Doctor's Reaction to Patient's Request (Discusses, Accepts, Encourages) and Agent of Death (Passive, Active) are statistically significant with regard to an APAS score formed by combining the scores of items 1 and 3 through 9 (F-Reaction = 48.88, $p < .01$; F-Agent = 9.22, $p < .01$) while the effects of Doctor's Action (Observes, Assists, Acts) are not (F-Action = .52, $p = .06$). These same patterns also hold for the individual items "Are Doctor's Actions Morally Right or Wrong?" (F-Doctor's Reaction = 67.64, $p < .01$,

F-Death Agent = 19.89, $p < .01$, F-Doctor's Action = .51, $p = .61$), and "Should Doctor's Actions be Regulated by Law?" (F-Doctor's Reaction = 51.84, $p < .01$, F-Death Agent = 18.54, $p < .01$, F-Doctor's Action = .74, $p = .48$). In addition they also hold for the six "Extenuating Circumstances" items, except for Doctor's Reaction with regard to Depression ($F = 3.75$, $p = .03$), and the nonsignificant effects of the Agent of Death with regard to Mental Incapacity ($F = 3.56, p = .06$), Depression ($F = 2.77, p = .10$) and Alternative Treatment ($F = 1.37, p = .25$).

The only significant interaction emerges between Doctor's Reaction and Agent of Death, and here only for the overall APAS score ($F = 4.27$, $p = .02$), Morality ($F = 11.62$, $p < .01$), Legality ($F = 10.32$, $p < .01$), and the single extenuating circumstance of Pain ($F = 5.86$, $p < .01$). The specific pattern is for the discrepancy between a Passive Agent of Death (more acceptable in all cases) and an Active Agent (less acceptable in all cases) is greater in the Doctor Discusses condition then in the Doctor Encourages condition. It is interesting to note that in the Doctor Encourages condition, a Passive means of death (removal of treatment) has become as unacceptable to the participants as a more Active one.

As can be seen in Table 2, there is an overall pattern of greatest approval to least approval across the conditions. Table 2A is deliberately arranged such that the conditions which created greatest approval are displayed to the left (Discussed/Passive/Acts) and conditions which created progressively less approval are displayed to the right. The perceived morality and legality of the suicide declines, first, with respect to the Doctor's Reaction to the Patient's Request (i.e.,—from Discusses to Accepts to Observes), second, with respect to the Agent of Death (from Passive to Active), and finally, with respect to the Doctor's Action (Committed Act to Assisted to Observed). Thus, the Discussed/Passive/Doctor Commits Act condition receives the most approval, and the Encouraged/Active/Doctor Observes condition receives the least support. As can be seen in Table 2, a cell mean can be included within a Zone of Acceptance if the cell mean was less than 3.5 (a lower score indicates greater acceptability) and within the Zone of Rejection if it was equal to 3.5 or more. Table 2B presents the significance level of the effects of differences due to the experimental conditions.

Looking first at the APAS score (created by averaging the answers for items 1 and 3 to 9), Passive/Discussed Assisted Suicide, or suicide in which the doctor discusses with the patient all the options and implications of the current situation, is seen as acceptable, ranging from 2.8 to 3.2. An Active Agent of Death is also seen as acceptable, but only if the doctor actually commits the act. If the doctor only assists or observes the patient carry out an active suicide, this is not seen as acceptable, nor is any other combination of conditions. In terms of the APAS score, then, discussion with the patient produces the strongest acceptance. The APAS score itself (for reliability, see below) is only an average across several individual items, and looking at the results for some of the individual items, although the overall pattern is very consistent, can still be useful.

Table 2A. Mean Responses and Zones of Acceptance

	Condition:					
	Doctor Discusses					
	Passive Agent			Active Agent		
	Acts	As'st	Obsv	Acts	As'st	Obsv
APAS Scale	2.8	2.9	3.2	3.0	3.5	3.6
Items						
1: Morality	1.8	2.3	2.3	2.4	3.6	3.1
3: Legality	1.8	2	2.3	2.3	3.2	3.2
Circumstances						
4: Pain	1.8	2.3	2.2	2.2	3.2	3.0
5: Terminal	2.4	2.3	2.8	2.4	2.8	3.0
6: Physical	2.7	3.0	3.2	2.8	3.1	3.4
7: Mental	3.6	3.3	3.7	3.7	3.4	3.9
9: Alternative	3.9	3.9	4.3	4.1	4.0	4.3
8: Depressed	4.3	4.4	4.8	4.4	4.7	4.7

Acts = Physician commits killing act himself. $n = 42$
As'st = Physician assists patient in killing self. $n = 38$
Obsv = Physician only observes without participation. $n = 37$

Items 1 and 3 will be examined first (items 2 and 10 are discussed under "Dichotomous Items," and 4 to 9 are discussed under "Mitigating Circumstances," below). For item 1 (Do you consider the doctor's actions to be right or wrong?) all forms of Discussed Suicide, by both Passive and Active means, are rated as being morally right, except when the doctor assists an active suicide. Only Doctor Discusses Suicide is morally right, all of the other conditions, including Doctor Accepts Suicide and Doctor Encourages Suicide, are seen as morally wrong (that is, they have an average rating of 3.5 or above on a 6-point scale). Doctor Discusses Suicide was also rated as "Should be Legal" (item 3), as was Doctor Accepts Suicide when the suicide is by a passive means and the doctor commits the act (but only just, the average rating was 3.3). No other combination of conditions was rated as "Should be Legal."

To summarize these results, the overall pattern when looking at the cell means is very clear: physician assisted suicide is only seen as morally right and rated as "Should be Legal" when the doctor discussed the issue carefully with the patient,

| Doctor Accepts | | | | | | Doctor Encourages | | | | | |
| Passive Agent | | | Active Agent | | | Passive Agent | | | Active Agent | | |
Acts	As'st	Obsv	Acts	As'st	Obsv	Acts	As'st	Obsv	Acts	As'st	Obsv
3.8	3.9	4.2	4.1	4.2	4.5	4.5	4.6	4.4	4.3	4.2	4.7
4.0	4.0	4.0	4.4	4.8	4.4	4.9	4.8	4.2	4.5	4.6	4.7
3.3	3.8	4.0	3.8	4.2	4.3	4.2	4.2	4.1	4.0	3.7	4.6
3.3	3.4	3.8	3.7	3.7	4.2	4.0	4.0	4.0	3.9	3.5	4.5
3.2	3.6	4.2	3.7	3.7	4.3	4.1	3.8	4.4	3.9	3.8	4.6
3.6	3.9	4.2	3.8	4.1	4.6	4.3	4.3	4.5	4.2	4.2	4.8
4.1	4.2	4.4	4.3	4.2	4.8	4.5	4.6	4.5	4.4	4.5	4.9
4.2	4.1	4.7	4.5	4.2	4.8	5.0	4.4	4.8	4.8	4.4	5.0
4.5	4.7	4.8	4.7	4.8	4.9	4.9	4.8	4.8	4.8	4.8	5.0

Table 2B. Significance Levels

	Attitude	Agent	Action	Attit × Agent	Attit × Action	Agent × Action	3-Way
APAS Scale	.00**	.00**	.60	.02*	.82	.38	.20
1: Morality	.00**	.00**	.61	.00**	.28	.25	.16
3: Legality	.00**	.00**	.48	.00**	.46	.38	.09
4: Pain	.00**	.00**	.54	.00**	.19	.29	.17
5: Terminal	.00**	.05*	.36	.30	.80	.77	.24
6: Physical	.00**	.05*	.42	.35	.91	.34	.80
7: Mental	.00**	.06	.73	.58	.72	.16	.31
8: Depressed	.03**	.10	.86	.55	.70	.62	.36
9: Alternative	.00**	.25	.50	.52	.57	.98	.56

Table 3. Percentages of Participants Giving Responses Below the Median
and Zones of Acceptance/Rejection
(Value indicates % who agree should be moral or legal)

Condition:						
	Doctor Discusses					
	Passive Agent			Active Agent		
	Acts	As'st	Obsv	Acts	As'st	Obsv
General Items						
1: Morality	91.2	80.6	84.6	78.8	56.7	60.0
3: Legality	88.2	83.9	76.5	81.8	61.3	52.0
Circumstances						
4: Pain	91.2	74.2	88.5	84.8	58.1	68.0
5: Terminal	67.6	80.6	65.4	72.7	66.7	64.0
6: Physical	64.7	61.3	57.7	63.6	63.3	56.0
7: Mental	41.9	51.6	46.2	42.4	60.0	40.0
8: Depressed	29.4	25.8	19.2	27.3	24.1	20.0
9: Alternative	44.1	48.4	30.8	33.3	41.4	36.0
Yes/No Items						
2: Regulated?	38.2	54.8	73.1	60.6	67.0	76.0
10: Do Same?	72.7	58.6	63.6	38.7	42.3	45.8

Between Subjects:

Acts = Physician commits killing act himself. $n = 34$

As'st = Physician assists patient in killing self. $n = 31$

Obsv = Physician only observes without participation. $n = 26$

and not when the doctor merely accepts the patients decision without question
and especially not when the doctor is presented as having encouraged the patient
to die. There is also some tendency to see passive modes of death as more
acceptable than active ones. The actual actions of the doctor, whether he simply
observed the suicide, assisted the suicide, or committed an act of euthanasia, is
not as important as the other two factors (Doctor's Reaction to Patient's Request
and Active or Passive Agent of Death). Nevertheless, the Doctor Act's condition
is often judged most favorably and the Doctor Observes condition least favorably.

Clearly, the doctor's approach toward the patients request (Discusses, Accepts,
or Encourages) was the most important factor in determining how moral or
legal each hypothetical assisted suicide situation was perceived to be. Across all

| Doctor Accepts | | | | | | Doctor Encourages | | | | | |
| Passive Agent | | | Active Agent | | | Passive Agent | | | Active Agent | | |
Acts	As'st	Obsv	Acts	As'st	Obsv	Acts	As'st	Obsv	Acts	As'st	Obsv
36.4	46.7	40.0	31.3	30.0	36.0	21.2	23.3	40.0	31.3	30.0	32.0
48.5	48.4	48.0	42.4	41.9	36.0	30.3	38.7	44.0	36.4	41.9	32.0
48.5	54.8	48.0	42.4	54.8	36.0	36.4	41.9	44.0	39.4	45.2	32.0
48.5	54.8	36.0	42.4	48.4	32.0	33.3	40.0	32.0	36.4	41.9	32.0
45.5	54.8	36.0	36.4	45.2	28.0	30.3	32.3	40.0	33.3	32.3	24.0
30.3	45.2	32.0	33.3	40.0	24.0	24.2	22.6	36.0	27.3	22.6	24.0
21.2	25.8	24.0	24.2	22.6	20.0	15.2	19.4	24.0	21.2	19.4	20.0
30.3	41.9	24.0	27.3	40.0	24.0	15.2	29.0	24.0	24.2	29.0	20.0
69.7	80.0	80.0	75.0	86.7	83.3	72.7	80.0	68.0	75.0	73.3	83.3
43.8	35.7	38.1	28.1	28.6	23.8	33.5	27.6	45.5	37.5	31.0	23.8

circumstances, Discusses was more acceptable than Accepts and Accepts more Acceptable than Encourages. Again without exception, a passive means of death is seen as more acceptable than an active one. The principal difference between Doctor's Reaction and the Agent of Death is that the Doctor Accepts and Doctor Encourages conditions are consistently seen as unacceptable (i.e.,—above the scale midpoint of 3.5). While an active agent of death does reduce the perceived acceptability of physician assisted suicide, it is not always seen as unacceptable (above the midpoint).

Zones of Acceptance and Rejection as Defined by Percentages

For descriptive purposes, a more sophisticated and meaningful "Zones of Acceptance" table can be created by substituting for the means in Table 2, the percentages of participants who answered an item below the mid-point of the scale (3.5). This method makes it clearer, for policy purposes, just what the degree of support is for each type of physician assisted suicide. As can be seen, the greatest acceptance of physician assisted suicide is found in the Doctor Discusses condition for both overall morality and legality of the doctor's actions, especially for a Passive Agent of Death.

Overall, an examination of this "Zones of Acceptance" table reveals that nearly all of the conditions in which more than 50 percent of the participants felt that the doctor's actions (killing the patient) should be moral or legal fall within the Doctor Discusses (patient's request with the patient) condition. In addition, higher percentages of participants endorsed assisted suicide in the Passive than in the Active mode. The highest levels of approval for assisted suicide occur when the Doctor discusses the implications of the patient's decision, and the mode of death is removal of treatment. These patterns of approval based upon percentages of participants correspond closely to the significant differences found for the means (see Table 2A).

The interaction between the reaction of the doctor and the agent of death is important. As mentioned above, the "Zones of Acceptance" table is deliberately arranged so that the greatest percentages of approving participants would appear on the left, and the lowest levels on the right. Thus the conditions range, starting at the left, from Discussed-Passive and Discussed-Active through Accepted-Passive and Accepted-Active to Encouraged-Passive and then Encouraged-Active suicide. What is revealed by displaying the data in this fashion is how narrow the Zone of Acceptance for physician-assisted suicide is: "Discussed" assisted suicide is perceived to be almost the only moral and legal category, causing more than 50 percent of the participants to endorse the option in all cases. Significantly, "Passive-Discussed" assisted suicide was the only category where more than 50 percent of the participants indicated that they would do the same as the patient (i.e., they would request to be killed).

Dichotomous Items

Finally, we examine the results for the two dichotomous dependent variables—items 2 and 10. Chi-square results for items 2 and 10 (yes/no items) are displayed in Table 4. Item 2 reads: "Should the actions of the doctor be regulated by law in any way?" Subjects also felt that physician assisted suicide should be regulated by law in every condition except Doctor Discusses/Passive Agent/Doctor Commits the Act, where the percent of subjects approving of legal regulation was still 48.8. Approval of legal regulation increases as approval decreases (see Tables 2 and 4). Thus, the great majority of the respondents feel that the doctor's actions should be regulated except for the Doctor Discusses/Passive Agent/Doctor Commits Act condition.

Table 4. Chi-Square Results

Experimental Conditions			Item 2: Should Law Regulate?						Item 10: Do Same As Patient?					
			Yes		No		Statistics		Yes		No		Statistics	
Doctor's Attitude	Death Agent	Doctor's Action	f	%	f	%	Chi-Sqr	Sig	f	%	f	%	Chi-Sqr	Sig
Discuss	Passive	Observe	19	73	7	27	5.54	0.02	14	64	8	36	1.64	0.20
		Assist	17	55	14	45	0.29	0.59	17	59	12	51	0.86	0.35
		Commit	13	38	21	62	1.88	0.17	24	73	9	27	6.82	0.01
	Active	Observe	19	76	6	24	6.76	0.01	11	46	13	54	0.17	0.68
		Assist	21	68	10	32	3.90	0.05	11	42	15	58	0.62	0.43
		Commit	20	61	13	39	1.48	0.22	12	39	19	61	1.58	0.21
Accept	Passive	Observe	20	80	5	20	9.00	0.00	8	38	13	62	1.19	0.28
		Assist	24	80	6	20	10.80	0.00	10	36	18	64	2.29	0.13
		Commit	23	70	10	30	5.12	0.02	14	44	18	56	5.00	0.48
	Active	Observe	20	83	4	17	10.67	0.00	5	24	16	76	5.76	0.02
		Assist	26	87	4	13	16.13	0.00	8	29	20	71	5.14	0.02
		Commit	24	75	8	25	8.00	0.00	9	28	23	72	6.13	0.01
Encourage	Passive	Observe	17	68	8	32	3.24	0.07	10	45	12	55	0.18	0.67
		Assist	24	80	6	20	10.80	0.00	8	28	21	72	5.83	0.02
		Commit	24	73	9	27	6.82	0.01	11	33	22	67	3.67	0.06
	Active	Observe	20	83	4	17	10.67	0.00	5	24	16	71	5.76	0.02
		Assist	22	73	8	27	6.53	0.01	9	31	20	69	4.17	0.04
		Commit	24	75	8	25	8.00	0.00	12	38	20	62	2.00	0.16

This pattern is parallel to that for item 10, which reads: "If you were the patient described in the story above, would you do the same thing?" A majority of the participants would make the same decision as the patient in the vignette (i.e., they would decide to die) only in the Discusses/Passive conditions. Agreeing that they would die decreases as approval of assisted suicide decreases.

Effects Due to Mitigating Circumstances

The effects of the mitigating circumstances items were averaged across the experimental conditions. Some of these mitigating circumstances (Physical Incapacity, Mental Incapacity, Depression, and Available Alternative Treatment) increase the unacceptability of assisted suicide above the midpoint of 3.5; and Constant Untreatable Pain actually decreased unacceptability to below the midpoint. The first three of these conditions were expected to reduce the acceptability of assisted suicide and can be termed "Negative Circumstances." The other circumstances (Pain, Terminality, and Physical Incapacity) were not expected to reduce the acceptability of assisted suicide and can be termed "Positive Circumstances." These results are displayed in Figure 2.

Returning to Table 2A, items 4 through 9 (the various mitigating circumstances), there is a very strong and consistent pattern. The three "Positive Conditions" (conditions not expected to decrease the acceptability of assisted suicide) were all rated as "Should be Legal" in the Discussed condition, as were the APAS score and the overall legality question (item 1). The three "Negative Conditions" (conditions expected to decrease the acceptability of suicide) were not rated as "Should be Legal," with the singular exception of mental incapacitation when the doctor discussed the situation with the patient and only assisted the patient in the act. Very few of the other possible conditions, even for the positive mitigating circumstances, were rated as either moral or legal.

The various "mitigating circumstances" items also show an interesting pattern when displayed in terms of the percentage of participants who responded below the midpoint (Table 3). In general, the hypothesis that constant pain, a terminal illness, and physical incapacitation would not decrease acceptance of assisted suicide was supported to the extent that these three conditions produced the least non-acceptance. Of the three conditions, only constant pain occasionally increases the percentage of participants who approve above that of the "overall legality" item (item 3). The other two usually produce lower levels of acceptance, although still higher than the three items which were hypothesized to decrease acceptance of assisted suicide (mental incapacity, depression, and the presence of an alternative treatment). Of these, severe clinical depression of the patient typically produced the lowest approval. To summarize, Pain, Terminality, and Physical Incapacitation resulted in higher acceptance than Mental Incapacitation, Alternative Treatments, or Depression. These results are displayed in Figure 2.

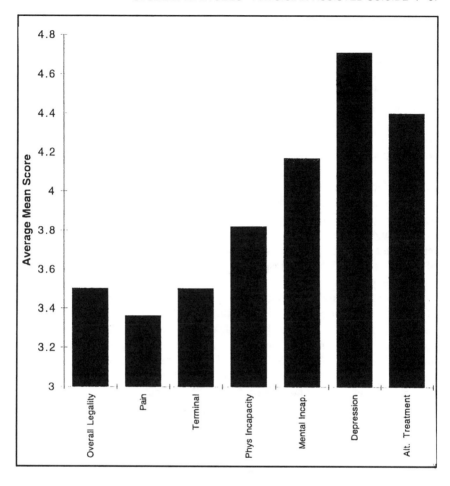

Figure 2. Mitigating circumstances.

DISCUSSION

A close analysis of these results lead to some very interesting conclusions. The Doctor's Reaction toward the patient's request to die appears to be the key factor which impacts the participants' attitudes toward the morality and legality of the doctor's actions. It seems far more important than the actual action of the doctor—whether observing or assisting the patient's suicide or actually performing euthanasia.

These results have profound implications for our understanding of the present debate on assisted suicide and social policy. It is not the purpose of this study to come down on one side or the other in the debate which is raging currently.

However, it is important to partisans of both sides to examine their assumptions in light of what is empirically known regarding public opinion. In a recent article (Cook et al., 1995) staff working at intensive care units were surveyed to determine what factors were important in deciding whether or not to give care to hypothetical critically ill patients. The findings revealed that there is a great range of variance in responses due to the values of the individual care provider. Thus, there seems to be a dangerous lack of consensus in terms of giving care to the critically ill. The issue of care for the critically ill and physician assisted suicide are related to the extent that there is any danger that assisted suicide comes to be seen as a cheaper substitute for other types of care, especially for terminally ill patients (Alpers & Lo, 1997).

The primary conclusion of our article is that, based upon this sample, the public does not regard assisted suicide as unthinkable, yet at the same time it feels that assisted suicide should be regulated by law. More importantly, the distinctions made by the participants in this study as the basis of their acceptance or rejection of assisted suicide do not correspond to the distinctions made either in law or in public policy.

At present, doctor-assisted suicide is legal only in Oregon. However, removal of life support is not only not illegal in any state, but is considered a basic right. One surprising conclusion is that in this study, removal of life support was considered unacceptable in most of the experimental conditions. "Passive Suicide" (defined in the survey materials as no longer wishing to receive the treatment that has been keeping the patient alive) was only acceptable to more than 50 percent of the participants in the "Discussed" condition. That is, the participants in this study considered cessation of life sustaining treatment acceptable only if the doctor "has a long discussion with this patient, in which they review a number of alternative solutions, the negative consequences of the patient's death for other people including family, and the patient's moral and ethical beliefs regarding suicide" (quoted directly from the vignette). How many laws regarding the removal of life support contain this clause?

On the other hand, doctor-patient discussion also seems to open the door to more extreme outcomes. Even "Active Suicide" (the patient "wishes to take a substance which will end his or her own life") is considered both moral and legal to more than 50 percent of the participants in the "Discussed" condition. In actual assisted suicides this does not always occur. Frequently in actual practice patients seeking advice from health professionals are actively encouraged to end their own lives, for example Dr. Kevorkian is documented as having done this (Betzold, 1993). According to Beauchamp (1996), the "mere assertion of a request cannot be binding." Desperation undermines a patient's autonomy, and trust in the doctor can lead to a vulnerability to persuasion or subtle coercion (Pellegrino, 1996). For the participants in this study, "Active-Encouraged" suicide was the least acceptable condition. The contrasting approach is perhaps best demonstrated by Dr. Quill, who engaged in extended dialog and discussion with one patient before prescribing what he knew would be a lethal overdose of pain killers (Quill, 1991).

The most likely explanation of these results would seem to be an empowerment perspective on the part of the participants. Respondents in this study seem less concerned with the moral culpability of the doctor than whether or not a rational, sound decision was made on the part of the patient. This is similar to the arguments of Batty who presents a Principle of Patient Autonomy enjoining doctors to respect a competent person's choice (Batty, 1994). Conditions which would tend to undermine such a decision, such as depression or mental incapacity, reduced acceptance of suicide. Conditions which made the decision seem less rational, such as the availability of an alternative treatment, also reduced acceptance. But the most significant factor in this regard appears to be whether or not the doctor discussed the implications of the patient's request. Accepting or actually encouraging the patient to die, as has been documented in some cases, was not acceptable to a majority of participants.

The present study is merely an exploration into this issue and further research is needed to extend and validate the results. The dynamics of the doctor-patient relationship need to be further studied. For example, various combinations of personality variables of the doctor, patient and research subject, such as locus of control or Eriksonian developmental level, could have important effects. Another important issue would be to compare the effect of emotional to physical pain on the part of the patient. In this study, constant pain of the patient was the one factor which actually increased the acceptability of assisted suicide in many conditions, but it is likely that the participants interpreted this as physical pain. Emotional pain was represented here as severe, clinical depression, which reduced acceptability, but more equivalent wording would allow a more direct comparison between these two conditions. Another factor is gender: what would be the effect of comparing different combinations of the gender of the patient, the doctor, the participant, and different mitigating circumstances? Would male participants have the same attitudes toward the suicide of male and female patients, and vice versa? Finally, the results here must be replicated with other populations than college students to be considered to have generalizability.

REFERENCES

Alpers, A., & Lo, B. (1997). Does it make clinical sense to equate terminally ill patients who require life-sustaining interventions with those who do not? *Journal of the American Medical Association, v277,* 1705-1708.

Batty, M. (1994). *The least worst death: Essays in bioethics on the end of life.* New York: Oxford University Press.

Betzold, M. (1993). *Appointment with doctor death.* Troy, MI: Momentum Books.

Boehm, F. (1997). *Physician Assisted Suicide* [On-line]. Available: http://dr-boehm.com/suicide.htm

Cook, D., Guyatt, G., Jaeschke, R., Reeve, J., Spanier, A., King, D., Molloy, D., Willan, A., & Streiner, D. (1995). Determinants in Canadian health care workers of the decision to withdrawn life support from the critically ill. *Journal of the American Medical Association, 273,* 703-708.

Glick, H. (1992). *The right to die: Policy innovation and it's consequences.* New York: Columbia University Press.

Hendin, H. (1995). *Suicide in America.* New York: W. W. Norton.

Pellegrino, E. (1996). Distortion of the healing relationship. In T. Beauchamp and R. Veatch (Eds.), *Ethical issues in death and dying.* New Jersey: Prentice Hall.

Pernick, M. (1996). *The black stork: Eugenics and the death of "defective" babies in American medicine and motion pictures since 1915.* New York: Oxford University Press.

Quill, T. (1991). Death and dignity: A case of individualized decision-making. *New England Journal of Medicine, 324,* 691-694.

Searles, N. (1995). *Silence doesn't obliterate the truth: A Manitoba survey on physician assisted suicide* [On-line]. Available: http://www.islandnet.com/deathnet/survey.html.

Wooddell, V., & Kaplan, K. (1998). *An expanded typology of suicide, assisted suicide, and euthanasia. Omega, 36,* 201-208.

DOCTOR ASSISTED SUICIDE: AN ANALYSIS OF PUBLIC OPINION OF MICHIGAN ADULTS

FLINT LACHENMEIER, PH.D.
Wayne State University

KALMAN J. KAPLAN, PH.D.
*Michael Reese Hospital and Medical Center
and Wayne State University*

DIANA CARAGACIANU, B.S.
Wayne State University

ABSTRACT

Michigan public opinion on Doctor Assisted Suicide (DAS) was assessed in January 1997 ($N = 603$). Asked if they would consider DAS for themselves, two-thirds would if being kept alive by a machine or were experiencing chronic pain; one-half would if they experienced a loss in mobility or independence, became a burden to others, or were diagnosed with a terminal disease; and one-third would if they were incontinent or going to a nursing home. A series of demographic and attitudinal comparisons were made for support for the concept of DAS and as a hypothetical consideration for oneself. The highest support for the concept of DAS was found among the following: men eighteen to twenty-four years old, some college education, $35-60,000/year income, Caucasian, Democrat, liberal, Protestant, and frequent church attendee. The highest self-consideration of DAS was found among the following: men, fifty to fifty-five years old, post-graduate education, $35-60,000/year income, Caucasian, Democrat, liberal, Protestant, and infrequent church attendee.

A majority of Americans seem to support some form of doctor assisted suicide (DAS). This support is also growing. A 1975 Gallup Poll showed that 41 percent of American's believed a person in great pain, without hope of improvement, had a moral right to commit suicide. By 1990 that figure had grown to 66 percent (Ames, Wilson, & Sawhill, 1991).

Some advocates have argued that the "right" to die is guaranteed by the first and fourteenth amendments to the Constitution (Cassel & Meier, 1990; Quill, 1991; Quill, Cassel, & Meier, 1992). Supporters, such as the American Civil Liberties Union and the Hemlock Society, use certain phrasing to make the issue of DAS seem to be a civil rights issue. Phrases like "right to die," "death with dignity," and "mercy killing" imply that helping people kill themselves is an issue of individual or civil rights.

There are also many opponents of DAS. Several professional organizations have come out publicly against legalizing this type of suicide. They are the American Medical Association, the American Geriatric Society, the American Bar Association (Koenig, 1993) and some religious organizations. It seems that public enthusiasm for the concept of legalizing DAS is not shared by the professionals that would be involved in carrying out the mandate. A recent article demonstrated that the phrases described above, such as "right to die," "death with dignity," and "existence without life" were used by Nazi doctors as euphemisms for state sanctioned murder (Mitchell, 1996).

Religious organizations are another group which are typically against DAS. This may be due to the traditional doctrines in the Biblical religions (Judaism, Christianity, and Islam) that stress that life belongs to God, rather than the individual, and oppose killing oneself to avoid pain and suffering. It is also true that a strong religious faith can serve to give a purpose to the pain and suffering by providing a framework in which it can have some meaning (Koenig, 1993).

Recently, the Hemlock Society has led ballot issues in California, Washington, and Oregon to legalize DAS. The issue narrowly failed in both California and Washington by the same 54 percent to 46 percent margin (Koenig, 1993). The initiative passed in Oregon, but was suspended pending appeal (Lee et al., 1996). The Supreme Court's refusal to hear this issue put the issue back into the lap of Oregon voters who voted to keep it legal by a 60 percent to 40 percent margin. In Oregon, fifteen people were assisted in committing suicide in 1998, the last year for which statistics are available (Chin, Hedberg, Higginson, & Fleming, 1999). Currently, Congress is considering legislation (the Pain Relief Promotion Act of 1999; Senate Bill 1272 and House Bill 2260) that would make it illegal to prescribe medication for the purposes of assisting in a suicide.

SUPPORT AND OPPOSITION TO DAS

Although as a group public opinion has become more favorable toward legalizing DAS, this is not true of all of people. The elderly have a very different position. A Harvard School of Public Health survey found that 79 percent of eighteen to thirty-four-year-olds supported DAS, this percentage continued to drop as age of participants increased (Lawton, 1991). Sixty-four percent of thirty-five to forty-nine-year-olds and 53 percent of fifty and older people supported DAS.

There is a clear downward trend of support with age. Perhaps by the time elderly persons find themselves in a situation in which they might consider DAS, a majority would likely not support it. This result could be due to several things. First, they are approaching the age when it becomes a real possibility rather than a hypothetical abstraction. Second, as a person ages they begin to realize how easy it would be to abuse the situation with themselves being the abused. The final reason may be that they begin to understand that a few aches and pains are not that bad, as they have had a long time to get used to their gradually increasing severity.

OPINIONS REGARDING DAS

Medical Profession Surveys

Cohen, Fihn, Boyko, Jonsen, and Wood (1994) surveyed doctors in Washington state regarding the legalization of DAS and euthanasia. They found that 48 percent agreed with the statement that euthanasia is never ethically justified (42% disagreed), 54 percent thought DAS should be legal in some situations, but only 33 percent said they were willing to perform euthanasia. Thirty-nine percent agreed that DAS was ethically justified, 50 percent disagreed. A slight majority felt that DAS should be legal in some situations (53%), but only 40 percent said they would participate. The survey was conducted after the defeat of Proposition 119 which would have legalized DAS and euthanasia.

Oregon doctors were also surveyed soon after the passage of the "Death With Dignity Act." Lee, Nelson, Tilden, Ganzini, Schmidt, and Tolle (1996) assessed doctors attitudes regarding DAS and other related issues. They found that 60 percent of doctors thought DAS should be legal in some situations and almost half (46%) would be willing to prescribe a lethal dose of medication if it were legal to do so. Another 31 percent would be unwilling to prescribe a lethal dose on moral grounds. Legalization of DAS is not required for it to be practiced by doctors or others, 21 percent of doctors said they had received a request to assist in a suicide and 7 percent admitted to complying with the request. A large percentage of doctors (83%) said that financial pressure seemed to play a major role in the requests for DAS

Duberstein, Conwell, Cox, Podgorski, Glazer, and Caine (1995) surveyed primary care physicians in New York state about their attitudes toward DAS. They found that 49 percent of surveyed doctors personally supported DAS in some form and in some circumstances. They also found that 31 percent supported legalization of DAS under some circumstances.

Doctors are not the only medical professional to deal with possible DAS patients. Perhaps nurses have even more contact than doctors with these patients. Asch (1996) surveyed critical care nurses regarding their attitudes toward and experience with assisted suicide. Asch found 17 percent of critical care nurses had received a request to perform assisted suicide. Almost all of those nurses who received requests to assist in a suicide did so (16%). Another 35 percent said they had hastened a patient's death by pretending to provide doctor-ordered treatment. A high dosage of opiate was the most commonly used assisted suicide method utilized by these nurses.

Bachman, Alcser, Doukas, Lichtenstein, Corning, and Brody (1996) conducted a survey of Michigan doctors and the public regarding their attitudes toward legalizing DAS and voluntary euthanasia. They found that 56 percent of doctors and 66 percent of the public supported legalization of DAS, 37 percent of doctors and 26 percent of the public preferred a ban on DAS, and 8 percent of each group were uncertain. When the doctor's choice was widened 40 percent preferred legalization, 37 percent preferred no law, 17 percent supported prohibition, and 5 percent were uncertain. This study suggests that most people and doctors would prefer little or no government interference in the issue.

Other Groups

Medical professionals are not the only group which has been surveyed about their attitudes toward DAS. Singer, Choudhry, Armstrong, Meslin, and Lowy (1995) explored Canadian public opinion regarding end-of-life decisions while manipulating the patients prognosis, type of practice, and the decision process. Eighty-five percent of the public supported a decision to forego life-sustaining treatment in a competent person if the patient was unlikely to recover. There was only 35 percent support if the patient was likely to recover. Public support remained high for an incompetent person, if they had expressed their wishes in advance in a living will (88%), higher even than for a competent patient (85%). If it was the family making the request then support for DAS dropped slightly to 76 percent.

Likely potential users of DAS have also been surveyed. Breitbart, Rosenfeld, and Passik (1996) surveyed ambulatory HIV-infected patients. The results showed 63 percent of patients supported the concept of DAS and a majority had considered the option for themselves (55%). Psychological distress was the highest predictor of interest in DAS for this group, followed by experience with a terminally ill family member or friend. Other predictors of support included race (Caucasian highest), low or no church attendance and low levels of perceived social support. Factors not related to support for DAS included severity of pain, pain-related functional impairment, physical symptoms, or extent of HIV disease.

One group that may have particular interest in DAS is the elderly. Seidlitz, Duberstein, Cox, and Conwell (1995) surveyed a sample of men and women over the age of sixty. A smaller percentage of this group expressed support for DAS legalization (41%) than in other surveys. There were many factors associated with support for some aspect of DAS including: increasing age, male sex, Caucasian, divorced/separated, higher income, and lower religiosity.

SLIPPERY SLOPE

If DAS is legalized there would be little justification to limiting the practice to terminal people. After all, mortality implies terminality. Once the terminally ill are allowed to seek DAS, there would be little to prevent those with less serious illness, physical impairments, and disabilities from seeking DAS as well. In fact, public pressure may mount to encourage these people to seek DAS as the amount we as a society spend on medical care and assistive technologies becomes widely known or budget pressures increase. It is not hard to imagine people of a certain age or physical capacity being carted off to the DAS center so that we can avoid costly Social Security or Medicare benefit disbursements (see the movies "Soylent Green" and, for an even more extreme case, "Logan's Run" where you were terminated at the age of 30, showing how arbitrary an age can become).

Koenig (1993) makes a point about "substituted judgments" (p. 177) easily replacing personal choice. A substituted judgment is when someone other than the person to be assisted seeks the act (i.e., a family member, friend, or government bureaucrat). It would be hard to establish the validity of these judgments with some patients, like those who are comatose or mentally incapacitated, leaving the door open to abuses.

Koenig also talks about a "generation effect" (p. 177) in which tolerance by one generation turns slowly into acceptance and then abuse by future generations. In other words, the policy becomes more liberally interpreted as time passes. This is clearly the case in U.S. jurisprudence, where the amount of and application of civil rights has expanded enormously since the U.S. Constitution was written. Another good case in point has to do with the American's with Disabilities Act, which was intended to reduce discrimination toward people with disabilities, but has been used to prevent overweight or persons with drug addictions from being fired from their jobs.

One of the reasons that this issue of DAS has been in the spotlight has to do with Dr. Jack Kevorkian. Dr. Kevorkian assisted at least ninety-two people to commit suicide in southeastern Michigan and has publicly claimed assisting over 130 people. He was tried four separate times, twice acquitted and one mistrial before finally being convicted in March 1999. He is currently serving a ten to twenty-five year sentence on the two convictions of second-degree murder and illegal delivery of a controlled substance. Prior to this conviction, over the preceding nine years, the Michigan legislature had attempted to pass legislation to stop him from assisting people to commit suicide. Local police departments distributed potential victim profiles to the local hotel and motel operators. Dr. Kevorkian had even been placed under police surveillance.

Local papers provided extensive coverage of Dr. Kevorkian. The continued publicity generated by Dr. Kevorkian's actions led to interest in pubic opinions on the issue of DAS. To explore these opinions, the Detroit Free Press has conducted a series of public opinion polls on DAS starting in 1990, after Dr. Kevorkian's first assisted suicide. It is the findings of one of the latest Detroit Free Press polls that is the subject of this study.

METHOD

Participants

Six hundred and three adults were randomly surveyed for the Detroit Free Press by EPIC/MRA, a public opinion survey organization based in Lansing, Michigan. The survey was conducted from January 15-20, 1997 and was composed of a representative sample of all adults in Michigan. The survey had an overall margin of error of ±4 percent.

PROCEDURE

A telephone poll was conducted by EPIC/MRA (Poll #47), January 15-20, 1997 for the Detroit Free Press. The sample was contacted as part of a larger survey covering various newsworthy and political issues of the time. The actual survey and demographic questions are as follows:

> Hello, my name is . . . from Michigan Researchers Associates. We're conducting a random survey with voters in Michigan about national, state and local issues. I'd like to take a few minutes of your time to include your opinions. (There were many issues researched in the same pole such as voter history, opinions of President Clinton and Governor Engler and aircraft safety).
>
> This past week, the Oakland County prosecutor said that he would not put Dr. Jack Kevorkian on trial again for assisting people to commit suicide, and the U.S. Supreme Court also heard arguments last week about whether assisted suicide should be legal in this country.
>
> 22. Do you favor or oppose the idea of allowing physician assisted suicide for people who are physically suffering or terminally ill, but mentally capable of requesting help to die?
>
> 23. Can you imagine any circumstance where you might consider the option of assisted suicide for yourself? If a yes response—ask questions 24-31.
>
> The 45 people that Dr. Jack Kevorkian assisted in suicide had many different reasons for seeking his help. Not all of them were considered terminally ill. I'm going to read a list of conditions some of these people or their families cited in making the decision to "draw the line" and ask for Dr. Kevorkian's help. For each condition that I describe, please tell me whether each is a condition that would cause you to consider physician assisted suicide? Questions 24-31 were rotated.
>
> 24. A medical diagnosis that you have less than 6 months to live.

25. Chronic pain that can only be managed with heavy medication.

26. Loss of mobility, not being able to get up and get around on your own.

27. Loss of independence, not being able to live on your own and care for yourself.

28. Incontinence, a loss of bladder and bowel control.

29. Prospect of going into a nursing home.

30. Becoming a burden on other people.

31. Being hooked up to machines that keep you alive.

Questions 32 and 33 were rotated.

32. When their life ends, some people will go to heaven if they lived a good life.

33. People who choose assisted suicide will not go to heaven?

Finally, I would like to ask you a few questions about yourself, for statistical purposes.

45. Do you think of yourself as pro-choice, meaning that you support allowing women to have the right to an abortion, or do you consider yourself pro-life, meaning that you oppose abortions except where it is necessary to save the life of the mother?

46. Could you please tell me in what year you were born?

47. What is your religion—Protestant, Roman Catholic, Eastern Orthodox, Jewish, Muslim or some other religion?

48. How often do you attend religious services—at least once a week, almost every week, more than half of the time, half of the time, less than half of the time, hardly ever, or never?

49. Do you or does any member in your household belong to a labor union or a teachers association?

50. Are you married, single, widowed, separated or divorced?

51. What is the last grade or level of schooling you completed?

52. What is your race—are you White, African-American, Hispanic or Asian?

53. Are there any school age children, age 18 years or under, living in your household?

55. On political issues, do you consider yourself a liberal, a conservative, or a moderate?

56. Generally speaking, do you consider yourself a Republican or a Democrat?

58. Would you please tell me into which of the following categories your total yearly household income falls—including everyone in the household?

61. Sex of respondent (By Observation Only)

The region that the respondent lived in was determined by the phone number.

ANALYSIS

Chi squares were computed for all demographics and the two attitude questions (32 and 33). Demographic and attitudinal effects were related to the questions regarding support for the concept of DAS (question 22) and a global consideration of DAS for oneself (question 23). Chi squares were also computed for the situational consideration of DAS for oneself variables (questions 24 through 31), but only for those participants who answered positively for the global consideration question.

Some demographic variables were split into two or more categories. Support for the concept of DAS and consideration of DAS for oneself were split into two categories—pro and con for each. The demographic variable of age was split into 4 categories: 18 to 29, 30 to 49, 50 to 64 and 65+. Education was also divided into four categories: kindergarten through high school graduate (K-12), some college courses, college graduate, and post graduate education. Income was divided into five categories: 0 to 25,000 (0-25K), 25,000 to 45,000 (25-45K), 45,000 to 75,000 (45-75K), more than 75,000 (75K+) and retired. Many different races were surveyed, however only two major groups could be formed for analysis purposes—white and other (including African-American, Hispanic, or Asian). Many religious denominations were surveyed, but only three categories had sufficient numbers for analysis: Protestant, Catholic, and other/none. Marital status was categorized as single, married, formerly married (which included separated, divorced, and widowed) and declined to answer.

Some of the attitudinal variables were as recategorized into two or more categories. Ideology was reclassified as liberal, moderate, conservative, and undecided/declined to answer. Party identification was split into four categories: Democrat, Independent, Republican, and other/declined. Church attendance was recoded as frequent, about half time, and seldom. Both of the two questions related to beliefs about heaven were categorized as agree, disagree, or undecided/ declined.

RESULTS

Initial analyses were centered around the responses to questions 22 and 23, support for the concept of DAS and consideration of DAS for oneself. As can be seen in Figure 1, these two variables are not identical ($r = .4474$). Although there is a certain amount of common variance ($r^2 = .200$), the remaining variance is unique. For example, there is greater support for the concept of DAS (61.9%) than there is for the personal application for oneself (45.3%; $\chi^2 = 164.3$, $p < .00001$). As we will see, this difference is maintained within various subgroups.

Figure 1 breaks this data into quadrants of favorability/unfavorability toward the concept of DAS crossed by favorability/unfavorability as a choice for oneself. As can be seen, 68.1 percent of those in favor of the concept also favor it for themselves ($\chi^2 = 164.3$, $p < .0001$). However, 31.9 percent of those who favor the concept do not apply it to themselves. Looking at this data the other way, 91.6 percent of those in favor of DAS for themselves also support it as a concept. Only, 8.4 percent of those supporting it for themselves are not in favor of it as a concept. In other words, support for the concept of DAS does not necessarily

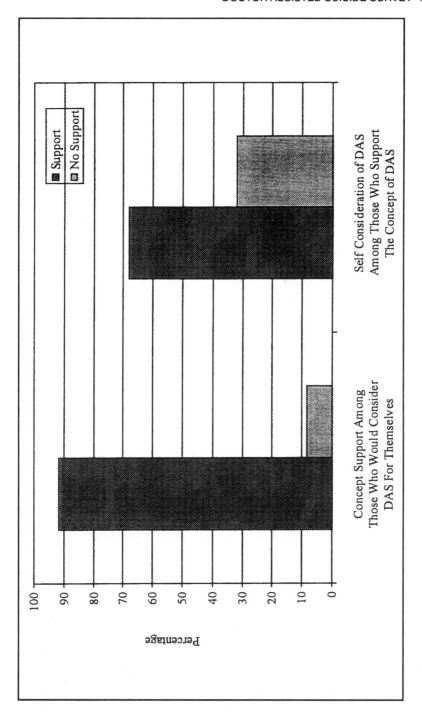

Figure 1. Support for the concept of DAS and as a consideration for oneself with respect to the other position.

imply personal application while support for personal application does imply support for the general concept.

Effects of Demographic Variables

We now examine each of these variables separately with regard to a number of demographic variables. The significant mean differences between groupings of the demographic variables are presented in Table 1 for both the general concept of DAS and personalized consideration of DAS for oneself.

Age

There was a significant age effect for both support of the concept of DAS ($\chi^2 = 12.5, p < .006$) and as a choice for oneself ($\chi^2 = 14.5, p < .002$). Concept support remained high at all age levels (68% or higher) except in the 65+ category where support dropped to 52.6 percent. Consideration of DAS for oneself was strongest in the middle age ranges of thirty to forty-nine (53.1%) and fifty to sixty-four (57.3%), and lowest for the extreme age categories of eighteen to twenty-nine (42.9%), and 65+ (36.7%).

Gender

There was a significant effect due to gender of the participant for both support of the concept of DAS ($\chi^2 = 6.5, p < .011$) and as a choice for oneself ($\chi^2 = 6.3, p < .012$). Men were stronger supporters of the concept of DAS than were women (70.1% v. 59.9%). Men were also more likely to consider it as an option for themselves (53.2%) than were women (42.8%).

Education

There was a significant education effect for support of the concept of DAS ($\chi^2 = 8.1, p < .043$), but not as a choice for oneself ($\chi^2 = 2.8, p = $ n.s.). Support for the concept grows with increasing amounts for education and a majority support the concept of DAS at all education levels. Fifty-eight percent of K-12, 64.6 percent of college attendees, 69.1 percent of college graduates, and 74 percent of those with some post graduate education support the concept of DAS.

Income

There was a significant income effect for both support of the concept of DAS ($\chi^2 = 16.2, p < .003$) and as a choice for oneself ($\chi^2 = 10.5, p < .032$). Among those making 0-25,000 58.4 percent support the concept of DAS and 49.5 percent would consider it for themselves. For those making 25-45,000 72.2 percent support the concept and 56.1 percent would consider it as an option for themselves. Support drops somewhat among those making 45-75,000, with 66.4 percent supporting the concept and 49 percent considering DAS for themselves. For those making more than 75,000 per year, 71.6 percent support the concept of

DAS, but only 48.4 percent would consider it for themselves. Support for both drops dramatically for the retired category, with only 38.7 percent supporting the concept and 23.3 percent considering DAS an option for themselves. Overall, it seems as if support for the concept of DAS increases with income level, but the relationship of income level and personal application of DAS is more varied.

Other Demographics

The other demographic categories of race ($\chi^2 = 2.7$, p = n.s., concept; $\chi^2 = 0.0$, p = n.s., self) religion $\chi^2 = 5.0$, p = n.s., concept; $\chi^2 = 5.1$, p = n.s., self), marital status $\chi^2 = 5.8$, p = n.s., concept; $\chi^2 = 0.8$, p = n.s., self) children living at home ($\chi^2 = 0.1$, p = n.s., concept; $\chi^2 = 0.6$, p = n.s., self), and geographic region ($\chi^2 = 8.0$, p = n.s., concept; $\chi^2 = 5.7$, p = n.s., self) did not produce significant effects for support of the concept of DAS or for consideration of DAS for oneself (see Table 1).

Effects of Attitudinal Variables

The relationships between personal attitudes and opinions and support for the concept of DAS and as a choice for oneself are presented in Table 2 and discussed below.

Political Ideology

Significant effects emerge between political ideology and both general ($\chi^2 = 24.3$, $p < .001$) and personal support for DAS ($\chi^2 = 21.9$, $p < .001$). Among those classified as liberals, 75.5 percent support the concept of DAS and 57 percent would consider it for themselves. Support for both DAS issues is similar among moderates with 70.1 percent supporting the concept and 53.8 percent considering it as an option for themselves. Among those identified as conservative, 50.6 percent support the concept and only 35.3 percent would consider it for themselves. For those who are undecided or who preferred not to name a political ideology, 58.6 percent favor the concept of DAS while only 30 percent favor DAS as a personal option.

Party Identification

Significant effects emerge between political party identification and both general ($\chi^2 = 11.0$, $p < .012$) and personal support for DAS ($\chi^2 = 14.9$, $p < .002$). Among those classified as Democrats 71.3 percent support the concept of DAS and 54.8 percent would consider it for themselves. Support for both DAS issues is similar among independents with 66.2 percent supporting the concept and 51.9 percent considering it as an option for themselves. Among those identified as Republicans, 56.7 percent support the concept and only 37.7 percent would consider it for themselves. For those who have other party identification or who prefer not to answer they party identification question, 67.6 percent favor the concept of DAS while 54.1 percent favor DAS as a personal option.

Table 1. Chi Square Results for Demographic Variables with Respect to Support for the Concept of DAS and Consideration of DAS for Oneself

Variable	Concept Support							DAS Consideration for Self						
	No	%	Yes	%	Total	χ^2	p	No	%	Yes	%	Total	χ^2	p
Age														
18-29	35	31.5	76	68.5	111	12.5	.006	64	57.1	48	42.9	112	14.5	.002
30-49	54	30.2	125	69.8	179			83	46.9	94	53.1	177		
50-64	44	30.8	99	69.2	143			61	42.7	82	57.3	143		
65+	63	47.4	70	52.6	133			81	63.3	47	36.7	128		
Gender														
Male	79	29.9	185	70.1	264	6.5	.011	123	46.8	140	53.2	263	6.3	.012
Female	126	40.1	188	59.9	314			178	57.2	133	42.8	311		
Education														
K-12	84	42.0	116	58.0	200	8.1	.043	111	56.9	84	43.1	195	2.8	.427
Some college	52	35.4	95	64.6	147			75	51.4	71	48.6	146		
College graduate	47	30.9	105	69.1	152			75	49.0	78	51.0	153		
Post graduate	20	26.0	57	74.0	77			38	48.7	40	51.3	78		
Income														
0-25K	42	41.6	59	58.4	101	16.2	.003	52	50.5	51	49.5	103	10.5	.032
25-45K	37	27.8	96	72.2	133			58	43.9	74	56.1	132		
45-75K	50	33.6	99	66.4	149			75	51.0	72	49.0	174		
75K+	25	28.4	63	71.6	88			47	51.6	44	48.4	91		
Retired	19	61.3	12	38.7	31			23	76.7	7	23.3	30		

Race														
White	187	36.7	323	63.3	510	2.7	.099	265	52.5	240	47.5	505	0.0	.963
Other	18	26.5	50	73.5	68			36	52.2	33	47.8	69		
Religion														
Protestant	106	34.5	201	65.5	307	5.0	.082	164	56.2	128	43.8	292	5.1	.078
Catholic	69	41.6	97	58.4	166			90	51.7	84	48.3	174		
Other/None	30	28.6	75	71.4	105			47	43.5	61	56.5	108		
Marital Status														
Married	140	37.3	235	62.7	375	5.8	.120	197	53.1	174	46.9	371	0.8	.848
Single	28	35.0	52	65.0	80			41	50.0	41	50.0	82		
Formerly Married	33	28.2	84	71.8	117			59	51.3	56	48.7	115		
Declined	4	66.7	2	33.3	6			4	66.7	2	33.3	6		
Children														
No	140	34.9	261	65.1	401	0.1	.730	213	53.5	185	46.5	398	0.6	.440
Yes	63	36.4	110	63.6	173			86	50.0	86	50.0	172		
Region														
Detroit	13	28.3	33	71.7	46	8.0	.154	22	47.8	24	52.2	46	5.7	.338
Outer Wayne	33	49.3	34	50.7	67			37	56.9	28	43.1	65		
Outer Metro	48	31.4	105	68.6	153			76	49.0	79	51.0	155		
Central	46	36.2	81	63.8	127			66	52.8	59	47.2	125		
West	52	36.1	92	63.9	144			82	58.6	58	41.4	140		
North	13	31.7	28	68.3	41			18	41.9	25	58.1	43		

Table 2. Chi Square Results for Personal Attitudes and Opinions Regarding Heaven and Suicide with Respect to Support for the Concept of DAS and Consideration of DAS for Oneself

Variable	Concept Support							DAS Consideration for Self						
	No	%	Yes	%	Total	χ^2	p	No	%	Yes	%	Total	χ^2	p
Ideology														
Liberal	24	24.5	74	75.5	98	24.3	.000	43	43.0	57	57.0	100	21.9	.000
Moderate	79	29.9	185	70.1	264			121	46.2	141	53.8	262		
Conservative	88	49.4	90	50.6	178			112	64.7	61	35.3	173		
Undecided/Declined	12	41.4	17	58.6	29			21	70.0	9	30.0	30		
Party Identification														
Democrat	66	28.7	164	71.3	230	11.0	.012	104	45.2	126	54.8	230	14.9	.002
Independent	27	33.8	53	66.2	80			38	48.1	41	51.9	79		
Republican	100	43.3	131	56.7	231			142	62.3	86	37.7	228		
Other/Declined	12	32.4	25	67.6	37			17	45.9	20	54.1	37		
Church Attendance														
Frequent	149	55.0	122	45.0	271	87.9	.000	197	75.2	65	24.8	262	104.4	.000
Half time	28	24.3	87	75.7	115			49	40.8	71	59.2	120		
Seldom	28	14.6	164	85.4	192			55	28.6	137	71.4	192		

	n	%	n	%	Total	χ^2	p	n	%	n	%	Total	χ^2	p
Good Go To Heaven														
Agree	133	35.5	242	64.5	375	9.0	.011	195	52.3	178	47.7	373	10.8	.005
Disagree	49	41.2	70	58.8	119			67	60.4	44	39.6	111		
Undecided/Declined	14	20.0	56	80.0	70			27	36.0	48	64.0	75		
Suicide Not Go To Heaven														
Agree	67	63.8	38	36.2	105	74.7	.000	74	71.8	29	28.2	103	48.1	.000
Disagree	74	21.6	268	78.4	342			135	40.2	201	59.8	336		
Other	60	48.4	64	51.6	124			87	68.0	41	32.0	128		
Abortion														
Pro-choice	36	11.6	275	88.4	311	176.5	.000	108	35.0	201	65.0	309	81.5	.000
Pro-life	155	66.5	78	33.5	233			172	74.1	60	25.9	232		

Church Attendance

Significant effects emerge between the frequency of church attendance and both general ($\chi^2 = 87.9$, $p < .001$) and personal consideration for DAS ($\chi^2 = 104.4$, $p < .001$). Among those who attend church frequently, 45 percent support the concept of DAS and 24.8 percent would consider it for themselves. Among those who attend church about half-time, 75.7 percent support the concept of DAS and 59.2 percent would consider it for themselves. Among those who seldom or never attend church, 85.4 percent favor the concept of DAS and 71.4 percent favor DAS as a personal option.

Belief that Good People Go to Heaven

Significant effects emerge between the belief that good people go to heaven and support for both the concept of DAS ($\chi^2 = 9.0$, $p < .011$) and for consideration of it for oneself ($\chi^2 = 10.8$, $p < .005$). Agreement that good people go to heaven is associated with higher support for the concept of DAS (64.5%) and for personal support of DAS (47.7%) than is disagreement with the idea that good people go to heaven (concept support, 58.8%; self consideration, 39.6%). Among those undecided as to the destiny of good people, 80 percent favor the concept of DAS and 64 percent favor DAS as a personal option.

Belief that Those Who Commit Suicide Go to Heaven

Significant effects emerge between the belief that suicides do not go to heaven and both general ($\chi^2 = 74.7$, $p < .001$) and personal support for DAS ($\chi^2 = 48.1$, $p < .001$). Among those who agree that suicides are excluded from heaven, 36.2 percent support the concept of DAS and 28.2 percent would consider it for themselves. Among those who disagree that suicides are excluded from heaven 78.4 percent support the concept of DAS and 59.8 percent would consider it for themselves. Among those undecided as to the destiny of suicides, 51.6 percent favor the concept of DAS while only 32 percent favor DAS as a personal option.

Attitudes toward Abortion

There was a significant relation between support of abortion rights and support for both the concept of DAS ($\chi^2 = 176.5$, $p < .001$) and for personal application of DAS ($\chi^2 = 81.5$, $p < .001$). Among those who label themselves as pro-choice on abortion, 88.4 percent favor the concept of DAS and 65 percent support DAS as a personal option. Among those who label themselves as pro-life on abortion only 33.5 percent support the concept of DAS and only 25.9 percent would choose DAS for themselves.

Yet the two issues are not identical. Only 65 percent of the sample are both pro-choice and pro-DAS as a personal option. Thus, we thought it useful to create four categories based on both respective positions toward abortion and DAS. An 2 × 2 ANOVA was performed on all demographic and attitude variables with respect to DAS concept support and personal consideration of DAS. No effects emerged with respect to personal application of DAS and these results will not be discussed further here.

The data regarding support for the concept of DAS did reveal significant differences with respect to one demographic variable and three attitudes. There was no difference in education level due to attitudes toward abortion among those who were against the concept of DAS ($M = 2.06$ for both groups, $F(1,540) = 5.85$, $p < .05$; increasing numbers indicated increasing amount of education). However, among supporters of DAS, a pro-choice position was associated with higher education ($M = 2.38$) than was a pro-life position ($M = 2.06$).

There was little difference in party identification among supporters of the concept of DAS between those who were either pro-choice ($M = 1.99$, $F(1,540) = 11.32$, $p < .001$; increasing values indicate more Republican identification) or pro-life ($M = 2.09$). However, a difference between those two groups does emerge among opponents of DAS. Republican leanings tend to be greater among supporters of abortion rights ($M = 2.45$), than among those opposed to it ($M = 1.58$).

Church attendance was highest among those opposed to both the concept of DAS and abortion rights ($M = 1.27$, $F(1,540) = 4.35$, $p < .01$; lower values indicate more frequent church attendance). Church attendance was almost equal among those who were against the concept of DAS and pro-choice ($M = 1.94$) and those who supported the concept of DAS, but were pro-life ($M = 1.95$). Church attendance was lowest among the one remaining group who were DAS concept supporters and also pro-choice ($M = 2.15$).

The highest disagreement with the belief that good people go to heaven was among supporters of the concept of DAS and abortion rights ($M = 1.50$, $F(1,527)= 5.31$, $p < .05$). There was slightly less disagreement with the belief that good people go to heaven among those who were pro-life, regardless of their position on the concept of DAS ($M = 1.43$; lower numbers indicate more agreement with the belief). The strongest agreement with the statement that good people go to heaven occurs among those who oppose the concept of DAS, but are pro-choice ($M = 1.14$).

Extenuating Circumstances

Figure 2 presents data regarding the mitigating effects of various extenuating circumstances on consideration of personal DAS. These mitigating circumstances included imagining that one was incontinent, becoming a burden to others, experiencing chronic pain, experiencing loss of independence, being diagnosed with a terminal illness (less than 6 months to live), being kept alive by a machine, becoming less mobile, and going to a nursing home.

Of special importance from a social policy point of view is which situations garner majority support for consideration of DAS for oneself. There was majority support for consideration of DAS for oneself in the hypothetical situations of

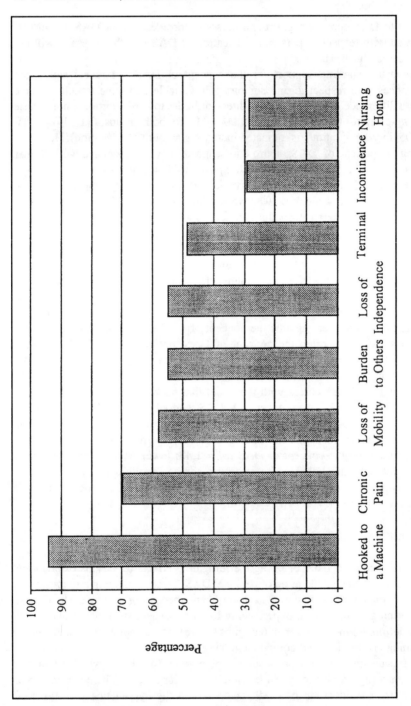

Figure 2. Consideration for DAS for oneself in various extenuating circumstances.

being hooked to a machine (94.2%), experiencing chronic pain (69.8%), personal loss of mobility (57.9%) being a burden to others (54.7%), and loss of independence (54.7%). There was *not* a majority sentiment of consideration of DAS for oneself given the hypothetical situations of having less than six months to live (terminality; 48.5%), experiencing a loss of bladder or bowel control (incontinence; 29.1%), or going to a nursing home (28.6%). However, the least supported situation still garnered almost 30 percent for consideration of DAS. These data should be measured against the 45.3 percent favorability percentage toward personal DAS in the absence of delineating specific extenuating circumstances.

These extenuating circumstances were then crossed with demographic and attitude variables discussed previously with regard to attitudes toward DAS for oneself with regard to the demographic variables presented in Table 3. The results with regards to attitudinal variables are presented in Table 4.

Being Hooked to a Machine

Being hooked to a machine accentuated the demographic effects of marital status ($\chi^2 = 14.9$, $p < .021$) and region ($\chi^2 = 19.7$, $p < .032$) and the attitude effects of political ideology ($\chi^2 = 17.5$, $p < .008$) and belief that suicides do not go to heaven ($\chi^2 = 9.8$, $p < .044$) on consideration of DAS for oneself. For marital status, 73.2 percent of single people, 88.6 percent of married people, 98.2 percent of those formerly married, and 100 percent of those who declined to answer would consider DAS for themselves if they were hooked to a machine that was keeping them alive. Consideration of DAS for oneself when hooked to a life sustaining machine was strong everywhere in the state of Michigan. The rates of consideration of DAS for oneself were for Detroit (91.7%), outer Wayne county (west of Detroit, 89.3%), outer metro (north of Detroit, 87.5%), central (Lansing area, 93.2%), west (Grand Rapids, 86.2%), and north (Traverse City, 80%).

For ideology, undecided/declined were most likely to consider DAS for themselves when hooked to a life sustaining machine (100%), followed by conservatives (95.1%), moderates (88%), and liberals (78.9%). Consideration of DAS for oneself when hooked to a machine was weakest among those who believe a suicide does not go to heaven (86.7%), followed by those who were unsure or declined to express an opinion (87.8%), and finally those who disagree with this idea (88.6%).

Experiencing Chronic Pain

There were significant differences for gender ($\chi^2 = 10.8$, $p < .005$), race ($\chi^2 = 6.7$, $p < .036$), and marital status ($\chi^2 = 22.1$, $p < .001$) in consideration of DAS for oneself when experiencing chronic pain. Women were more likely to avoid DAS when experiencing chronic pain (57.1%) then were men (42.9%). Whites were more likely to consider DAS for themselves when in chronic pain (60.2%) than were other racial groups (51.5%). Consideration of DAS for oneself when

Table 3. Chi Squares for Demographic Variables with Respect to Extenuating Circumstances

Demographic	Hooked to a Machine χ^2	p	Chronic Pain χ^2	p	Loss of Mobility χ^2	p	Burden to Others χ^2	p
Age	5.3	n.s.	5.0	n.s.	15.0	.020	8.5	n.s.
Gender	4.4	n.s.	10.8	.005	1.0	n.s.	7.7	.022
Education	8.3	n.s.	5.6	n.s.	4.7	n.s.	.6	n.s.
Income	12.0	n.s.	3.2	n.s.	8.4	n.s.	13.2	n.s.
Race	3.1	n.s.	6.7	.036	5.2	n.s.	1.6	n.s.
Religion	5.9	n.s.	1.7	n.s.	3.2	n.s.	2.5	n.s.
Marital Status	14.9	.021	22.1	.001	9.0	n.s.	12.5	.051
Children	2.1	n.s.	.1	n.s.	3.2	n.s.	3.1	n.s.
Region	19.7	.032	11.3	n.s.	20.2	.030	8.6	n.s.

Demographic	Loss of Independence χ^2	p	Terminal χ^2	p	Incontinence χ^2	p	Nursing Home χ^2	p
Age	7.0	n.s.	9.2	n.s.	5.3	n.s.	6.8	n.s.
Gender	4.5	n.s.	.2	n.s.	6.2	.046	2.5	n.s.
Education	1.3	n.s.	24.5	.000	7.9	n.s.	8.3	n.s.
Income	8.7	n.s.	11.7	n.s.	14.4	n.s.	8.4	n.s.
Race	.2	n.s.	.8	n.s.	.8	n.s.	.7	n.s.
Religion	.9	n.s.	3.1	n.s.	4.6	n.s.	2.6	n.s.
Marital Status	8.0	n.s.	9.9	n.s.	15.3	.018	4.6	n.s.
Children	3.4	n.s.	2.9	n.s.	11.3	.003	11.6	.003
Region	6.6	n.s.	22.2	.014	14.1	n.s.	12.4	n.s.

Table 4. Chi Squares for Attitude Variables with Respect to Extenuating Circumstances

Attitude	Hooked to a Machine		Chronic Pain		Loss of Mobility		Burden to Others	
	χ^2	p	χ^2	p	χ^2	p	χ^2	p
Ideology	17.5	.008	5.8	n.s.	5.9	n.s.	1.7	n.s.
Party Identification	5.8	n.s.	19.4	.004	7.3	n.s.	3.8	n.s.
Church Attendance	1.4	n.s.	4.1	n.s.	14.5	.006	6.9	n.s.
Good Go To Heaven	1.8	n.s.	2.3	n.s.	5.0	n.s.	7.4	n.s.
Suicide Not To Heaven	9.8	.044	7.0	n.s.	5.5	n.s.	6.0	n.s.
Abortion Rights	4.2	n.s.	.1	n.s.	5.9	.052	5.4	n.s.

Attitude	Loss of Independence		Terminal		Incontinence		Nursing Home	
	χ^2	p	χ^2	p	χ^2	p	χ^2	p
Ideology	7.9	n.s.	7.5	n.s.	5.5	n.s.	5.4	n.s.
Party Identification	7.7	n.s.	7.2	n.s.	11.7	n.s.	14.1	.028
Church Attendance	7.3	n.s.	6.6	n.s.	8.4	n.s.	10.8	.030
Good Go To Heaven	1.9	n.s.	9.4	.052	1.4	n.s.	12.2	.016
Suicide Not To Heaven	10.3	.036	4.1	n.s.	7.1	n.s.	5.3	n.s.
Abortion Rights	4.6	n.s.	.8	n.s.	1.1	n.s.	1.0	n.s.

experiencing chronic pain was highest among formerly married individuals (67.9%), followed by currently married individuals (63.4%), and those who are single (31.7%).

Only one attitude had a significant impact on consideration of DAS for oneself when experiencing chronic pain and that was political party identification ($\chi^2 = 19.4, p < .004$). Those who's party affiliation was Democratic showed the highest personal consideration of DAS when in chronic pain (63.5%), followed by independents (56.1%), Republicans (56.3%), and finally those who had other than a mainstream party affiliation (50%).

Loss of Mobility

Loss of mobility accentuated the demographic effect of age ($\chi^2 = 15.0$, $p < .020$) and region ($\chi^2 = 20.2$, $p < .030$) and the attitude effect of church attendance ($\chi^2 = 14.5$, $p < .006$) and position on abortion rights ($\chi^2 = 5.9$, $p < .052$) on consideration of DAS for oneself. Consideration of DAS for oneself when experiencing a loss of mobility was highest among eighteen to twenty-nine (56.3%), followed by 65+ (55.3%), thirty to forty-nine year-olds (47.4%), and finally fifty to sixty-four (43.9%). Consideration was highest in terms of geographic region in central Michigan (61%), followed by Detroit (54.2%), northern Michigan (52%), western Michigan (46.6%), outer Wayne (46.4%), and finally outer metro (41.3%).

Consideration of DAS when experiencing a loss of mobility was highest among those who seldom attend church (54.7%), followed by half-time attendees (50%), and frequent attendees (36.9%). Among abortion rights supporters, consideration of DAS when experiencing a loss of mobility was 52 percent and among pro-life supporters it was 43.3 percent.

Being a Burden to Others

Becoming a burden to others accentuated the demographic effect of gender ($\chi^2 = 7.7$, $p < .022$) and marital status ($\chi^2 = 12.5$, $p < .051$). Women would consider DAS for themselves at a higher rate (53.4%) if they became a burden than would men (44 percent). For marital status, the highest rates of consideration when becoming a burden occur for those who are formerly married (55.4%), followed by those who are currently married (49.1%), and single (39%).

Loss of Independence

Loss of independence accentuated the effects for the attitude that suicides do not go to heaven ($\chi^2 = 10.3$, $p < .036$) on consideration of a personal DAS. Support was highest for the consideration of DAS for oneself among those who disagree that suicides do not go to heaven (48.3%), followed by those who were unsure of the fate of suicides with respect to heaven (41.5%) and those that agreed that suicides do not go to heaven (40%). There were no significant demographic effects.

Terminality

Terminality accentuated the effects on two demographic factors in the consideration of DAS for oneself when told that you have six months or less to live (terminal) and one significant attitude difference. There was a clear downward trend in consideration of DAS for oneself with increasing levels of education ($\chi^2 = 24.5$, $p < .001$) with support at the following levels: K-12, 53.6 percent; some college, 45.8 percent; college graduate, 30.8 percent; and post graduate education, 30 percent. Support for consideration of DAS for oneself was highest in northern Michigan (60%), followed by Detroit (50%), western Michigan (44.8%), central Michigan (40.7%), outer metro areas (37.5%), and outer Wayne county (25%; $\chi^2 = 22.2$, $p < .014$).

Terminality also accentuated the effect of the attitude that good people go to heaven on consideration of DAS as an option for oneself. Consideration was highest at 45.8 percent among those who agreed that good people go to heaven, followed by those who disagreed that good people go to heaven (43.2%) and those who were undecided or declined to answer (22.9%; $\chi^2 = 9.4$, $p < .052$).

Incontinence

Incontinence accentuated the effects of three demographic variables on consideration of DAS for oneself. Women would consider DAS for themselves when experiencing incontinence (27.1%) at a higher rate than men (25.5%; $\chi^2 = 6.2$, $p < .046$). Those who are formerly married had the highest rates of consideration of DAS when experiencing incontinence (39.3%), followed by single (31.7%), and currently married (21.1%; $\chi^2 = 15.3$, $p < .018$). Among those with no children living at home, support for consideration of DAS for oneself when experiencing incontinence was 29.7 percent and only 19.5 percent of those with children currently living at home would consider DAS for themselves ($\chi^2 = 11.3$, $p < .003$).

Going to a Nursing Home

Going to a nursing home accentuated the effect of having children at home on consideration of DAS for oneself among those who would be facing going to a nursing home ($\chi^2 = 11.6$, $p < .003$). Again, having no children living at home increased consideration of DAS for oneself (27%) as compared to having children at home (21.8%).

Going to a nursing home accentuated the effects of three attitude variables on consideration of DAS for oneself. Among those who's party identification was independent, support for DAS for oneself when going to a nursing home was highest (36.6%), followed by those who had no party affiliations or who declined to answer (35%), Democrats (23%), and finally Republicans (20.7%; $\chi^2 = 14.1$, $p < .028$). Consideration of DAS for oneself when going to a nursing home was highest among those who frequently attend church (29.2%) and those who seldom attend church (28.5%), followed by those who attend church services about half the time (15.3%; $\chi^2 = 10.8$, $p < .030$). Consideration of DAS for oneself when faced with moving to a nursing home was highest among those who were uncertain about whether good people go to heaven or those who declined to answer (31.3%) and those who disagree that good people go to heaven (31.8%), followed by those who think good people do go to heaven (21.2%; $\chi^2 = 12.2$, $p < .016$).

DISCUSSION

This survey shows that there is greater support for the general concept of DAS than for personal application to oneself. The wider acceptance of the general concept as opposed to personal application suggests that society considers DAS in relation to others rather than to themselves. The effect on age illustrates this principle. While people of middle-age support the general concept of DAS (because they don't see themselves as targets of the concept), there is a sharp decline in support among the elderly. The demarcation line between the general acceptance and personal application of DAS thins out with age.

The results on income and education further reflects the undeniable danger of DAS becoming a procedure advocated or even imposed by some people on others. The general concept received more support in the middle and upper classes, but only the 25 to 45,000 income category showed a majority of support for personal application. This may be due to societal pressure concerning cost and the biased illusion our culture has derogating any dependency.

Support for the concept but not for the personal application grows with increasing education. The pattern with regard to conceptual attitudes reflects the historic pattern of the better educated to be morally nuanced (Bayet, 1922) with respect to general suicide and thus be more tolerant of it. The nonsignificant pattern with regard to personal application suggests, in addition, a kind of elitism. It is a solution for others but not for oneself, or, alternatively, a playing with the idea of suicide without direct ramifications to oneself. This data is critical because it highlights the danger of potential abuse of DAS where it is selectively employed against certain classes of people. The greater support of the general concept of DAS as opposed to its personal application contains a disquieting undertone. Members of society are quick to apply DAS to other groups (but not themselves) which society is quick to judge have poor "quality of life."

This undertone is also evident for both genders. Men were very strong supporters of the concept (70.1%), but show lesser support for personal application (53.2%). Women score lower on both (59% for concept and 42.8% for self). This illustrates the willingness of both genders to apply DAS to groups other than themselves. This can be paralleled to Kevorkian's patients. Most Kevorkian cases were women (which is a discrepancy from the data given by the survey showing that only a minority of women would support self-application), but it would not be surprising that those supporting and maybe recommending the application of DAS were men.

A variety of factors have been linked to life-taking attitudes, including degree of religiosity and denomination (Beswick, 1970; Granberg, 1978; Harris & Mills, 1985; Jelen, 1984; Kalish, 1963; Kearl & Harris, 1981; Rhodes, 1985), attitudes toward women (Kyes, 1980), education level (Granberg, 1978), gender (Deluty, 1988) and ethnicity, age and personal experiences (Feifel & Shaq, 1980). A God-ownership orientation to one's life is a stronger predictor of a person's attitudes toward abortion, suicide, and assisted suicide than either religion or political orientation (Ross & Kaplan, 1993). Beswick (1970) makes the point that taking a person's life is a complex issue with different domains producing different attitudes for the same person.

For example, although the Hebrew Bible clearly prohibits suicide (Gen. 9:5-6) it is more ambivalent about abortion, making a clear legal distinction between the unintentional killing of a fetus and that of a pregnant woman as a result of a quarrel between two nearby men (Exo. 21:22-23). The death of the fetus is compensated for in damages paid to the woman's husband. The death of the mother, in contrast, calls for the death penalty.

This data also illustrates the important role played by extenuating circumstances, such as being hooked to a machine, experiencing chronic pain, personal loss of mobility, incontinence, being a burden to others, and loss of independence. The data reported here reflects hypothetical extenuating circumstances as opposed to the actual situations experienced by patients in the above survey (Breitbart, Rosenfeld, & Passik, 1996).

In our hypothetical situations, experiencing chronic pain served as a major factor in consideration of DAS for oneself (69.8%). But in HIV-infected patients actually experiencing chronic pain (Breitbart et al., 1996) the severity of pain or pain-related functional impairment were not a factor related to consideration of DAS for themselves. This was also true for the Kevorkian patients previously discussed (Kaplan, Lachenmeier, Harrow, O'Dell, Uziel, Schneiderhan, & Cheyfitz, 1999-2000), where psychological distress seemed more important, especially among the women.

ACKNOWLEDGMENTS

The authors would like to thank Ron Dwonkowski and Brian Dickerson of the Detroit Free Press for making the data in this poll available for analysis.

REFERENCES

Ames, K., Wilson, L., & Sawhill, R. (1991). Last rites. *Newsweek, 26,* 40-41.

Asch, D. A. (1996). The role of critical care nurses in euthanasia and assisted suicide. *The New England Journal of Medicine, 334* (21), 1374-1379.

Bachman, J. G., Alcser, K. H., Doukas, D. J., Lichtenstein, R. L., Corning, A.D., & Brody, H. (1996). Attitudes of Michigan physicians and the public toward legalizing physician-assisted suicide and voluntary euthanasia. *The New England Journal of Medicine, 334* (5), 303-309.

Bayet, A. (1922). *La suicide et moral.* Paris, France: F. Alcan.

Beswick, D. G. (1970). Attitudes toward taking human life. *Australian and New Zealand Journal of Sociology, 6,* 120-130.

Breitbart, W., Rosenfeld, B. D., & Passik, S. D. (1996). Interest in physician-assisted suicide among ambulatory HIV-infected patients. *American Journal of Psychiatry, 153* (2), 238-242.

Cassel, C. K., & Meier, D. E. (1990). Morals and moralism in the debate over euthanasia and assisted suicide. *The New England Journal of Medicine, 323,* 750-752.

Chin, A. E., Hedberg, K., Higginson, G. K., & Fleming, D. W. (1999). Legalized physician-assisted suicide in Oregon—The first year's experience. *New England Journal of Medicine, 340,* 577-583.

Cohen, J. S., Fihn, S. D., Boyko, E. J., Jonsen, A. R., & Wood, R. W. (1994). Attitudes toward assisted suicide and euthanasia among physicians in Washington state. *The New England Journal of Medicine, 331* (2), 89-94.

Deluty, R. H. (1988). Factors affecting the acceptability of suicide. *Omega, 19,* 315-326.

Duberstein, P. R., Conwell, Y., Cox, C., Podgorski, C. A., Glazer, R. S., & Caine, E. D. (1995). Attitudes toward self-determined death: A survey of primary care physicians. *Journal of the American Geriatrics Society, 43* (4):395-400.

Feifel, H., & Shaq, D. (1980). Death outlook and social issues. *Omega, 11,* 201-215.

Granberg, D. (1978). Pro-life or reflection of conservative ideology? An analysis of opposition to legalized abortion. *Sociology and Social Research, 62,* 414-429.

Harris, R. J., & Mills, E. W. (1985). Religion, values and attitudes toward abortion. *Journal for the Scientific Study of Religion, 24,* 137-153.

Jelen, T. G. (1984). Respect for life, sexual morality and opposition to abortion. *Review of Religious Research, 25,* 220-229.

Kalish, R. A. (1963). Some variables in death attitudes. *The Journal of Social Psychology, 59,* 137-145.

Kaplan, K. J., Lachenmeier, F., Harrow, M., O'Dell, J., Uziel, O., Schneiderhan, M., & Cheyfitz, K. (1999-2000). Psychosocial versus biomedical risk factors in Kevorkian's first forty-seven physician-assisted deaths. *Omega, 40* (1), 109-163 (this issue).

Kearl, M. C., & Harris, R. (1981). Individualism and the emerging "modern" ideology of death. *Omega, 12,* 269-280.

Koenig, H. G. (1993). Legalizing physician-assisted suicide: Some thoughts and concerns. *The Journal of Family Practice, 37* (2):171-179.

Kyes, K. B., (1990). *Attitudes toward abortion as an indicant of attitudes toward sex.* Paper presented at the 36th meeting of the Southeastern Psychological Association, Atlanta, Georgia, April 1990.

Lawton, K. (1991). The doctor as executioner. *Christianity Today, 16,* 50-52.

Lee, M. A., Nelson, H. D., Tilden, V. P., Ganzini, L., Schmidt, T. A., & Tolle, S. W. (1996). Legalizing assisted suicide—Views of physicians in Oregon. *The New England Journal of Medicine, 334* (5), 310-315.

Mitchell, B. (1996). Nazi Germany's euphemisms. In J. F. Kilner, A. B. Miller, & E. D. Pellegrino (Eds.), *Dignity and dying: A Christian appraisal.* Grand Rapids, MI: William B. Eerdmans.

Quill, T. E. (1991). Death and dignity: A case of individualized decision making. *The New England Journal of Medicine, 324,* 691-694.

Quill, T. E., Cassel, C. K., & Meier, D. E. (1992). Care of the hopelessly ill: Proposed clinical criteria for physician-assisted suicide. *The New England Journal of Medicine, 327,* 1380-1384.

Rhodes, A. L. (1985). Religion and opposition to abortion reconsidered. *Review of Religious Research, 27,* 158-167.

Ross, L. T., & Kaplan, K. J. (1993-94). Life ownership orientation and attitudes toward abortion, suicide, doctor-assisted suicide, and capital punishment. *Omega, 28* (1), 17-30.

Seidlitz, L., Duberstein, P. R., Cox, C., & Conwell, Y. (1995). Attitudes of older people toward suicide and assisted suicide: An analysis of Gallup Poll findings. *Journal of the American Geriatrics Society, 43* (9), 993-998.

Singer, P. A., Choudhry, S., Armstrong, J., Meslin, E. M., & Lowy, F. H. (1995). Public opinion regarding end-of-life decisions: Influence of prognosis, practice and process. *Social Science and Medicine, 41* (11), 1517-1521.

PHYSICIAN-ASSISTED SUICIDE AND EUTHANASIA: THE PHARMACIST'S PERSPECTIVE

MARK E. SCHNEIDERHAN, PHARM.D., BCPP
University of Illinois at Chicago
College of Pharmacy

ABSTRACT

Pharmacists are in a critical position when pharmaceutical agents are prescribed for the purpose of physician-assisted suicide and/or euthanasia and they may need to decide whether dispensing a lethal dose of a medication is ethically and morally acceptable for a patient. In many cases, pharmacists may not even be aware that prescriptions are intended for physician-assisted suicide and/or euthanasia. Pharmacists have a special responsibility to protect patients who are contemplating end-of-life decisions such as physician-assisted suicide and euthanasia. Pharmaceutical care ("Responsible provision of drug therapy for the purpose of achieving definite outcomes that improve a patient's quality of life . . . ") requires that the pharmacist not only understands the medications but also the individual patient and the complexities of their lives and suffering. Only in this way can pharmacists provide safe and effective use of medications for the patients they serve.

What is and what should be the role of the pharmacist in physician-assisted suicide? Pharmacists are in a critical position when pharmaceutical agents are prescribed for the purpose of physician-assisted suicide and/or euthanasia and they may need to decide whether dispensing a lethal dose of a medication is ethically and morally acceptable for a patient. In many cases, pharmacists may not even be aware that prescriptions are intended for physician-assisted suicide and/or euthanasia.

The purpose of this discussion is to describe the role of the pharmacist in physician-assisted suicide. Euphemisms and terminology such as "Physician aid-in-dying," "Death-with-dignity," "Pharmaceutically assisted death,"

"Deliverance," "Physician-assisted-death," and "Physician-assisted-dying" are commonly used terms to describe physician-assisted suicide. These terms can confuse and de-emphasize the meaning of physician-assisted suicide/euthanasia or justify the intended activity. For purposes of consistency, the term *physician-assisted suicide* and *euthanasia* will be used throughout this discussion.

PHARMACY PRACTICE

The practice of pharmacy has evolved dramatically in the last thirty years. Consumers typically view pharmacists as dispensers of medications and educators. Historically, pharmacists were responsible for compounding certain medications. Today pharmacists perform less compounding because the pharmaceutical manufacturers formulate the majority of commonly used dosage forms. Most importantly, pharmacists are readily accessible to the public to answer healthcare related questions. As a result, the public perceives pharmacists as being very trustworthy.

Today, pharmacists are increasingly accepting the responsibilities of the direct outcome of medication treatment of the patient. The shift from the emphasis on pharmaceutical products (i.e., medications) to direct patient care is becoming the standard of pharmacy practice. Hepler and Strand (1990) described the concept of pharmaceutical care as the responsible provision of drug therapy for the purpose of achieving definite outcomes that improve a patient's quality of life including: 1) cure of a disease, 2) reduction or elimination of symptoms, and 3) preventing disease progression or symptomatology. In addition, unwanted outcomes may be experienced if a medication is: 1) inappropriately prescribed, 2) not accessible to the patient or not administered appropriately, 3) not taken correctly by the patient, 4) causing unwanted side effects, and 5) not closely monitored for efficacy or side-effects. As a result of the current trends, professional organizations such as the American Society of Health-System Pharmacists and American Pharmaceutical Association have adopted the following statement: "The mission of pharmacy is to serve society as the profession responsible for the appropriate use of medications, devices, and services to achieve optimal therapeutic outcomes" (American Society of Hospital Pharmacists, 1993).

As stated above, a goal of pharmaceutical care is to improve the quality of life of an individual. Unfortunately, the literature is very vague in defining quality of life and often relies on subjective opinion or on certain established rating scales. Quality of life rating scales are used to assess a patient's perception and beliefs regarding their general health by assessing daily activities, problems (physical or emotional) that interfere with social activities, and overall well-being over a specified time frame. Quality of life rating scales are typically self-rating scales as compared to interview rating scales. An important disadvantage to self-rating scales is the dependence on the patient's insight into their illness and judgment to provide accurate self-assessments. Insight and judgment are often impaired in many psychiatric disorders. A thorough mental status examination and psychiatric history is often needed to assess the patient's insight and judgment. Another limitation is that the results of quality of life rating scales are valid only over the specified time period. The validity of the results cannot be assured before or after the specified period that is being assessed. Therefore, a single rating can only provide information over the tested time frame and should not be extrapolated beyond the time period. Finally, quality of life scales cannot replace the aspects of personal dialogue and "getting to know the patient." Dixon and Keir describe the interplay of mercy, pharmaceutical care and quality of life (Dixon & Keir, 1998)

> Assessments of quality of life are subjective and richly personal. An apprecia-
> tion of these issues requires extensive interactions and meaningful discus-
> sions. To understand individuals' perception of a minimally adequate or a
> good quality of life is to come to know how they define themselves, identify
> meaningful activities, or pare down a unique existence to its bare essentials. If
> you begin to understand why a suffering person wishes to die, you begin to
> understand the ways in which unresolved pain, horrifying symptoms, and
> unaddressed needs have destroyed the person's identity and way of life.
> Concern for the quality of life thus brings an understanding of suffering to
> those who practice pharmaceutical care (p. 581).

Determining what is considered responsible provision of drug therapy or the appropriate use of medications sometimes requires judgment that goes beyond the pharmacology, pharmacodynamics, or pharmacokinetics of a drug product. The moral and ethical issues that involve the appropriate use of medications cannot be overlooked. The moral and ethical issues that pharmacists face are often the products of the interrelationship between intent of prescribed medications and the "quality of life" of an individual patient. Defining "quality of life" for another individual will directly influence decisions regarding futility of medical care and the need for physician-assisted suicide. Such decisions can be often influenced by the degree of helplessness, anxiety and uncertainty among the patient, family members, and healthcare providers (Ross & Kaplan, 1993). Conflicts may occur as the result of disagreement, feelings of helplessness and anxiety among the patient, family members, and healthcare providers. In addition, disagreements may occur among the caregivers or family members when the physician determines that continued treatment is futile and limits are placed on the level of care. Ethical concerns can erupt when the emphasis shifts from the preservation of life to a focus on death. Essentially, pharmacists providing pharmaceutical care must carefully balance beneficence and the patient's autonomy (Strand, Cipolle, & Morley, 1992). The fine balance of beneficence, trust, awareness of patient's autonomy, and desire for self-determination are the essence of the doctor-patient relationship.

Pharmacists may not be privy to certain aspects of the doctor/patient relationship which plays an essential role in the end-of-life decision process. The level of involvement of the physician and autonomy of the patient can directly influence the outcome of the end-of-life decisions. In the last decade, the role of individual autonomy especially in medical decisions has become an integral aspect of the patient-doctor relationship (Emanuel & Emanuel, 1992). Once again, conflicts can be expected to arise when the values of physicians, pharmacists, and patients are not in harmony and perhaps in discord. Healthcare practitioners such as pharmacists may not appreciate the subtle differences that may result from various levels of physician involvement and desire of the patient to end his or her life.[1]

PHARMACISTS ETHICAL DILEMMA

Pharmacists will most likely be caught in a front-line position because medications are the primary means of assisting the death of a patient. Because of this, pharmacist's attitudes about issues surrounding physician-assisted suicide have been recently studied. Rupp and Isenhower (1994) conducted a pharmacist survey ($n = 534$) that included a majority of male respondents (72.5%) with baccalaureate training. The median age of the respondents was forty-two years old and half (53.3%) were between the age of twenty-six and forty-five years old.

A majority (72.6%) of pharmacists believed that patients might be justified in wanting to end their own lives. This is consistent with popular opinion that individuals should be able to make end-of-life issues for themselves. Not surprisingly, a majority of pharmacists (70.9%) thought that prescription drugs are an appropriate means for physicians to use when assisting a patient's suicide/euthanasia. Almost half (48.6%) of pharmacists felt that it may be sometimes appropriate for a physician to actively assist a patient to end his or her life. Interestingly, religious conviction was a statistically significant factor among pharmacists who opposed physician-assisted suicide.

Pharmacists were less enthusiastic about becoming involved in this practice especially if they are not informed. Over half (53.8%) of the respondents with a statistically significant greater number of younger (less than 42 years old) pharmacists wanted to know the purpose of the prescriptions dispensed especially

---

[1] Wooddell and Kaplan (1998) describe the psychological and legal dynamics of the patient/ physician dyad that is necessary in defining the End-of-Life actions. Wooddell and Kaplan (1998) define the End-of-Life actions by matching the level of physician involvement with the decisions made by the patient. Three possible scenarios exist for Physician-Assisted Suicide and euthanasia and largely depend on the decision of the patient. The patients decisions may be influenced by the physician's discussion of alternatives (Discussed Assisted-Suicide) or by the absence of discussed alternatives (Accepted Assisted-Suicide), or by the direct or subtle encouragement by the physician (Encouraged Assisted-Suicide). Likewise, the patient's decision for euthanasia may be discussed, accepted, or encouraged (i.e., Discussed Voluntary Euthanasia, Accepted Voluntary Euthanasia, Encouraged Voluntary Euthanasia). Obviously the most objectional scenario is the patient who is overtly or covertly encouraged by the physician, family, or third party into assisted suicide or euthanasia.

if they were to be used in physician-assisted suicide. A majority of pharmacists (66.6%) thought that it was not appropriate for a physician to involve the pharmacist in a patient's euthanasia/suicide without the knowledge and consent of the pharmacist.

Interestingly the surveyors appeared biased toward physician-assisted suicide. The authors, in an attempt to provide directions to the respondents about physician-assisted suicide, included the following directions prior to the survey questions: "The following guidelines have been suggested to help physicians and others evaluate the appropriateness of suicide/euthanasia: 1) An explicit, repeated request by the patient to die; 2) Severe mental or physical suffering, with no prospect of relief; 3) An informed, free, and consistent decision by the patient; and 4) The lack of other treatment options and/or the failure of those available." The authors stated that the information was abstracted from current practice in the Netherlands. The authors also admitted that they might have introduced a pro-assisted-suicide bias to the survey. In actuality, the Netherlands experience with physician- assisted suicide is not quite equivalent to the interpretation of Rupp and Isenhower. For example, in 1984, the Royal Dutch Medical Association issued the following guidelines (underlined sections highlight the differences): 1) The patient must be a mentally competent adult. 2) The request for euthanasia needs to be voluntary, consistent and repeated. 3) The patient must be suffering intolerably with no help or relief, although, the disease need not be terminal. 4) The physician must consult with another physician who is not involved in the case.

Anecdotal reports suggested violations of the above guidelines including euthanasia among the psychiatrically ill and sometimes without the patient's request (Kimsma, 1996). Overall, the background information failed to describe the potential problems or the current problems with physician-assisted suicide and euthanasia in the Netherlands.

In a study of Michigan pharmacists, seven out of ten participants agreed that a patient has a legal right to commit suicide and half of the participants agreed that a patient has an ethical or moral right to commit suicide (Vivian, Slaughter, & Calissi, 1993). Nine out of ten pharmacists also agreed that physician assisted suicide is acceptable in terminal patients with thirty days to live. Comparatively, only five out of ten pharmacists agreed that physician-assisted suicide is acceptable in non-terminal cases. Additionally, six out of ten respondents agreed that a physician or other healthcare professional might participate in an assisted suicide. The study also indicated that age and religion were important factors influencing the decisions of pharmacists which was consistent with the previous study. Finally, a national survey conducted by Pharmacy Times indicated that over half of pharmacists supported physician-assisted suicide of patients in certain situations (Buckley, 1994).

Overall, a majority of pharmacists feel that patients can be justified in making a decision for physician-assisted suicide. A majority of pharmacists also feel that prescription medications are the appropriate means for physician-assisted suicide. However, a majority of pharmacists also feel that they have the right to know the intent of the prescription, especially in the case of a physician-assisted suicide. Because of the uncertainty arising from a lack of information, a majority of pharmacists were unable to commit to an involvement in physician-assisted suicide. In addition to ethical and therapeutic influences that weigh pharmacists' decisions, legal issues involving physician-assisted suicide will also influence pharmacists' involvement in this area.

LEGAL ISSUES AFFECTING PHARMACISTS

The Supreme Court recently ruled that there is no constitutional right for physician-assisted suicide but seemed to open the way for each state to control legislation. In other words, the Supreme Court has delegated authority to the individual states in the regulating of physician-assisted suicide. In a recent landmark decision, the people of Oregon State voted to legalize the right of an individual to choose a physician-assisted suicide (Measure 16, the Oregon Death with Dignity Act). Ethical conflict among pharmacists may be inevitable where physician-assisted suicide is legalized. Oregon's Measure 16 is the first law that allows assisted suicide or euthanasia in the United States. The ethically conflicted pharmacist may choose to conscientiously object physician-assisted suicide but may suffer the consequences of losing their job or creating internal tension among colleagues (Mullans, Allen, & Brushwood, 1996; Brushwood & Allen, 1996).

Certain immunities listed in Measure 16 state "no person" shall be subject to legal action for participating in the procedure (Mullans, Allen, & Brushwood, 1996). However, it is less clear for pharmacists who refuse to dispense medications for physician-assisted suicide cases. South Dakota Governor, William Janklow signed a measure that will protect pharmacists who conscientiously object to dispensing medications for physician-assisted suicide, euthanasia, mercy killing and abortions (ASHP Newsletter, 1998).

The Oregon Death with Dignity Act does not define who administers the lethal prescription; therefore, Measure 16 allows for physician-assisted suicide or euthanasia. If the patient is able to self-administer the lethal medication then the pharmacist may have an important role by providing the medication directly to the patient. Conversely, if the physician or the nurse administers the lethal medication (i.e., euthanasia), the pharmacists may be involved with dispensing the medication without knowledge of the purpose. Under the Oregon Death with Dignity Act, prescribers are not required to discuss the prescribed use of medications with the pharmacist. In addition, the pharmacist may not be able to ensure that the requirements for a lethal prescription are met. The Oregon Death with Dignity Act requires the following (Wittenburg, 1995):

*The patient is at least 18 years old, a resident of Oregon, has an incurable disease that will lead to death within six months.

*The patient has made both oral and written requests for life-ending medication, with two witnesses and a 15-day span between requests.

*The patient has been informed of the diagnosis, the prognosis, the risks associated with the medication to be prescribed, the probable result of taking the medication, and the feasible alternatives (e.g., comfort care, hospice care, and pain control); the patient has been offered opportunities to rescind the request.

*A second physician has confirmed the diagnosis and confirmed the patient is capable and acting voluntarily.

*The patient is requested to notify the next of kin.

*The following are documented in the medical record: all oral and written requests, diagnosis and prognosis; verification that the patient is capable, acting voluntarily, and making an informed decision; and a statement from the attending physician indicating that all requirements under the act have been met and describing the steps taken to carry out the request, including the medication prescribed.

In efforts to clarify Measure 16, the Oregon Board of Medical Examiners (BME) on April 7, 1998, proposed a ruling that a pharmacist will be made aware of the purpose of any prescription written pursuant to the Death With Dignity Act in order that they will have the opportunity to participate or not and to appropriately consult with the physician and counsel the patient. The Oregon Board of Pharmacy is currently waiting on the final ruling of the following proposal.

DIVISION 015 **GENERAL LICENSING RULES, RELATING TO CONTROLLED SUBSTANCES**

Attending physicians prescribing medications to physician assisted suicide patients 847-015-0035

Attending physicians prescribing medications pursuant to ORS 127.800 - 127.897 shall:

(1) Dispense medications directly, including ancillary medications intended to facilitate the desired effect to minimize the patient's discomfort, provided the attending physician is registered as a dispensing physician with the Board of Medical Examiners, has a current Drug Enforcement Administration (D.E.A.) certificate, and complies with the provisions of ORS 677.089, OAR 847-015-0015 and OAR 847-015-0025; or (2) With the patient's written consent: (a) Contact a pharmacist, and inform the pharmacist of the purpose of the prescription, and (b) Deliver the written prescription personally or by mail to the pharmacist who will dispense the medications to either the patient, the attending physician, or an expressly identified patient's agent.

Statutory Authority: ORS 677.265 Stats. Implemented: ORS 127.815

Interestingly, the proposal requires the patient's consent prior to contacting the pharmacist. Patient consent is not typically required for physicians and pharmacists to discuss patient medical issues together. The well-being and safety of the patient (i.e., medication indications/contraindications, drug- interactions, allergies) can be discussed without patient consent. The requirement of consent may prevent the pharmacist from realizing the true purpose of a lethally prescribed medication. In certain contexts, patients may be fearful to consent to have their physician discuss the purpose of the medication with the pharmacist. However, this interferes with the professional courtesy of communication that commonly occur between physicians and pharmacists to ensure safe and optimal medication usage and treatment of a patient.

THE PHARMACIST'S ROLE

The Oregon Society of Hospital Pharmacists expressed the concerns that a pharmacist may not be able to ensure that the requirements are met for a physician to issue a lethal prescription (Wittenburg, 1995). Most likely, pharmacists will receive orders and unknowingly dispense lethal prescriptions to critically ill patients. Without access to patient's medical history, diagnosis and physician intent, pharmacists may unknowingly participate in a physician-assisted suicide. The pharmacist is legally required to consult the patient regarding medications. However, without the correct information, the pharmacist may falsely reassure the patient of the palliative effects of a medication being prescribed to end a patient's life. To ensure appropriate use of medications, the pharmacist should be familiar with a patient's disease state, target symptoms, and current treatment.

Currently, there are no medications that are uniquely indicated for euthanasia or physician-assisted suicide. Among the medications used in euthanasia and assisted suicide, the most frequently used include controlled substances such as opioid narcotics such as morphine and sedatives or barbiturates. The opioid narcotics are commonly used to treat pain and comfort patients. For example, a typical starting dose of Morphine Sulfate may be between 5-30 mgs per dose given orally every three to four hours around the clock until acute pain is controlled and then may be given as needed for pain (Baumann, 1997). The dose should be initiated at the lowest dose and carefully titrated up to response with frequent assessments to monitor and manage side effects. Opioid narcotic dosages may vary based on the patient's age, weight, respiratory distress, tolerance to opioids, and severity of pain (Baumann, 1997). Typically, elderly patients are more sensitive to the analgesic effects (AGS Panel on Chronic pain in Older Persons, 1998) and likewise more susceptible to side effects such as respiratory depression and respiratory arrest (cessation of breathing) if the dosage is greater than the tolerance level of the patient. For example, the pharmacist may be alerted if the initial morphine dosage is greater than 60 mg in twenty-four hours for a debilitated elderly patient. The pharmacist is responsible for reviewing the clinical indications and prescription for the above morphine order prior to dispensing. However, if a dose appears acceptable, pharmacists may not question the prescribed medication when he or she is not aware of the physician's intent.[2]

The pharmacist is responsible for evaluating the physician's order prior to dispensing the medication to the patient. If the pharmacist is aware of the physician's intention to assist a suicide, the pharmacist then must decide whether he or she will participate in the dispensing or administration of the medications. Studies indicate that pharmacists may be hesitant in participating in euthanasia or assisted suicide unless they are well informed. From an emotional perspective, the pharmacist would be among the healthcare professionals most likely to have the last contact with the patient. If disagreements emerge regarding the treatment of the patient, a pharmacist may be forced to conscientiously object to dispensing or administering medications to a patient based on their clinical judgment. Aside from the problems of conscientious objections as described above, pharmacists may be at a disadvantage because of the lack of training to effectively assess the use of the lethal medication. Currently, there is very little scientific literature to support use or effectiveness of medications for physician-assisted suicide or euthanasia.

The defining role of the pharmacist is essential to understanding the physician-assisted suicide dilemma faced by the pharmacist. Pharmacists must sometimes act in the best interest of the patient. Moreover, the act of beneficence on the part of the pharmacist may directly effect the autonomy of the patient making end-of-life decisions. However, freedom of choice does not always justify physician-assisted suicide. The pharmacist's main role is to first begin to understand the patient and his or her unique situation. The variables involved in end-of-life decisions can be complicated and difficult to comprehend, including many factors that have little to do with biomedical factors (i.e., losing control or independence, becoming a financial burden, and suffering from loneliness, and/or depression) (Kaplan, Lachenmeier, Harrow, O'Dell, Uziel, Schneiderhan, & Cheyfitz, 1999-2000). The most disturbing variable affecting the patient's decisions are the direct influences, opinions, and motives of physician, family, and friends involved in advocating end-of-life decisions.

Even chronic pain, commonly found in the elderly is estimated to be untreated in 45 to 80 percent of nursing home residents (AGS Panel on Chronic pain in Older Persons, 1998). Consequences of chronic pain among the elderly can

---

[2] For example, opioid narcotics are usually indicated to treat pain and comfort the suffering hospitalized patient. However, the patient's death may be likewise hastened by the hospital administration of opioids to treat the pain. The activity is known as "Double Effect." From a legal perspective, the physician does not directly intend to cause death, but rather provides treatment to the patient that may hasten death. The legal aspects are primarily concerned with the physician's intent and level of involvement and assume that the patient's decisions are informed and voluntary.

include depression, decreased socialization, sleep disturbances, impaired ambulation, and increased healthcare utilization, and costs (AGS Panel on Chronic pain in Older Persons, 1998). Because of the myriad of variables influencing patients, pharmacists have a responsibility to assess the patient who is confronted with end-of-life decisions. With specialized training, the pharmacist may be able to determine if psychiatric consultation is indicated. Psychiatric assessments may uncover symptoms of depression underlying the motives as to why a patient wishes to end his or her life. The pharmacist's intervention may prove life-saving when dealing with a patient who is potentially suicidal.

Pharmacists interested in palliative care and hospice may consider providing consultations to organizations that provide support for patients who are considering physician assisted-suicide. One such organization started in 1993 is called "Compassion in Dying" in Seattle, Washington. "Compassion in Dying" provides information, consultation, and support to patients and involved family members who are deciding how to end their lives (Coombs, 1998). The organization opposes the criminalization of physician-assisted suicide and argues that patients die alone because family members are afraid of prosecution or patients are forced to commit a violent suicide, although there are no studies to support this. The organization emphasizes palliative care is an important option; however when palliative care fails, the organization counsels the patient on how to ask the doctor to assist in their suicide. Pharmacists can have an integral role in evaluating and determining why palliative care strategies fail. Palliative care may fail because of noncompliance, inadequate pain management, or because of underlying psychiatric illness. Therefore, specially trained pharmacists are in a unique position to provide the necessary recommendations to improve patient care.

In conclusion, pharmacists have a special responsibility to protect patients who are contemplating end-of-life decisions such as physician-assisted suicide and euthanasia. A realization of the complexity surrounding end-of-life decisions and associated variables that occur within the context of the patient/doctor relationship will serve to guide the pharmacist in assessment strategies and subsequent medication usage. Pharmaceutical care requires that the pharmacist not only understands the medications but also the individual patient and the complexities of their lives and suffering. Only in this way can pharmacists provide safe and effective use of medications for the patients they serve.

REFERENCES

American Geriatrics Society (AGS) Panel on Chronic Pain in Older Persons (1998). The management of chronic pain in older persons. *Journal of the American Geriatrics Society, 46*, 635-651.

American Society of Hospital Pharmacists (1993). ASHP statement on pharmaceutical care. *American Journal of Hospital Pharmacy, 50*, 1720-1723.

American Society of Health-System Pharmacists (1998). South Dakota approves sweeping conscience clause. *American Journal of Health-System Pharmacy Newsletter, 31* (5), 2.

Baumann, T. J. (1997). Pain management. In J. Dipiro, R. Talbert, G. Yee, et al. (Eds.), *Pharmacotherapy: A pathophysiologic approach (3rd ed.)* (pp. 1259-1277) Stamford, CT: Appleton & Lange.

Brushwood, D. B., & Allen, W. L. (1996). Constitutional right to pharmaceutically assisted death. *American Journal of Health-System Pharmacy Newsletter, 53,* 1797-1799.

Buckley, B. (1994). Pharmacists offer their views on reimbursement, illicit drugs, suicide. *Pharmacy Times, 60,* April, 43-44, 46.

Coombs, B. (1998). The aid-in-dying perspective. *American Journal of Health-System Pharmacy, 55,* 547-550.

Dixon, K. M., & Keir, K. L. (1998). Longing for mercy, requesting death: Pharmaceutical care and pharmaceutically assisted death. *American Journal of Health-System Pharmacy, 55,* 578-585.

Emanuel, E. J., & Emanuel, L. L. (1992). Four models of the physician-patient relationship. *Journal of the American Medical Association, 267,* 2221-2226.

Hepler, C. D., & Strand, L. M. (1990). Opportunities and responsibilities in pharmaceutical care. *American Journal of Hospital Pharmacy, 47,* 533-543.

Kaplan, K. J., Lachenmeier, F., Harrow, M. O'Dell, J. C., Uziel, D., Schneiderhan, M., & Cheyfitz, K. (1999-2000). Psychosocial versus biomedical risk factors in Kevorkian's first forty-seven physician-assisted deaths. *Omega , 40* (1), 109-163 (this issue).

Kimsma, G. K. (1996). Euthanasia and euthanizing drugs in the Netherlands. *Journal of Management of Pain and Symptom Control, 4,* 193-210.

Mullans, K., Allen, W. L., & Brushwood, D. B. (1996). Conscientious objection to assisted death: Can pharmacy address this in a systematic fashion? *The Annals of Pharmacotherapy, 30,* 1185-1191.

Ross, L. T., & Kaplan, K. J. (1993). Life ownership orientation and attitudes toward abortion, suicide, doctor-assisted suicide and capital punishment. *Omega, 28,* 17-30.

Rupp, M. T., & Isenhower, H. L. (1994). Pharmacists' attitudes toward physician-assisted suicide. *American Journal of Hospital Pharmacy, 51,* 69-74.

Strand, L. M., Cipolle, R. J., & Morley, P. C. (1992). Pharmaceutical care: An introduction. *Current Concepts.* Kalamazoo, MI: The UpJohn Company.

Vivian, J. C., Slaughter, R. L., & Calissi, P. (1993). Michigan pharmacists' attitudes about medically-assisted suicide. *Journal of Michigan Pharmacists, 31,* 490-495.

Wittenburg, A. S. J. (1995). Oregon's Death with Dignity Act lacks pharmacist's perspective. *American Journal of Health-System Pharmacy, 52,* 131-136.

Wooddell, V., & Kaplan, K. J. (1998). An expanded typology of assisted suicide and euthanasia. *Omega, 36,* 201-208.

POTENTIAL PSYCHODYNAMIC FACTORS IN PHYSICIAN-ASSISTED SUICIDE

STEPHEN H. DINWIDDIE, M.D.
Finch University of Health Sciences/The Chicago Medical School
North Chicago, Illinois

ABSTRACT

A number of assumptions underlying the debate over physician-assisted suicide (PAS) deserve closer scrutiny. It is often implicitly assumed that decisions as to the competency of the patient to request PAS can be accurately made, and that the treating physician's values and intrapsychic conflicts can be successfully separated from the decision to accede to or reject the patient's request. This article argues that in such an emotionally-laden decision, such factors may play a significant role, and that even were PAS to gain widespread acceptance, ignoring them may lead to errors in classifying patients either as appropriate or inappropriate for PAS.

The debate over the ethical justification of physician-assisted suicide (PAS) shows no signs of abating. Those framing the argument in terms of respect for individual autonomy generally note that rational patients have traditionally been allowed to decline treatment, even if such a decision might hasten or cause death. They further point out that physicians traditionally have been empowered to withhold futile treatment, and that any distinction between hastening death by inaction (withholding treatment) and actively assisting in a patient's demise is at best a subtle one which cannot be distinguished on the basis of intent. In this schema, the principle that one should be free to make one's own choices (even if others might disagree with them) is considered paramount (Dinwiddie & Yutzy, 1997).

Those taking the opposite side, point out that self-determination is not equivalent to a right to demand assistance in terminating one's life, and that while it is permissible to provide treatment which may secondarily result in an increased risk of death or more rapid demise, the purposeful taking of life runs contrary to basic principles of medicine (Dinwiddie & Yutzy, 1997).

But even if this fundamental ethical question were ultimately to be resolved in favor of physician-assisted suicide, physicians must operate in the realm of practical decision making. On that level, I believe there are a number of irreducible uncertainties which, particularly given the magnitude of harm caused by an erroneous decision, may render the larger ethical question moot.

I have elsewhere (Dinwiddie, 1992) argued that, as in every other medical endeavor, some degree of classification error as to who might be appropriate for PAS is inevitable, and have suggested some areas in which such errors are likely to occur. While consultation or case review might lower the rate of error, regardless of whatever "safeguards" are put into place, given a high enough volume of cases, some patients in fact inappropriate for PAS would be wrongly classified as appropriate, and *vice versa.*

For example, while it may be comforting to assume that mandating a requirement that patients must be clinically judged as "competent" to request PAS will assure that the decision is rational, how the clinician might go about assessing competency in such cases remains unaddressed. Studies of diagnostic concordance in other areas of medicine demonstrate that even careful, well-trained clinicians using explicit criteria and objective data often disagree (Landis & Koch, 1977); in such a difficult clinical determination, without access to such aids, it seems unlikely that disagreement between clinicians will be less frequent—and in such disagreements, one will inevitably be wrong. In such cases, whose opinion should prevail? (Agreement is, of course, no guarantee that a "correct" decision is made, either: Both might be wrong.)

As an aside, it is interesting to note that in the debate over PAS, there appears to be little enthusiasm on either side for involving the judicial system, even though one of its roles in society is precisely to deal with problems which have no clear-cut medical or scientific solution to a conflict of opinion. While admittedly imperfect, the judicial system's approach to life-and-death issues, characterized by an adversarial approach, requirement of very high standards of proof, and multiple levels of review suggests a willingness to tolerate at least the temporary "incorrect" preservation of life as an unavoidable cost of preventing the greater wrong of its erroneous termination.

Unfortunately, the subjectivity of judgments as to degree and cause of suffering, absence of significant intercurrent psychiatric illness such as depression which might subtly influence decision making, rationality of the choice, and freedom from coercion implies that some degree of assessment error is inevitable. Such subjectivity further suggests that it would be perilous to ignore those factors within the physician-patient relationship which have the potential of profoundly affecting the way in which such a decision might be reached. As I shall argue, the existence of such factors would seriously undermine the confidence which can be placed in the correctness of any decision favoring physician-assisted suicide.

UNCONSCIOUS FACTORS IN ASSISTED SUICIDE

Proponents agree that physician-assisted suicide should be restricted to those who voluntarily request it, who are cognitively competent to make such a decision, and who are suffering intolerably (Angell, 1988). This formulation therefore requires at a minimum that the patient is aware of the procedure and its alternatives and has not been unduly pressured by family, physicians, or society to opt for it, and implies that once these standards are found to be met the physician's ethical duty is discharged.

Such a "rationalistic" standard ignores research findings which indicate that the desire for death is not common among terminally ill patients in general (Breitbart, Rosenfeld, & Passik, 1996; Brown et al., 1986). Given the well-established connection between suicide and depression, the first consideration might be that the desire for death found in these patients is related to affective illness. It has been found that 11 to 31 percent of medically ill patients report pronounced feelings of depression (Glass et al., 1978; Kathol & Petty, 1981; Rodin & Voshart, 1986); among some severely medically ill groups the rate may be even higher (Bukberg, Penman, & Holland, 1984; Noyes & Kathol, 1986). Research further indicates that in this population, all too often the low mood is considered without further evaluation to be a rational, understandable reaction to situational factors, while treatment if initiated at all is not pursued vigorously enough (Callies & Popkin, 1987; Keller et al., 1982). This is a puzzling outcome, since palliation of other forms of suffering in the terminally ill is seen as a high priority. Moreover, while low mood may be an understandable reaction to severe pain without possibility of relief, the possibility also exists that other dynamics within the patient and the caregiver play a large and unrecognized role in the undertreatment of depression and the acceptance of suicide as an option.

The first consideration, of course, is that the suicidality may be a reaction not to the physical illness and associated pain, but rather a reflection of what these mean to the individual: The loss of significant objects (impending loss of family or friends) or a blow to self-esteem due to being unable to work or perhaps even to care for oneself. Thus, while pain or the lack of a hopeful prognosis may be cited by the patient as reasons to die, these may be rationalizations, rather than being based in logic.

Alternatively, rather than a manifestation of grief over this impending loss, the dysphoria and suicidal thoughts might represent anger at the prospect of being deprived of these objects. Finally, to the extent that the patient feels responsible for causing or contributing to his illness, suicide might represent an act of atonement, relieving guilt feelings arising from the patient's perception of the grief felt by family members.

Most importantly of all, the request for assisted suicide may represent a covert message to the physician, and in that sense might be seen as equivalent to any other suicide threat or gesture. Such a request could represent a plea for help, an entreaty that the physician acknowledge or take more seriously the patient's feelings of isolation, helplessness, and despair at facing a life-threatening disease. It might also be an expression of anger at the physician for not curing the patient—saying in effect that the physician's failure caused his death—or for distancing himself from the patient. Communication of desire for assistance in suicide might also be seen as a way for the patient to find the physician's true feelings: Will the physician be willing to stand by the patient until the very end, or will he be rejected and death hastened as a result?

COUNTERTRANSFERENCE ISSUES

These possibilities might be broadly considered to be transference distortions, that is, arising from the patient's feelings toward the physician and the treatment situation. Countertransference issues must be considered as well. The most obvious pitfall, of course, is for the physician to identify too closely with the patient's depression: Unconsciously accepting the patient's melancholy outlook and allowing him to act on it is a well-known peril in the treatment of depression whether or not concomitant physical illness is present. Clinicians who have treated patients with severe depression are often struck, not only by their evident anguish, but also by how cogent and reasonable a case these patients can present to explain why they are hopeless and desire death. The chance of amelioration is rejected, palliative measures are denigrated, and the prospect of relief of their depression is not accepted. Far from appearing incompetent to make treatment decisions, depressed patients may appear exquisitely aware of their situation and eminently logical.

Indeed, it is probably the rare physician who, despite recommending treatment, has not to some extent feared that the patient was correct and that acceding to their expressed wish to die might indeed be the more compassionate course. But in such a situation, the physician who acquiesces in assisting a patient's suicide, risks doing the patient harm by an unreflective trust in the patient's rationality. Patients with severe depression often do recover, and when they do no longer desire death; many express shock that they could have desired it in the first place. Retrospectively it seems that the appearance of competence was spurious, that in fact the patient's thinking was strongly colored by the cognitive distortions of depressive illness (Gutheil & Bursztajn, 1986).

If the physician has unresolved feelings, for example due to having lost a family member to a lingering illness, he might be more vulnerable to such projective identification. But over-identification with the patient's feelings of hopelessness is not the only potential countertransference distortion. Not only might the physician over-identify with the patient's suffering (Goodwin, 1991); unadmitted hostility directed toward the patient might literally result in "killing him with kindness." Such hostility could stem from the physician's frustration at his inability to cure the patient or as a way of preventing the patient from making more demands on his time; it might also arise more circuitously as a defense against the physician's unacknowledged feelings of inadequacy for not being able to effect a cure.

Finally, the physician faced with such a request also runs the risk of acting out family members' aggressive feelings, which again may stem from a variety of sources: over-identification with the patient's suffering, covert (or not so covert) hostility, exhaustion from dealing with a terminally ill family member, and so on (Wasserman, 1989).

It hardly needs pointing out that, as with any other medical intervention, the decision to administer or withhold treatment is ultimately the physician's, not the patient's. Some physicians refuse to provide services, such as abortion, which are legal and widely (if hardly universally) accepted but to which they are personally opposed. More generally, it is a commonplace in practice to decline to provide certain therapies requested by the patient because the physician believes it to be medically inappropriate in that specific case. Rather, in such situations (ideally, if not always in practice) the patient is educated about better treatment alternatives, or the request is clarified as being an expression of less overt problems: A plea for narcotics is identified as a manifestation of drug addiction and chemical dependency treatment offered, or a desire for cosmetic surgery is discovered to be based on unrealistic expectations or needs which might be better dealt with by other interventions. Similarly, in the case of a request for PAS, final responsibility can hardly be abdicated to the patient. Given that the physician, as noted above, may not be able to easily identify some of his own motivations, it is far from certain that he can be adequately assured that his motives have not been confused with the patient's.

OTHER FACTORS

It is evident that the exposition has been completely one-sided up to this point, concentrating on factors which might lead the physician to agree to assist in a patient's suicide. What of those forces which might act to prevent the physician from agreeing that a patient's request for suicide is in fact rational? For that matter, what of intrapsychic forces which might prevent a patient from realizing his situation is truly hopeless and that he should rationally choose to end his life in a painless and convenient manner?

It is clear that physicians and other healthcare providers differ considerably in how they assess a given patient's physical suffering (Lebovits et al., 1997; Sjostrom et al., 1997) and stubbornly refusing to admit that a patient is suffering intolerably, in the face of overwhelming evidence to the contrary, may well be a reflection of denial on the part of the physician. Obviously, refusing to try to alleviate a patient's pain—physical or psychic—is poor medicine, and it is incumbent on the physician caring for such a person to ensure that this own feelings are not preventing him from delivering adequate care. One may argue that the risk of erroneously accepting a patient's appearance of rationality and participating in his suicide outweighs the potential wrong done by falsely believing the patient to be incompetent to request assisted suicide. But even if that argument is not accepted, the considerations noted above remain.

The second question is fundamentally more disturbing. Logically, the possibility exists that unconscious forces might prevent terminally ill patients from realizing the hopelessness of their situation, thereby preventing suicide. But, as the existentialists might point out, the same is true for anyone, terminally ill or not. Furthermore, a therapy whose purpose would be to eliminate the factors blocking the patient from considering suicide would seem to be inherently a contravention of medical ethics. If physician-assisted suicide were generally accepted, however, one might nonetheless conceive of a situation in which "therapy" would be directed in this manner.

SUMMARY

I have argued elsewhere (Dinwiddie, 1992) that even if PAS could be justified on the basis of ethical theory, on practical grounds it inherently runs a high risk of violating fundamental medical principles, since despite any possible safeguards, some errors of assessment would be made. Some patients who were incompetent to make the decision or who could have been effectively treated otherwise would be put to death, and it is not clear that this fundamental ethical difficulty can be counterbalanced on utilitarian principles. But as the foregoing discussion indicates, there is another consideration as well: Significant but unrecognized distortions in the physician-patient relationship have the potential to bias determination of fitness to request assisted suicide, potentially causing the wrongful death of a patient.

At this time, such concerns are purely theoretical, even speculative in nature. Over the last few years, empirical studies of issues fundamental to the debate over PAS have begun to appear, for example, investigations into the base rate of suicidal feelings among the elderly (Skoog et al., 1996), interest in PAS among patients with HIV (Breitbart, Rosenfeld, & Passik, 1996), psychiatric diagnoses among completed suicides who had been diagnosed with cancer (Henriksson et al., 1995), and studies of attitudes toward PAS by physicians and the general public (Bachman et al., 1996; Back et al., 1996; Lee et al., 1996). However, there has been no comparable study of issues such as interrater agreement as to "competency" to request PAS or clinicians' rating of presence or absence of intercurrent psychiatric illness among those requesting PAS. Moreover, the role of the psychological issues mentioned above has yet to be studied, even though such dynamics might well influence the physician's response to a patient's request for assisted suicide. It is incumbent on the physician to be convinced that these processes have not affected the decision-making process, either on the part of the patient requesting it or on the part of the physician who might acquiesce—but the subtle nature of these forces all but guarantees that they will be missed at least on occasion, while at other times the physician will actively deny that they play any role at all. In effect, the physician who contemplates assisting a patient in suicide would be required to guarantee a negative. These uncertainties about motive, without possibility of definitive resolution, make a difficult and ethically perilous decision even less tenable when clinical decisions must be made.

REFERENCES

Angell, M. (1988). Euthanasia. *New England Journal of Medicine, 319* (20), pp. 1348-1350.

Bachman, J. G., Alcser, K. H., Doukas, D. J., Lichtenstein, R. L., Corning, A. D., & Brody, H. (1996). Attitudes of Michigan physicians and the public toward legalizing physician-assisted suicide and voluntary euthanasia. *New England Journal of Medicine, 344,* 303-309.

Back, A. L., Wallace, J. I., Starks, H. E., & Pearlman, R. A. (1996). Physician-assisted suicide and euthanasia in Washington state. *Journal of the American Medical Association, 275* (12), 919-925.

Breitbart, W., Rosenfeld, B. D., & Passik, S. D. (1996). Interest in physician-assisted suicide among ambulatory HIV-infected patients. *American Journal of Psychiatry, 153* (2), 238-242.

Brown, J. H., Henteleff, P., Barakat, S., & Rowe, C. J. (1986). Is It Normal for Terminally Ill Patients to Desire Death? *American Journal of Psychiatry, 143* (2), 208-211.

Bukberg, J., Penman, P., & Holland, J. C. (1984). Depression in hospitalized cancer patients. *Psychosomatic Medicine, 46,* 199-212.

Callies, A. L., & Popkin, M. K. (1987). Antidepressant treatment of medical-surgical inpatients by nonpsychiatric physicians. *Archives of General Psychiatry, 44* (2), 157-160.

Dinwiddie, S. H. (1992). Physician-assisted suicide: Epistemological problems. *International Journal of Medicine and Law, 11* (5/6), 345-352.

Dinwiddie, S. H., & Yutzy, S. H. (1997). Ethical issues in psychiatric practice. In S. B. Guze (Ed.), *Adult psychiatry* (pp. 445-453). St. Louis: Mosby-Year Book.

Glass, R. M., Allan, A. T., Uhlenhuth, E. H., Kimball, C. P., & Borinstein, D. I. (1978). Psychiatric screening in a medical clinic. *Archives of General Psychiatry, 35,* 1189-1195.

Goodwin, J. S. (1991). Mercy killing: Mercy for whom? *Journal of the American Medical Association, 265* (3), 326.

Gutheil, T. G., & Bursztajn, H. (1986). Clinicians' guidelines for assessing and presenting subtle forms of patient incompetence in legal settings. *American Journal of Psychiatry, 143* (8), 1020-1023.

Henriksson, M. M., Isometsa, E. T., Hietanen, P. S., Aro, H. M., & Lönnqvist, J. K. (1995). Mental disorders in cancer suicides. *Journal of Affective Disorders, 36,* 11-20.

Kathol, R. G., & Petty, F. (1981). Relationship of depression to medical illness. *Journal of Affective Disorders, 3,* 111-121.

Keller, M. B., Klerman, G. L., Lavori, P. W., Fawcett, J. W., Coryell, W., & Endicott, J. (1982). Treatment received by depressed patients. *Journal of the American Medical Association, 248* (15), 1848-1855.

Landis, J. R., & Koch, G. G. (1977). An application of hierarchical kappa-type statistics in the assessment of majority agreement among multiple observers. *Biometrics, 33,* 363-374.

Lebovits, A. H., Florence, I., Bathina, R., Hunko, V., & Fox, M. T. (1997). Pain knowledge and attitudes of healthcare providers: Practice characteristics differences. *Clinical Journal of Pain, 13* (3), 237-243.

Lee, M. A., Nelson, H. D., Tilden, V. P., Ganzini, L., Schmidt, T. A., & Tolle, S. W. (1996). Legalizing assisted suicide—Views of physicians in Oregon. *New England Journal of Medicine, 334,* 310-315.

Noyes, R., & Kathol, R. G. (1986). Depression and cancer. *Psychiatric Developments, 2,* 77-100.

Rodin, G., & Voshart, K. (1986). Depression in the medically ill: An overview. *American Journal of Psychiatry, 143* (6), 696-705.

Sjostrom, B., Haljamae, H., Dahlgren, L. O., & Lindstrom, B. (1997). Assessment of postoperative pain: Impact of clinician experience and professional role. *Acta Anaesthesiology Scandinavica, 41* (3), 339-344.

Skoog, I., Aevarsson, O., Beskow, J., Larsson, L., Palsson, S., Waern, M., Landahl, S., & Östling, S. (1996). Suicidal feelings in a population sample of nondemented 85-year-olds. *American Journal of Psychiatry, 153* (8), 1015-1020.

Wasserman, D. (1989). Passive euthanasia in response to attempted suicide: One form of aggressiveness by relatives. *Acta Psychiatrica Scandinavica, 79,* 460-467.

PSYCHOSOCIAL VERSUS BIOMEDICAL RISK FACTORS IN KEVORKIAN'S FIRST FORTY-SEVEN PHYSICIAN-ASSISTED DEATHS

KALMAN J. KAPLAN, PH.D.
Wayne State University and Michael Reese Hospital and Medical Center

FLINT LACHENMEIER, PH.D.
Michael Reese Hospital and Medical Center

MARTIN HARROW, PH.D.
University of Illinois College of Medicine

JYLL C. O'DELL, MA
John Jay College of Justice

OREN UZIEL, BA
New York University School of Law

MARK SCHNEIDERHAN, PHARM.D.
*University of Illinois College of Pharmacy
and Michael Reese Hospital and Medical Center*

KIRK CHEYFITZ
Free-Lance Journalist

ABSTRACT

This article examines biomedical and psychosocial data on the first forty-seven cases of physician-assisted suicides (PAS) of Kevorkian as collected by means of both a physical autopsy and a preliminary psychological autopsy. The following patterns emerge: 1) The physical condition of these PAS patients was not typical of the conditions that lead to death in the United States. 2) Consistent with the above findings, our pilot data indicate that only 31.1 percent of these patients were terminal. While 73.9 percent were described as reporting pain, only 42.6 percent were revealed at autopsy to have a specific anatomical basis for their pain. However 36 percent were described as depressed, 66 percent as having some disability, and perhaps of key importance, 90 percent expressed a fear of dependency. Most important, our pilot data suggest the possibility of large gender differences, since 3) 68.1

percent of these forty-seven PAS's are women and only 31.9 percent are men. This represents the reverse of the gender pattern for completed suicides in the United States in 1995, resembling instead the approximate pattern for unsuccessful suicide attempts. 4) Approximately 75 percent of both men and women in the above sample were described as reporting pain. Men were almost twice as likely to have had an anatomical basis for the pain and three times as likely to be terminal. Our pilot data indicate PAS women are more likely to be described as depressed and twice as likely to have had a history of previous unsuccessful suicide attempts. 5) Kevorkian's patients were older than the typical unaided suicides in America. Reported pain decreases with age as does depression; however anatomical basis for pain increases slightly with age, and no age effect emerges for terminality. 6) Approximately two-thirds of these physician-assisted suicides were at middle SES levels. History of disability was the biggest risk factor for the low SES patients and fear of dependency for the high SES patients.

A number of studies have cited physical illness as a risk factor for suicide, especially in later life (Chynoweth et al., 1980; Dorpat et al., 1968; Robins et al., 1959; Sainsbury et al., 1955; Steward, 1960). Many of these elderly suicides were unlikely to have ever used mental health services, though the majority visited their family physician within weeks or months before their death. A number of organizations in the United States and elsewhere (e.g., The Hemlock Society in America and the Voluntary Euthanasia Society in the United Kingdom) have advocated the legalization of the right of these sick people to obtain aid in ending their lives. Central to these advocacy groups is the assumption that physically ill people attempt suicide because of biomedical factors associated with their illness, for example, terminality, physical immobility and intractable physical pain. Thus, the decision to die can be seen as a "rational suicide."

The emerging data, however, suggest that the case is far more complicated. As far back as 1972, Fawcett pointed to the mediating role of depression in the relationship between physical illness and suicide. Whitlock (1978) found that persons aged fifty and over dying from suicide were found at autopsy to be more likely to have had malignant neoplasms and benign intracranial tumors than were a matched control group of persons dying from other violent causes. Murphy (1997) discovered that no evidence of cancer could be found at autopsy in any of his several forensic autopsy cases in which a person had reportedly been "told" by a physician or "knew" personally that he "had cancer," and shortly afterward committed suicide. In a later study of eight suicides, Conwell et al. (1990) found no evidence of malignancy in three of the four cases in which autopsies were conducted. However, they found evidence of major depression in five of the eight cases, a history of alcohol abuse in a sixth and intoxication on prescribed opiates in a seventh. Only one of the eight cases was without psychiatric diagnosis. Conwell et al. suggest that "having cancer may become the metaphor for the hopelessness that drives them to end their lives" (p. 1337).

The critical role of psychosocial suicide risk factors among the physically ill is not limited to cancer. A landmark study by Brown et al. (1986) of hospice patients diagnosed with terminal illness, found only a small percentage who expressed a wish to die, all of whom met criteria for major depression. In a second study, Horton-Deutsch et al. (1992) conducted a psychological autopsy of fourteen cases of suicides in older adults who had experienced chronic dyspnea in the months or weeks before death. Most of these patients had a diagnosable psychiatric disorder, although none had previous contact with a mental health professional. Other common characteristics were chronic or terminal heart or lung disease, recent contact with a primary physician, prior experience of self or significant other suffering a debilitating disease, and a fiercely independent and inflexible personality type. In a third study, Berman and Samuel (1993) compared twenty-four people with multiple sclerosis who completed suicide with twenty-two who made nonfatal attempts and a matched group of twenty-two nonsuicidal persons with multiple sclerosis. Results indicated that completers were more likely to use a gun, be male, unemployed and experiencing financial stress, more likely to be severely disabled, at a later phase of MS and to report unbearable psychic pain. They were also less able to express feelings, ask for help, and were more likely to withdraw from potential supports.

In another study of terminally ill patients Chochinov et al. (1995) reported that only seventeen (8.5%) of 200 patients terminally ill with cancer acknowledged a serious and pervasive wish for a hastened death. This desire for a hastened death was associated with ratings of presence of pain and low levels of family support, but most significantly with measures of depression. Specifically, the prevalence rate of depression among these patients who wished a hastened death was 58.8 percent compared to 7.7 percent among the patients who did not have this wish. Similar results were found in several other studies, one with oncology patients (Emanuel et al., 1996) and another with HIV patients (Breitbart, Rosenfeld, & Passik, 1996). Both these studies attested to the important role of depression in the desire for a hastened death. In contrast, a more recent study by Ganzini et al. (1998) examined the attitudes of patients with ALS toward physician-assisted suicide (PAS) per se. Here it was hopelessness that seemed to be a predictor of a specific desire for PAS rather than depression (cf. Minkoff et al., 1973). Specifically, hopelessness scores were higher for those amyotrophic lateral sclerosis (ALS) patients willing to consider PAS for themselves as compared to those who were not.

Psychosocial risk factors also emerged as important in Harris and Barraclough's (1994) review on mortality in the sixty-three medical diagnoses (ICD9) identified in the literature as having altered suicide risk. They conclude that only a few of these conditions had an increased risk of suicide, including HIV/AIDS, Huntington disease, malignant neoplasms, multiple sclerosis, peptic ulcer, renal disease, spinal cord injury, and systemic lupus erythematosus. Most of these were associated with mental disorder, substance abuse, or both. All these factors lead Clark (1992) to question whether the suicide of people with terminal conditions or disabilities is truly "rational" or the product of a temporary psychiatric illness. More generally, the question emerges as to whether people who commit suicide with physical illness do so primarily because of biomedical aspects of their illness or psychosocial factors.

A unique sample to test this question has emerged in a new phenomena in America, labeled by the media "physician-assisted suicide." It started June 4th, 1990 with the involvement of Dr. Jack Kevorkian in the death of Janet Adkins, fifty-four, who had been diagnosed with Alzheimer's disease one year earlier. An invention of Dr. Kevorkian's, called the "suicide machine," was used. The device consists of three IV bottles attached to a single intravenous needle. One bottle contains saline and is used to keep the intravenous needle open. The second bottle contains a powerful muscle relaxant, which is opened into the intravenous flow by the patient when he/she is ready to commit suicide. The final bottle contains potassium chloride and is temporarily sealed with a clamp. One end of a tightly pulled string is attached to the clamp, the other end to the "patient's" upright arm. As the muscle relaxant takes effect, the patient's arm relaxes and falls, pulling the clamp from the potassium chloride bottle. The potassium chloride causes heart failure almost instantaneously. This is how Janet Adkins died.

Kevorkian claims to have aided about 130 people in committing suicide (since 1990). This study scientifically examines in detail for the first time, the first forty-seven known Kevorkian-assisted deaths. Specifically, this study examines these people who were aided in dying by Kevorkian between June 4th, 1990 and February 2nd, 1997. These details, mostly provided by The Detroit Free Press and the Medical Examiner's Office in Oakland, Wayne, Macomb, and Leelanau Counties,[1] include family history, medical history, and demographics.

METHODS

Sample

The sample for this study consists of the first forty-seven acknowledged-assisted deaths of Dr. Jack Kevorkian, a retired Michigan pathologist. The subjects are described in Appendix A, Table A1. All forty-seven of these decedents were assisted in their death June 4, 1990 and February 2, 1997.

Measures

Most of the data analyzed here was collected and provided by The Detroit Free Press with the advice of the senior author (Kaplan) and one junior author

---

[1] The authors would like to offer their gratitude to the medical examiners of Oakland County (Drs. L. J. Dragovic, Kanu Virani, and Bernardino Pacris), Wayne County (Drs. Sawait Kanluen and J. Scott Somerset) and Macomb County (Dr. Werner U. Spitz). All deaths investigated in Oakland County have been classified as euthanasia. The patients' names are public record and have been previously published in newspapers and books (*The Detroit Free Press*, 1997) and are accessible on the Website of the Hemlock Society on the Internet.

(Cheyfitz). The Free Press employed a modified and informal psychological autopsy technique to interview those most closely involved and knowledgeable about the patients in an attempt to reconstruct aspects of the patient's life. The measures collected included demographic, biomedical, and psychosocial factors as well as consultation history, drug history, experience with Kevorkian, and circumstances of death.

In some cases, information on the diagnosis of existing conditions and medical drug treatments used was provided by the patient's doctor or a specialist treating the patient provided. When the doctor was unavailable or unwilling to comment on their patients, the Free Press utilized other sources familiar with the patient's history. These people could include close family members or close friends, but in any case people who would have had an intimate knowledge of what types of treatments the patients received, their medical condition, and the drugs they had been prescribed. These non medical informants were of great value in obtaining information as to psychosocial issues regarding a patient's life. To ensure accuracy, a positive symptom or piece of information required the agreement of two to three informants who knew the proband well (see the work of Clark & Horton-Deutsch, 1992).

Demographic Factors

Education was defined by presence of some college education. Parental status was defined by the presence of older age children and those under eighteen. Social economic status was defined as lower (less than $25,000/year), middle ($25-75,000/year), and upper class (more than $75,000/year). Occupation was defined as the occupation that filled the bulk of the patient's working life. It was divided into helping-type jobs, homemaker or other. Patient's religious affiliation was defined by his family of origin's traditional religious identification unless the patient specifically had adopted another faith or spiritual practice. Overall living arrangements were defined by being a Michigan resident or not, and by whether one was a homeowner or not.

Biomedical Factors and Physical Limitations

A positive history of physical disease was determined at the physical autopsy as was terminality (less than 6 months to live) and an anatomical basis for pain. A psychological history of psychosis and/or depression and sleep disorder was based only on interviews with mental health professionals as part of the psychological autopsy. Reported pain was measured through interviews with friends and relatives. A functional definition was applied to ability to work, walk, and drive. Ability to go to the toilet by oneself was defined as mobility to get to the toilet, undo one's own clothing and position oneself without help. A history of disability referred not to qualification for Social Security Disability Benefits but to functional limitations in day-to-day life. Incontinence was a medical condition—medically incontinent or wearing a ileostomy or colostomy bag.

Psychosocial History

Living arrangement was defined by whether at the time of death, the decedent lived alone, with a spouse or partner, or with children or other family or live-in or periodic paid care. A patient's expressed fear of dependency was also determined through interview with friends and relatives. Information with regard to insurance history was also obtained. A deteriorating financial condition was defined as one where the patient had sustained a substantial loss of income in the five years preceding their death, had been forced to move to a smaller house or apartment or had one's savings depleted to pay for medical costs. A professional or financial reversal was defined as one not arising from the patient's illness. A history of loss and trauma with regard to death and separation from immediate family and friends was obtained both at one and five years preceding the patient's suicide. A positive history of physical, sexual, and substance abuse, alcoholism, and suicide attempts and family history of suicide was determined by interviews with friends and relatives as well.

Consultation History Before or During Kevorkian

A patient's consultation history with a mental health professional, religious figure, and family and his acceptance/rejection of medical treatment including pain medication refers to contact with these professionals *before* Kevorkian was contacted. Consultation about the patients wish to die may or may not have occurred before Kevorkian was contacted. This is also true of a history of a patient's rejection of medical treatment designed to extend his life and a history of insufficient pain medication.

Toxicology and Drug History

Drug history was assessed in two different ways: first by a history of prescription and illicit drugs obtained through the interviews of health professionals, friends, and relatives, and second, toxological assays of drugs present in the patient's blood serum at the time of death as part of the medical examiner's procedure. Categories of drugs were divided into antidepressants, anti-psychotics, anti-seizure drugs, muscle relaxants and nonpiods, opiates, sedatives/hypnotics, and stimulants.[2]

Experience with Kevorkian

Kevorkian's contact times refer: 1) to the time between Kevorkian receiving an initial communication from the proband or his/her family and Kevorkian's attempt at a response, or 2) the time between Kevorkian's initial face-to-face meeting with the patient and the patient's death. Kevorkian's consultation with

---

[2] The drug treatment classifications were made by one of the authors, Mark Schneiderhan (Pharm.D., University of Illinois College of Pharmacy, Chicago, Illinois).

the patient's physician, a specialist, a pain relief consult, or psychiatrist refers to actual interchange taking place, not simply an attempt by Kevorkian to make contact. An attempted contact of the patient's physician was scored if Kevorkian merely tried to contact him, whether or not he was successful. A family member or friend had to display significant opposition, not just voice a passing concern, in order to be coded as opposing the contact with Kevorkian.

Circumstances of Death

Circumstances of death was measured by location, the presence of others, the identity of the informant, the county in which death occurred, the cause of death (by method), and the disposal of the body (cremation, burial, or entombment).

Phase

The forty-seven deaths were divided into four distinct time periods or phases defined by significant legal-political events encountered by Kevorkian in Michigan. We selected three critical cutoff points differentiating the four time periods:

1. December 15, 1992—Michigan Governor John Engler signs into law a temporary ban on physician-assisted suicide.
2. May 14, 1996—Kevorkian is acquitted on murder charges in the deaths of Marjorie Wantz and Sherrie Miller, the last pending case against him.
3. August 6, 1996—Kevorkian's nemesis, Richard Thompson is defeated in the Republican primary in his bid for re-election as Oakland County Prosecutor. David Gorcyca, the victorious Republican candidate in the heavily Republican district of Oakland County, publicly stated that he would not prosecute Kevorkian under existing Michigan common law.

These four distinct time periods can be delineated as follows:

1. June 4, 1990 through December 15, 1992, entitled the "honeymoon" phase;
2. December 16, 1992 through May 14, 1996 entitled the "prosecution" phase;
3. May 15, 1996 through August 6, 1996 entitled the "revenge" phase;
4. August 7, 1996 through February 2, 1997 entitled the "business as usual" phase.

Analysis

Overall frequencies were examined in all forty-seven decedents with regard to the above factors: demographic, biomedical, psychosocial, consultation, drug history, experience with Kevorkian, and circumstances of death. In addition, Chi-Square analyses were conducted with regard to the effects of gender, age, marital status, socioeconomic status, ancestry, and phase on the above variables.

RESULTS

The data on Kevorkian's first forty-seven deaths are massive. First, we present overall frequencies with regard to the total sample, beginning with demographic variables, and then moving on to biomedical history, psychosocial history, consultation history, experience with Kevorkian, and circumstances of death. In the second section of the results we compare frequencies within each of five demographic categories: 1) gender, 2) age, 3) marital status, 4) socioeconomic status (SES), and 5) ancestry. Finally, we present patterns with regard to the four phases into which we divide Kevorkian's first forty-seven suicides.

Overall Frequencies

Kevorkian's first forty-seven acknowledged physician-assisted suicides are listed and briefly described in Appendix A, Table A1. Once again we want to emphasize that the patient names are public record and have been previously published (see Footnote 1).

Demographics

The first forty-seven of the Kevorkian decedents represent an interesting cross section of people. Thirty-two of the first forty-seven patients were women (68.1%), while only fifteen were men (31.9%). Their average age was 58.1 years (SD = 13.4; Minimum = 27; Maximum = 82). There was no difference in age between males (M = 60.3 years; SD = 16.6) and females (M = 57.1 years, SD = 11.7; t = .75, df = 45, p = n.s.).

Seven were single (14.9%), seventeen married (36.2%), seventeen divorced (36.2%), and six widowed (12.8%). Most of his patients were middle class (27; 62.8%), with a fairly even split of the remainder between lower (9; 20.9%) and upper class (7; 16.3%). The income of four people was not known. The ancestry breakdown is as follows: fifteen English, Scottish, or Irish (31.9%); twelve Russian, Polish, or Lithuanian (25.5%); nine German or Dutch (19.1%); five American or Canadian (10.6%); three Swedish or Norwegian (6.4%); two Middle Eastern (4.3%); and one Hispanic (2.1%). Forty-six out of the first forty-seven patients (97.9%) were Caucasian and thirty-two were categorized as White Anglo-Saxon Protestant (English, Scottish, Irish, German, Dutch, American, Canadian, Swedish, and Norwegian).

As can be seen in Appendix A, Table A2, 59.6 percent of these patients had at least some college education, 80.9 percent had one or more children and only 8.5 percent had minor children (under the age of 18) at the time of their death. Only 19.1 percent of the people were homemakers, but 40.4 percent had a job in the helping professions. Only 36.2 percent of these people resided in Michigan and 66 percent of them resided in their own homes.

Biomedical History

Appendix A, Table A3 presents overall frequencies with regard to biomedical precipitants as reported by informants. With regards to consultation history 27.7 percent of the patients were described as having more than one condition while 72.3 percent were reported as having only one condition. The number of patients with each condition is as follows: fourteen (31%) had some form of cancer, ten (22.2%) had multiple sclerosis (MS), eight (17%) had Lou Gehrig's disease (ALS), two (4%) had heart or lung disease, one (2%) had Alzheimer's, four (9%) had multiple conditions, and seven (15%) had other medical conditions (Figure 1). Causes of death in the United States provide an interesting comparison. In 1995 heart disease accounted for 31.9 percent of all deaths, cancer 23.3 percent, stroke 6.8 percent, lung disease 4.5 percent, and accidents 4 percent (Anderson, Kochanek, & Murphy, 1997). All other causes of death accounted for less than 4 percent of total deaths. Chronic nonterminal but disabling diseases such as multiple sclerosis were over-represented in the Kevorkian sample as

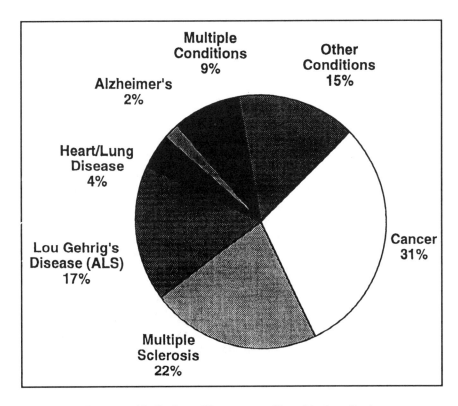

Figure 1. Medical conditions among Kevorkian's patients.

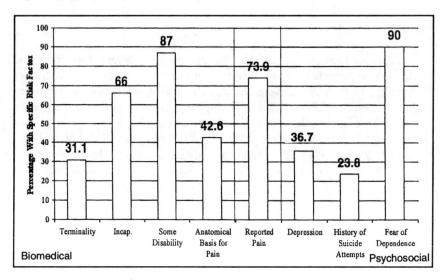

Figure 2. Biomedical vs. psychosocial risk factors for Kevorkian's
first forty-seven suicides.

compared to national mortality statistics while heart and lung disease were
under-represented.

Over one-quarter (27%) of these patients were described as being mentally
incapacitated (Figure 2). While only 2.9 percent were described as having a
history of psychosis, 36.7 percent were described as having a history of depression, and 9.1 percent as having a history of sleep disorders.[3] With regard to
symptomatology, 87 percent reported a history of disability, 66 percent were
physically incapacitated (incontinent, not able to walk, or to work) and 47.5
percent had a functional physical limitation (not able to walk or work). Almost
half (45.2%) had a history of incontinence, 57.8 percent were defined as being
unable to go to the toilet alone, 60.9 percent were defined as being unable to
walk, 84.8 percent as unable to drive. Only 10.6 percent were able to work and
only 4.3 percent were working at the time of their death.

Almost three-fourths (73.9%) of the patients reported experiencing pain, but
only 42.6 percent were described by medical authorities as having an underlying
anatomical condition likely to cause this pain. Finally, only 31.1 percent of
Kevorkian's patients were considered terminal as defined as having less than
six months to live as judged by the medical examiner or another qualified professional (Figure 2).

---

[3] A proband could be scored positively in multiple categories.

Psychosocial History

Appendix A, Table A4 presents overall frequencies with regard to psychosocial history as reported by informants. Living arrangements seem very important. At the time of death of the first forty-seven patients, less than half (40.9%) were described as having a surviving spouse or children. Moreover, 70.2 percent were reported living with someone else. Of these, 40.4 percent were reported as living with a spouse/partner, 29.8 percent living with children, and 12.8 percent were living with other family members, these three categories not necessarily being mutually exclusive. In addition 34.1 percent were described as living with periodic paid help at the time of their death and 4.3 percent with live-in, around-the-clock paid help. Only 29.8 percent lived alone at the time of death. Fully 90 percent of the patients were described by informants as having expressed a fear of being or becoming dependent (see Figure 2).

The Free Press reporters were able to uncover life insurance information with regard to only twelve of the forty-seven patients. The beneficiary was the spouse in only six of these twelve cases (50%). Recent losses and traumas were also examined. Informants indicated that 30 percent of patients experienced a deterioration in their standard of living in years immediately prior to their death and 14.3 percent were reported as experiencing financial or professional reversal within five years of death. Twenty-two point five percent were reported as experiencing the death of a parent within five years, 13 percent were reported as divorcing or separating during this period, 4.4 percent reported the death of a child during this period, 4.3 percent reported the death of a spouse, and 3.6 reported the death of a friend. Only 2.5 percent reported being the victim of a crime while 17.1 percent were described of being a victim of another trauma during the preceding five year period.

The data are also interesting in regard to personal and family history of suicide, physical abuse, and substance abuse. One-quarter of the decedents (23.8%) were described as having a history of previous suicide attempts and 9.4 percent as having a history of suicide in their immediate family (including parent, grandparent, aunt, uncle, sibling, spouse, or child) 11.4 percent were purported as having a history of substance abuse and only 4.3 percent were portrayed as having any history of alcoholism. Finally, 8.1 percent of the first forty-seven patients seemed to have a history of physical abuse and only 2.6 percent of sexual abuse per se.

Consultation History Before Kevorkian

Appendix A, Table A5 presents overall frequencies with regard to consultation history as reported by informants.

Most patients (91.3%) consulted with family members about their wish to die, 24.1 percent with a religious figure, and 28.1 percent with a mental health professional. Doctors were reported as providing insufficient pain relief by the informants of 29.3 percent of the decedents and were reported as having rejected additional medical treatment designed to extend their lives in 28.9 percent of the cases while 11.6 percent of the decedents were described as having declined pain medication.

Drug History

Appendix A, Table A6 presents overall frequencies with regard to drugs used during medical treatment and those present at the time of death. The purpose of reviewing the medications during medical treatment and upon autopsy, provides insight into the severity and treatment of underlying diseases and the possible addition of adjunctive medications (i.e., sedative/hypnotic medications) used during or prior to the end-of-life procedure.

Drugs Used During Medical Treatment

Most patients (63.8%) were reported by informants as taking at least one drug during treatment prior to coming to Kevorkian. Over one-third (34%) were described as using opiates, 21.3 percent were described as using muscle relaxants, 19.1 percent used sedatives or hypnotics, 12.8 percent were described as being on anti-depressants, 4.3 percent were described as being on anti-seizure drugs, 2.1 percent used stimulants while none were described as being on anti-psychotics. Over a quarter of the patients (27.7%) used drugs not falling within the above seven categories.

Drugs Assayed at Autopsy

A different pattern emerged with regard to drugs assayed at autopsy at the time of death. Almost three-fourths of the sample (72.3%) showed the presence of more than one drug in the system at autopsy. Over half (51.1%) showed presence of sedatives and hypnotics at the time of death, 36.2 percent showed signs of opiates, 10.6 percent showed signs of muscle relaxants and non-opiates, 8.5 percent showed signs of stimulants, 6.4 percent showed signs of anti-depressants, 4.3 percent showed signs of anti-seizure medication and none showed signs of anti-psychotics. Only 4.3 percent showed the presence of other drugs at autopsy.

Experience with Kevorkian

This section presents data on the experience of the first forty-seven patients with Kevorkian himself. Appendix A, Table A7 presents overall frequencies with regard to experiences with Kevorkian as reported by informants. In 69.2 percent of the cases, the patient made the initial contact, in 30.8 percent of the cases an intermediary made the initial contact. In 60.6 percent of the cases, Kevorkian himself was first contacted, in the remaining 39.4 percent of the cases another person (Geoffrey Fieger, Janet Good, The Hemlock Society, etc.) was contacted.

In 34.3 percent of the cases, contacts were initiated on the telephone. In the remaining 65.4 percent of the cases the initial contact was made on another modality (letter, Internet, etc.). In 25.6 percent of the cases, a friend or family member was opposed to the patient meeting Kevorkian.

The entire process went very quickly. In 74.5 percent of the cases, Kevorkian responded to the patient's initial inquiry less than one day. In 29.8 percent of the cases the time from the patient's first contact (i.e., by whatever modality) with Kevorkian and his death was one day or less. In 63.8 percent of the cases, the time between the patient's first face-to-face interview with Kevorkian and his or her death was one day or less. In 48.6 percent of the cases only one face-to-face contact was reported. In 17.1 percent of the cases, the time between a patient's initial diagnosis by his primary care physician and his assisted suicide by Kevorkian was less than six months.

Finally, we examined Kevorkian's consultation with other professionals. There was evidence of Kevorkian trying to contact the treating physician in almost one-third of the cases. However, he only succeeded in contacting the treating physician in 11.8 percent of the cases. In 26.9 percent of the cases, Kevorkian consulted with a psychiatrist; in 25 percent of the cases he consulted with a specialist with regard to the patient's disease; and in only 7.1 percent did Kevorkian consult a pain relief specialist.

Circumstances of Death

We conclude this section by describing the actual circumstances of the patient's death (Appendix A, Table A8). Thirty-nine of the first forty-seven patients died in Oakland County, Michigan, four in Wayne County, one in Macomb County (these three counties comprise the metro Detroit area), two in Leelanau County, and one in Ionia County. Next we will describe the location where thirty-four of the forty-seven suicides took place (thirteen were unknown). Ten suicides took place in the patient's home, seven suicides occurred in area motels, three took place in either Kevorkian's home or Janet Good's home (his assistant and later patient), and fourteen took place in other locations including Kevorkian's van, local state parks, rented buildings, and other assorted locations. A friend or family member was present with the patient at the moment of death in 84.4 percent of the cases. The spouse notified authorities in 41.3 percent of the cases. The Oakland County medical examiner processed the body in 80.8 percent of the cases. Across counties, homicide was listed on the death certificate in 71.7 percent of the cases and suicide was listed on 13 percent of the death certificates. The cause of death was carbon monoxide poisoning in 68.1 percent of the cases and was potassium chloride in 31.9 percent of the cases.

Finally, and strikingly, 87.2 percent of the bodies were cremated. This figure was four times as great as the overall cremation figure of Michigan suicides (23.6%) in 1995 and twice as great as the cremation figure for suicides in Michigan (40%) that same year.

Gender Effects

Demographics

A number of important differences emerge between the fifteen men and thirty-two women among Kevorkian's first forty-seven patients (see Appendix A, Table A9; Figure 3). It should be noted that the preponderance of women to men in this sample reverses the national trend of unaided completed suicides in 1995, but resembles that of unsuccessful attempted suicides.

Starting with demographic data it might be expected that women would have different types of jobs than men—and Kevorkian's list provides no exception. Women are more likely to be homemakers (28.1%) than are men (0%, $\chi^2 = 5.22$, $p < .02$) and are also more likely to have a helping-type job (53.1% to 13.3%' $\chi^2 = 6.71, p < .01$).

Biomedical History

Several important gender differences emerged. For men the following medical conditions were present: 46.7 percent with cancer, 20 percent with multiple sclerosis (MS), none with Alzheimer's, 13.3 percent with ALS, and 6.7 percent each for heart or lung disease, multiple conditions, or an uncategorized miscellaneous condition. For women the following conditions were present: 22.6 percent with cancer, 22.6 percent with MS, 3.2 percent with Alzheimer's, 19.4 percent with ALS, 3.2 percent with heart or lung disease, 9.7 percent with multiple conditions, or 19.4 percent with an uncategorized miscellaneous condition.

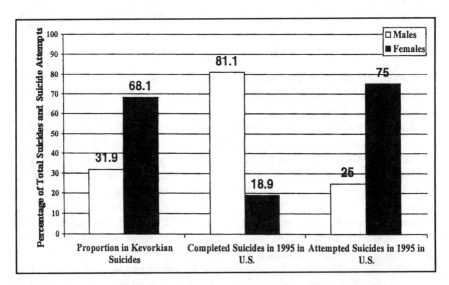

Figure 3. Gender differences in Kevorkian's first forty-seven suicides and the 1995 National Suicide Statistics.

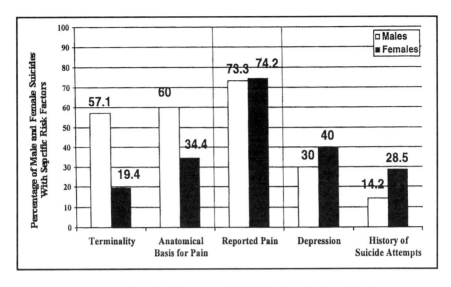

Figure 4. Gender differences in risk factors for Kevorkian's
first forty-seven suicides.

Although approximately three-quarters of the sample of both men and women report pain, evidence supplied by the medical examiner indicates a dramatic difference in whether the two genders have a specific anatomical basis for their pain. Sixty percent of the men show such an anatomic-physiological basis, but only 34 percent of the women (Figure 4).

A number of differences emerge between men and women with regard to physical limitations. 28.6 percent of the men were able to drive at the time of their death, and only 9.4 percent of the women. Over one-quarter (26.7%) percent of the men were able to work, but only 3.1 percent of the women ($\chi^2 = 5.95$, $p < .02$). 13.3 percent of the men actually were working and none of the women ($\chi^2 = 4.46$, $p < .03$). Finally, 57.1 percent of the men were considered by the medical examiner to be terminal (life expectancy less than or equal to 6 months) at the time of their own death, but only 19.4 percent of the women ($\chi^2 = 6.43$, $p < .01$).

Psychosocial History

Sixty percent of the men both had surviving spouse or children at the time of their death and were living with a spouse or partner. Only 31 percent of the women had surviving spouse/children and were living with them ($\chi^2 = 3.5$, $p < .06$).

No difference emerged between men and women with regard to death of a friend or family divorce or separation or being the victim of a crime or disaster. With regard to other unspecified traumas, a difference did emerge between men and women. No men were reported as experiencing such trauma in the year before their death, but 20.8 percent of the women were reported as experiencing trauma ($\chi^2 = 3.13, p < .08$).

Consultation History/Treatment Before Kevorkian

Almost three times as many women were described as having multiple conditions at the time of their death (34.4%) as were men (13.3%). Only one significant difference emerged with regard to drugs reported in the patient's system either during treatment or at the time of death. Almost twice as many women (59.4%) had sedatives/hypnotics in their system at the time of death as did men (33.3%).

Experience with Kevorkian

Seventy-two percent of the women made their initial contact with Kevorkian himself as opposed to 25 percent of the men who were more likely to contact someone else in the Kevorkian entourage ($\chi^2 = 5.61, p < .02$). Kevorkian seemed to act more quickly with his male patients than his female patients. With 46.7 percent of the men, less than one day (24 hours) elapsed between initial contact and death. Only 21.9 percent of the women were dispatched so quickly ($\chi^2 = 3.00, p < .08$).

Circumstances of Death

All of the women for whom data were available died in the presence of a friend or family member but this was true for only about half (54.5%) of the men ($\chi^2 = 11.31, p < .001$). The informant was the spouse for 66.7 percent of the men, but only 29 percent of the women ($\chi^2 = 5.91, p < .02$). Men were more likely to be killed with carbon monoxide (80%) than were women (46.9%) who were more likely to be given a lethal injection ($\chi^2 = 4.58, p < .03$).

Finally, more women died in Oakland County (93.8%) than did men (60%, $\chi^2 = 8.24, p < .01$). This resulted in several spurious effects due to different definitional systems employed by the Medical Examiners in the different counties. First, homicide was more likely to be listed as cause of death on the death certificate for women (81.3%) than men (50%, $\chi^2 = 4.69, p < .03$). Suicide, in contrast, was more likely to be listed as the cause of death for men (35.7%) than for women (3.1%, $\chi^2 = 9.12, p < .01$).[4]

---

[4] Examination indicated that this was a function of the different definitions employed by the different medical examiners. Dr. L. J. Dragovic, Chief Medical Examiner of Oakland County, does not accept the definitional category of physician-assisted suicide. In a letter to Michigan State Senator William VanReganmorter (September 11, 1997), Dr. Dragovic argues that assisted-suicide is a paradoxical term misconstruing the reality of physician-assisted death or homicide.

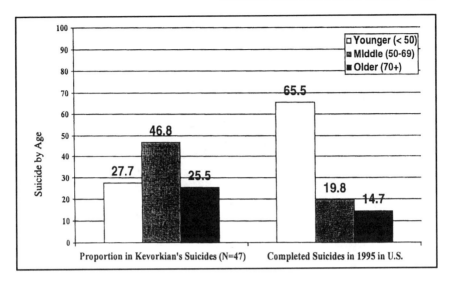

Figure 5. Age differences in Kevorkian's first forty-seven suicides and the 1995 National Suicide Statistics.

Age Effects

Age was trichotomized for the analysis in this section into three categories: forty-nine or younger, fifty through sixty-nine, and seventy or older (see Appendix A, Table A10; Figure 5).

Demographics

A significant age effect emerged with regard to middle class income. The percentage of patients at middle class income increased with age ($\chi^2 = 8.30$, $p < .08$). The percentage of patients with children also increased with age ($\chi^2 = 9.30$, $p < .01$) while patients with minor children (under age 18) tended to decrease with age. The percentage of patients who were married at the time of death shows a curvilinear relationship with age, being highest for ages sixty to sixty-nine and lower for the younger and older groups.

Biomedical History

Incontinence, surprisingly, decreased with age ($\chi^2 = 83.0$, $p < .02$), as did reported pain ($\chi^2 = 45.9$, $p < .05$; Figure 6). Significantly, anatomical basis for pain was unaffected by age (between 30% and 40% for all age groups), suggesting that older people had developed an increased pain threshold. No differences in terminally or physical limitations emerged for the three age groups.

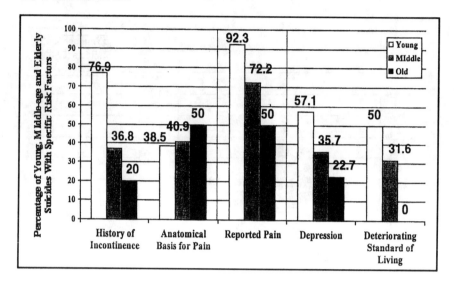

Figure 6. Age differences in risk factors for Kevorkian's
first forty-seven suicides.

Psychosocial History

The percentage of patients living alone is surprisingly unaffected by age, although the percentage of patients living with a spouse/partner is higher for a middle age decedent (54.5%) than for a younger (23.1%) or older (33.3%) one. Living with children is unaffected by age (hovering between 25% and 30%) although the direction of the psychological dependency is clearly different for younger and older patients. Living with family members other than parents or children (e.g., siblings) does decrease with age, however ($\chi^2 = 5.8, p < .05$).

A deteriorating financial condition significantly decreased with age with fully half of the patients under fifty reflecting this and none over 70 ($\chi^2 = 6.1, p < .04$; Figure 6). Likewise the recent death of a parent also decreased with age whether in the previous year ($\chi^2 = 7.6, p < .02$) or the previous five years ($\chi^2 = 7.5, p < .02$). Finally, younger patients were more likely to have experienced a financial/professional reversal within the last five years.

Consultation History/Treatment Before Kevorkian

Tendency to consult with a mental health professional declined with age ($\chi^2 = 5.6, p < .06$) while tendency to consult with a religious figure was greatest for the middle aged patients ($\chi^2 = 7.8, p < .02$). Tendency to reject medical treatment also increased with age, being lowest for the youngest patients ($\chi^2 = 6.7, p < .03$).

Older patients were reported less likely to have had drugs in their system during treatment ($\chi^2 = 7.3$, $p < .03$). Younger patients were more likely to have stimulants in their system at the time of death ($\chi^2 = 5.5$, $p < .06$) and less likely to have drugs other than the main categories of antidepressants, anti-psychotics, anti-seizure medications, muscle relaxers, opiates, and sedative/hypnotics in their systems at the time of death (15.4%, 0%, 0%, $\chi^2 = 5.4$, $p < .06$).

Experience With Kevorkian/Circumstances of Death

Length of time between first diagnosis of the condition and death decreased with age, with the proportion of patients dying within six months of their initial diagnosis increasing with age ($\chi^2 = 5.4$, $p < .07$). Finally, the likelihood that the informant was the spouse tended to increase with age.

Marital Status Effects

Appendix A, Table A11 presents analyses comparing the effects of being married at the time of death versus not being married (which here refers to being single, divorced or widowed; Figure 7).

Demographics

A number of significant and non-significant demographic effects emerge in relation to marital status. First, suicides younger than fifty and older than seventy

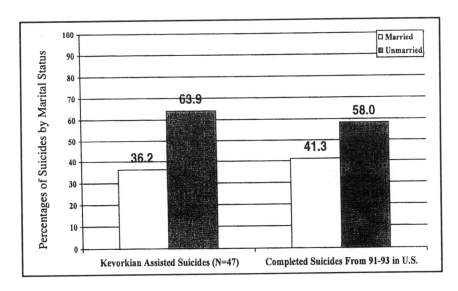

Figure 7. Marital status differences in Kevorkian's first forty-seven suicides and the 1991-1993 National Suicide Statistics.

were more likely to be single than married. However, suicides between fifty and seventy were equally likely to be married or unmarried at the time of their death. There is a higher proportion of married decedents from WASP background (82.4%) then there is of unmarried decedents (60%). All seventeen of the patients married at the time of death had children as compared to 63 percent of the patients unmarried at the time of death (χ^2 = 6.31, p < .01). No surprises here. The next effect is somewhat more interesting. A higher proportion of married patients were likely to have held helping type jobs (58.8%) than were unmarried patients (30%, χ^2 = 3.74, p < .05). Finally, another unsurprising demographic effect. A greater number of married patients lived in a house at the time of their death (88.2%) than did unmarried patients (55.2%, χ^2 = 5.33, p < .02).

Biomedical History

Marital status interacts with several biomedical variables. First, married suicides are two times more likely to be described as mentally incapacitated (40%) than are patients unmarried at the time of death (18.2%). Although the proportion of patients reporting pain is similar in the unmarried (79.3%) and married groups (64.7%, n.s.), a physiological anatomical basis for the pain emerges more often in the unmarried (53.3%) than the married group (23.5%, χ^2 = 3.95, p < .05; Figure 8). Perhaps being married provides permission for complaining about free-floating pain or phantom pain with no specific anatomical basis. In line with this interpretation, a greater proportion of unmarried patients

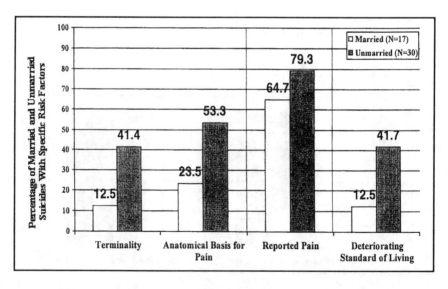

Figure 8. Marital status difference in risk factors for Kevorkian's first forty-seven suicides.

were reported as terminal (41.4%) than were married patients (12.5%, $\chi^2 = 4.01$, $p < .05$). This will be treated in greater detail in the discussion section.

Psychosocial History

Only a few significant psychosocial effects emerged with regard to marital status. First, none of the patients married at the time of death were living alone. However, 46.7 percent of the unmarried patients lived alone at the time of death ($\chi^2 = 11.3$, $p < .001$). Similarly, all seventeen of the married suicides lived with their partner at the time of death, but only 6.7 percent of the unmarried patients lived with a significant other ($\chi^2 = 39.25$, $p < .001$). A practically identical effect occurs with regard to the presence of surviving spouse/children ($\chi^2 = 32.5$, $p < .001$). A slightly more interesting effect occurs with regard to life insurance policies. All of the six unmarried suicides with life insurance policies left them to a non-spouse while all of the six married suicides left them to a spouse ($\chi^2 = 32.45$, $p < .001$). Finally, a higher proportion of unmarried people reported deteriorating financial conditions (41.7%) than did married people (12.5%, $\chi^2 = 3.84$, $p < .05$; Figure 8). A higher proportion of unmarried people experienced the death of a parent within the previous five years (30.8%) than did unmarried patients (21%, $\chi^2 = 2.91$, $p < .09$).

Consultation History/Treatment Before Kevorkian

Married patients are twice as likely to have multiple conditions at time of death (41.2%) than are unmarried patients (20%, $\chi^2 = 2.43$, $p < .12$). Married decedents were more likely to have used anti-seizure drugs during treatment than were single patients (0%, $\chi^2 = 3.65$, $p < .05$).

Circumstances of Death

The death of sixteen of the seventeen married patients (94.1%) was reported by the surviving spouse/partner. Partners reported the deaths of unmarried patients in only 10.3 percent of the cases ($\chi^2 = 31.02$, $p < .001$). This difference, while highly significant, seems more a function of their living situation than anything else. With no spouse, someone other than a spouse must report the death.

Socioeconomic Status Effects

Appendix A, Table A12 presents analyses comparing the effects of three levels of socioeconomic status—lower, middle and higher (Figure 9).

Demographics

The greatest number of upper class decedents were between the ages of fifty and seventy (57.1%). The same pattern held for middle class decedents (48.1%). The greatest number of lower class patients (66.7%), in contrast, tended to be under the age of fifty ($\chi^2 = 8.28$, $p < .08$). As expected, the proportion of patients

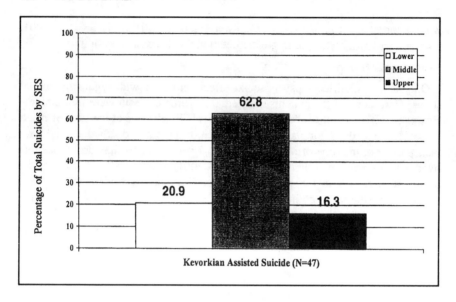

Figure 9. Social class differences in Kevorkian's first forty-seven suicides.

with at least some college education tended to increase with higher SES. Being married also tended to increase with higher socioeconomic status as did living in a house (χ^2 = 7.43, p < .02).

Biomedical History

A history of disability (χ^2 = 7.97, p < .02; Figure 10) and incontinence (χ^2 = 8.15, p < .02) decreased with social class as did physical incapacitation (χ^2 = 5.60, p < .06) and tendency for functional physical limitation. No significant differences in terminality or reported pain occurred across social economic class nor was there any difference in anatomical basis for that pain. Finally, proportion of decedents working at time of their death increased with higher social class (χ^2 = 10.79, p < 004).

Psychosocial History

Tendencies toward using periodic paid care tended to be lower for middle class patients than for those at either end of the socioeconomic scale. The likelihood of having a surviving spouse or children increased with social class (χ^2 = 6.84, p < .03) as did tendencies to have been divorced or separated within the past five years (χ^2 = 7.44, p < .02). Likelihood of experiencing a deteriorating financial condition was lowest for the middle class patients (χ^2 = 8.31, p < .02; Figure 10). A history of substance abuse decreased with increasing social class (χ^2 = 14.73, p < .02).

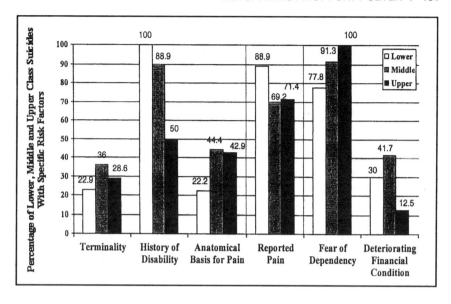

Figure 10. Social class differences in risk factors for Kevorkian's
first forty-seven suicides.

Consultation History/Treatment Before Kevorkian

Patient acceptance of medical treatment tended to decline with increasing social class, but tendency to consult a psychiatrist increased ($\chi^2 = 4.90$, $p < .08$). Use of antidepressants tended to decrease with lower social class as did use of sedatives/hypnotics ($\chi^2 = 8.28$, $p < .02$). Drugs other than the main category were most used by upper and lower class patients ($\chi^2 = 5.02$, $p < .08$). The presence of both anti-seizure medication ($\chi^2 = 10.79$, $p < .005$) and opiates at autopsy both increased with high social class.

Experience with Kevorkian/Circumstances of Death

Speed of time from first contact to death increased with higher social class ($\chi^2 = 6.50$, $p < .04$) as did tendency for the informant to be a spouse ($\chi^2 = 6.30$, $p < .04$) as well as have had death classified as a suicide ($\chi^2 = 6.97$, $p < .03$) though this latter effect might well be a function of the particular medical examiner. Finally, tendency toward having someone (friend or family) with them at the time of death was greatest for the middle class patients ($\chi^2 = 6.97$, $p < .03$).

Ancestry Effects

Appendix A, Table A13 presents analyses comparing the 32 patients coming from White, Anglo-Saxon Protestant ancestry (WASP) with the remaining fifteen coming from non-WASP backgrounds.

Demographics

Only one demographic interaction approaches significance. A greater proportion of WASP patients tended to be married at the time of their death (43.7%) than
did non-WASP patients (20%).

Biomedical History

None of the twenty-seven WASP patients for whom data was available showed
any sign of psychosis, while one of eight (12.5%) non-WASP patients with data
showed such signs ($\chi^2 = 3.47, p < .06$). WASP patients had a lesser proportion
(3.8%) of a history of sleeping disorders than did non-WASP patients (28.6%,
$\chi^2 = 4.08, p < .04$). Fully one-third of the WASP patients are portrayed as
mentally incapacitated while only 10 percent of the non-WASP patients are
similarly portrayed. Over half (53.6%) of the WASP suicides show signs of
functional physical limitation while only one-third of the non-WASP patients
tended to show such signs. WASP patients were less likely (34.4%) to be able to
go to the toilet than were non-WASP patients (61.5%, $\chi^2 = 2.80, p < .09$).

Finally, contrary to the popular stereotype, WASP patients report pain to
the same degree as do non-WASP patients (about 75%), but tend to have
much less anatomical-physiological basis for this pain (34.4% to 60%). In
line with this, the WASP patients were less likely to be terminal than were
non-WASP patients.

Psychosocial History

WASP patients were less likely to be alone at the time of death (18.8%) than
were non-WASP patients (53.3%, $\chi^2 = 5.84, p < .02$). Specifically, WASP patients
were more likely to be living with a spouse/partner (50% to 20%, $\chi^2 = 3.82$,
$p < .05$) but less to be living with paid help (0% to 13.3%, $\chi^2 = 4.32, p < .04$)
than were non-WASP patients. Non-WASP patients were generally more likely
to have experienced recent traumas/losses than were WASP patients. For
example, non-WASP patients were more likely than WASP patients to have
experienced, within the five years prior to their suicide, the death of a spouse
(13.3% to 0%, $\chi^2 = 4.48, p < .03$), of a child (13.3% to 0%, $\chi^2 = 4.19, p < .04$)
or within one year prior to death a financial/professional reversal (23.1% to 3.6%,
$\chi^2 = 3.84, p < .05$).

Consultation History/Treatment Before Kevorkian

WASP patients were less likely than non-WASP patients to have consulted a
pain relief specialist (0% to 28.6%, $\chi^2 = 6.46, p < .01$) or a religious figure
(16.7% to 60%, $\chi^2 = 4.24, p < .04$), but more likely to consult members of their
family about their wish to die (96.9% to 78.6%, $\chi^2 = 4.1, p < .04$). WASP patients
were also less likely to have used sedative/hypnotics during treatment (9.4% to

40%, $\chi^2 = 6.1$, $p < .01$) or for that matter any drugs other than the main categories described previously (62.5% to 93.3%, $\chi^2 = 4.85$, $p < .03$).

Experience with Kevorkian

Kevorkian was less likely to have contacted a treating physician for WASP patients (20%) than for non-WASP patients (66.7%, $\chi^2 = 4.7$, $p < .03$) and was less likely to have only one face-to-face meeting with WASP patients (40.7% to 75%, $\chi^2 = 2.90$, $p < .09$).

Circumstances of Death

The death of WASP patients was more likely to be reported by the spouse (50%) than was that of non-WASP patients (21.4%, $\chi^2 = 3.28$, $p < .07$). However, this is probably a function of the higher marriage rate among the WASP patients. The last finding regarding death is quite interesting, however; WASP patients have a significantly higher proportion of cremations (93.8%) than do non-WASP patients (73.3%, $\chi^2 = 3.8$, $p < .05$; Figure 11). Ancestry is the only one of the demographic effects presented in this article to affect this tendency. Cremation rates for Kevorkian suicides were abnormally high to begin with at 87.2 percent, in comparison to the 1995 Michigan rate of cremations for all deaths of 23.6 percent and 40 percent for suicides in particular. For patients of White, Anglo-Saxon background, the rate is even higher!

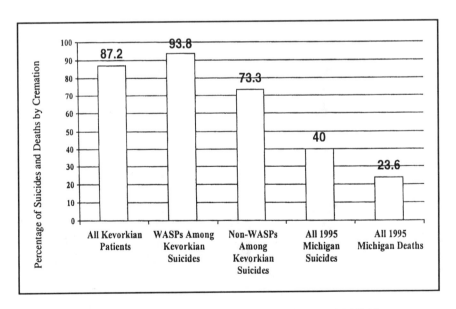

Figure 11. Cremation rates among Kevorkian and 1995 Michigan suicides and deaths.

Phase Effects

Appendix A, Table A14 describes the breakdown in gender, age, marital status, SES, and ancestry for each of these four phases as defined in the methods section. A dramatic phase effect emerges with regard to gender (Figure 12). The "honeymoon" phase (June 4, 1990 through December 15, 1992) was composed of only women (8 total). In the second phase (December 16, 1992 through May 14, 1996) or "prosecution" phase was composed of an almost exactly even number of men and women (11 vs 9). The "revenge" phase (May 15, 1996 through August 6, 1996) repeats the pattern of the honeymoon phase—100 percent women (6 total). Finally in the "business as usual" phase (August 7, 1996 through February 2, 1997), Kevorkian resumes the overall male/female ratio of about two females for each male (30.8% to 69.2%, $\chi^2 = 11.5, p < .009$).

No significant phase effects emerge with regard to the other major demographics factors (age, marital status, or ancestry). The ancestry pattern, however, does resemble the gender patterns described above, with an equal number of WASP and non-WASP decedents emerging during the first and third phases and a preponderance of WASP suicides (75% and over) occurring during the first and third phases. This pattern is interesting given the absence of significant differences in the proportion of WASPs among men (73.3%) and women (65.6%).

Several other demographic effects do emerge for phase, however. Over time, a greater proportion of Kevorkian's patients came from outside of Michigan

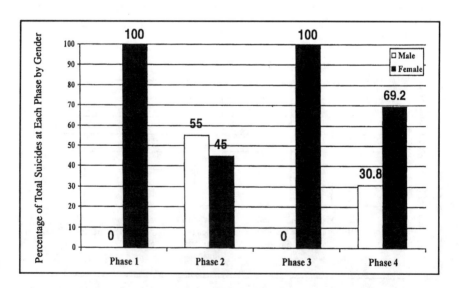

Figure 12. Phase differences in gender ratio among Kevorkian's
first forty-seven suicides.

($\chi^2 = 19.9, p < .01$). In the first phase, 75 percent came from Michigan, in the second phase 50 percent, in the third phase none out of six and in the fourth phase only one out of thirteen (7.7%) came from Michigan. Another interesting demographic pattern is the county in which the patient's body was found: whether Oakland county, the seat of Kevorkian's nemesis Richard Thompson, or another county in Michigan. In only the second phase (when Kevorkian was in the greatest legal difficulty) was there a distribution of deaths across counties. In the first and third phases, all the patients' bodies were found in Oakland county. In the fourth phase (after Thompson was defeated), twelve of the thirteen deaths were found in Oakland county ($\chi^2 = 8.25, p < .04$).

A number of other disturbing phase effects occur as well, largely dealing with the amount of care given to each patient, in terms of consideration of alternatives and time spent making and thinking about the decision. To begin, there are no significant phase effects with regard to terminality, reported pain, or anatomical basis for pain. However, in percentages, the proportion of terminal patients declined from 37.5 percent in phase one to 15.4 percent in phase four.

History of depression actually declined over time (from 80% in the first phase to 10% in the fourth; $\chi^2 = 7.28$, $p < .06$) as did mental incapacitation and opposition to the suicide from friends and family (62.5% to 27.5%; $\chi^2 = 8.42$, $p < .05$). Ability to work was actually greater in the later phases ($\chi^2 = 7.88, p < .05$), but the proportion of those actually working did not increase with phase. However, financial/professional reversal ($\chi^2 = 8.47, p < .04$) and deterioration of financial condition ($\chi^2 = 8.97, p < .03$) were less in the first phase than in the later phases.

The number of face-to-face meetings between Kevorkian and the patients decreased with time (Figure 13). The patients in the first phase (from whom information was available) met with Kevorkian only once. This same pattern held in phase two where only 26.7 percent of his patients (4 out of 15) met with Kevorkian only once. In the later phases this pattern totally reversed, with 80 percent of the patients in phase three and 90 percent of the patients in phase four meeting Kevorkian only once. ($\chi^2 = 16.5, p < .001$). Correspondingly, decreasing with phase was the length of time from the initial contact with Kevorkian until the patient's death ($\chi^2 = 7.49, p < .06$) and the time from the first face to face meeting with Kevorkian and the patient's death ($\chi^2 = 11.7, p < .01$). No patients in the initial phase died on the day of the first contact with K, while only 25 percent died on the day of their first face-to-face meeting with him. By the fourth phase both of these figures had drastically increased 53.8 percent of the patients dying on the day of first contact with Kevorkian and 84.6 percent dying on the day of the first face-to-face meeting with him.

Also declining over time was Kevorkian's tendency to consult another medical professional, whether the treating physician ($\chi^2 = 17.5, p < .001$), a pain relief specialist ($\chi^2 = 7.90, p < .05$), a specialist ($\chi^2 = 11.5, p < .01$) or a psychiatrist; Figure 14). Significantly, the proportion of patients dying in a motel dramatically

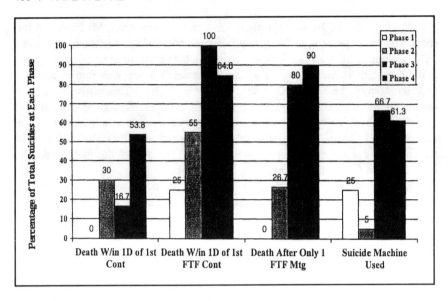

Figure 13. Phase differences in speed of death among Kevorkian's
first forty-seven suicides.

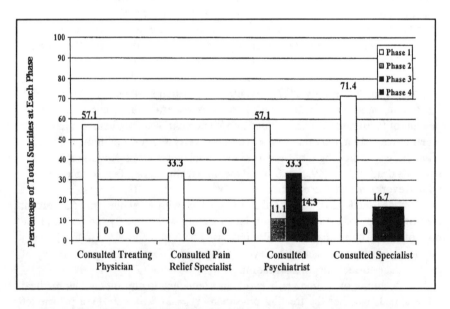

Figure 14. Phase differences in Kevorkian consultation history among
Kevorkian's first forty-seven suicides.

increased in time from 0 percent to 80 percent (χ^2 = 29.1, p < .01), as did those dying on the "suicide machine" rather than with carbon monoxide, increasing from 25 percent in phase one to 61.5 percent in phase four (χ^2 = 15.4, p < .001) and patients being given sedative and hypnotics at the time of death increased from 50 percent in phase one to 100 percent in phase three and remaining high in phase four as well (χ^2 = 9.88, p < .02).

DISCUSSION

We have presented data regarding Kevorkian's first forty-seven acknowledged suicides. Some of the more important effects will be discussed in more detail in this section.

Terminality, Disability, and Fear of Dependency

We are struck first by the low proportion of terminality (31.1%), but high proportion of physical incapacitation (66%) and disability (87%), and an even higher fear of dependency (90%) among the patients. This raises the question of whether disability or fear of dependency plays a greater role in these cases than terminality per se and what can be done by society to better enable people with physical incapacitation and disabilities to live more full lives. Central to this may be the phobia against dependency in our highly individualistic society.

An example of this phobia leaps out from the letters written to the senior author by one of Kevorkian's later (post-47) suicides. Martha Wichorek, a physically healthy eighty-two-year-old woman, advocated for a state euthanasia clinic for those in a "miserable existence stage" (cannot do anything for yourself or others). She argued that this "stage of the life-death cycle" can last weeks, months, or years and is the most dreaded of human experiences. Among the indignities of the miserable existence stage are 1) nursing home and hospital testing procedures, 2) living with children, 3) hospice, 4) in-home and visiting nurse arrangements, 5) living wills, and 6) committing suicide without the help of a doctor (Kaplan & Leonhardi, 1997, 1999-2000).

Pain, Depression, and History of Suicide

We are also struck by the discrepancy between the proportion of patients reporting pain (73.9%) and those described as having an anatomical basis for this pain (42.6%). One possible explanation for this discrepancy is the sizeable proportion of depression (36.7%) and history of suicide attempts (23.8%) among these patients. This suggests that a considerable number of these patients may be experiencing psychologically-based pain or phantom pain rather than anatomically-based pain. This effect becomes even more pronounced when we consider gender differences. Males and females are reported as experiencing pain at about the same rate (approximately 75%), but men are described as having almost twice the rate of anatomical basis for pain (60%) as women (34.4%) and are much more likely to be terminal (57.1%) than women (19.4%). History of depression is slightly higher for women (40%) than for men (30%) and history of prior suicide attempts is twice as high for women (28.5%) than for men (14.2%), though neither of these latter effects is significant.

What does one make of these patterns? One does not want to question the sincerity of the reported pain. However, treatment of the pain requires knowing the basis for that pain, be it physical or psychological. Consider some individual cases. Doctors could find no physical reason for Marjorie Wantz's vaginal pain. No sign of multiple sclerosis emerged in the autopsy of Rebecca Badger. Judith Curren reportedly was suffering from Chronic Fatigue Syndrome Immunodeficiency Disorder, but no sign of any disease was present at autopsy. Furthermore, she was reported to have been hit by her husband several weeks prior to her death.

Gender, Completed Suicide, and Attempted Suicide

These data suggest that some women may have considered physician-assisted suicide because of psychosocial rather than biomedical reasons. Particularly relevant here is the high proportion of women among Kevorkian's first forty-seven suicides (68.1%) and their relatively less frequent objective indices of pain (i.e., anatomical bases for pain) and terminality. We should remember the national differences in gender on attempted and completed suicides. In the year 1995, four men completed suicide for every woman, yet three women attempted suicide for each man. This pattern suggests that Kevorkian's assisted-suicides may be more similar to attempted suicides in the general population than to completed suicides. These attempted suicides may intend to draw attention to their feeling of misery rather than being certain in their desire to die.

Also interesting in this regard is that nearly three times as many of the women (72%) than the men (25%) contacted Kevorkian himself as opposed to one of his associates. These results suggest Kevorkian may have served as an important psychological figure for the women. Kevorkian helps them carry out plans about which they may be initially ambivalent. Kevorkian's first suicide, Janet Adkins, was in the very early stages of Alzheimer's disease and had been told by her family physician that she had a number of quality years ahead. She had defeated her son in tennis three days earlier. Yet Kevorkian agreed with Adkin's husband that she was "terminal in a mental sense." Rather than explore the reasons for Janet wanting to die, Kevorkian frames the discussion in terms of "autonomy and self-determination" and praises Janet as a heroine for dying because this is the first time this has happened since classical Greece.[5]

---

[5] This, for someone of Kevorkian's intelligence, is no idle reference. Ancient Greece was a fatalistic society, permissive if not encouraging toward suicide and infanticide (especially with regard to baby girls). Examine the many suicides, especially women, who are almost all altruistic (killing themselves to meet other's expectations) in Greek tragedies (see Kaplan, 1991).

The greater reliance of women's decision to die on social support is illustrated by the fact that 100 percent of the women had family or friends present at the moment of their death as compared to 54.5 percent of the men. Finally, wives of male patients are more than twice as likely (66.7%) to inform the authorities of their spouses' death as were husbands of female patients (29%).

Age, Pain, and Stressors

Although anatomical basis for pain was unaffected by age differences in Kevorkian's patients (between 30 and 40% for all age groups), reported pain significantly decreased with age (92% to 50%), suggesting older people developed a greater tolerance for pain. This tendency is supported by the greater tendency of older people to reject medical treatment.

Terminality did not vary systematically with age, although a history of depression decreased with age. This suggests that people may learn how to deal better with life stressors as they grow older. Alternatively, younger people may simply have been experiencing more stressors. This position is supported in that younger patients were more likely to have recently experienced a professional or financial reversal and to be experiencing a deteriorating standard of living.

Marriage as a Buffer or a Precipitant to Stressors

Several interesting results emerged with regard to the marital status of Kevorkian's patients. Married and unmarried (single, divorced, and widowed) patients were equally likely to report pain (about 70% of the people in both conditions). However, unmarried people were more likely to have an anatomical basis for this pain (53.3%) than were married people (23.5%) and were more likely to be terminal (41.4%) than married people (12.5%). They were also more likely to have experienced a deteriorating standard of living (41.7%) than married people (12.5%). Yet they complained less. Perhaps being married provides a kind of permission to complain about free-floating or phantom pain which has no specific anatomical base or life stressor. However, unmarried patients are also less likely to be mentally incapacitated (18.2%) than married patients (40%). Perhaps mental incapacitation is tolerated more in marriage—or is it sometimes a consequence of an unhealthy mental dynamic?

Unmarried people among Kevorkian's suicides seemed to be better able to handle life's stressors whether physical or psychological than married people. In this way, they seem to be behaving similarly to men and older people in this population. At the same time, though, we must not forget that thirty of the forty-seven suicides were unmarried at the time of their death. Marriage may provide some buffer against suicide.

Social Class, Disability, and Fear of Dependency

Social class was not associated with terminality, reported pain, or the presence of an anatomical base for the pain. However, a history of disability, physical incapacity and limitation, and incontinence decreased with rising social class, as did not working. The advantage of high social economic class seems obvious. Financial security helps make roughly equivalent physical conditions less disabling and more manageable. However, fully 100 percent of the upper class patients expressed a fear of dependence, more than any other group.

Although a minority of the suicides were upper class (7 out of 47), the data suggest that upper class patients who do suicide, do so not because of disability per se (which is less than for middle and lower class suicides), but out of a phobic reaction to dependency. Again we are reminded of Martha Wichorek's equation of "life" with independence! Indeed, acceptance of medical treatment was less for the upper classes and the proportion of patients who killed themselves within one day of their first contact with Kevorkian was more. Once they decided to exercise their "freedom to die," upper class patients seemed to proceed unimpeded upon this quest.

Anxiety, Pain, and Cremation

Contrary to popular stereotypes, WASP patients in this sample do not keep a "stiff upper lip." They report the same proportion of pain as do non-WASP patients (about 75%), but with much less of an anatomical basis (34.4% to 60%). They are also less likely to be terminal than non-WASP patients, again suggesting a different underlying motivational dynamic. WASP patients may not like the inconvenience of illness and do not seem to tolerate it as well. This distaste is perhaps reflected in their 93.8 percent cremation rate: significantly higher than the 73.3 percent rate for non-WASP's.

The overall cremation rate was 87.2 percent. This figure was four times as great as the overall rate of Michigan deaths in 1995 and twice as great as the 1995 cremation rate for suicides. Several explanations are possible. 1) Cremation is a cost-effective way of disposing of the remains ($1000 as opposed to $4400 for a burial), especially when the person is away from home. 2) Cremation is a way to dispose of "evidence" and prevent further investigation. 3) Cremation itself was a popular means of body disposal in ancient Greece, perhaps reflecting an anti-Biblical body-soul dualism. 4) Cremation may involve a hatred of the body which an ill patient may feel has betrayed him or her. 5) Traditional Biblical religions have been reluctant to bury a suicide within the grounds of the synagogue/church, although this taboo is probably much less today.

WASP suicides may accentuate some of these cremation tendencies as compared to more religiously traditional non-WASP suicides and may, along with upper class patients, reflect in purest form the phobic reaction against dependency and imperfection underlying our highly individualistic culture. For these people, suicide represents freedom, echoing the words of the Roman stoic Seneca (De Ira 3.15.3-4), and is not necessarily the result, as popularly assumed of an impossible biomedical situation. It seems clear the Kevorkian patients vary widely in the gravity of their situations and that over time, Kevorkian has proceeded much more quickly, impulsively and arbitrarily.

Phase, Patient Selection, and Care

Two disturbing patterns emerge from our analysis of the time phase data (from Kevorkian's first 47 patients). First, Kevorkian's selection of patients seems highly influenced by extra-medical considerations. Second, his level of care and compliance with his own stated criteria seems to have declined dramatically with time.

With regard to the issue of patient selection, one cannot help but be struck by one pattern. In the "honeymoon" and "revenge" phases, all of Kevorkian's acknowledged suicides were women. These phases once again denote respectively, the "honeymoon" period before Governor Engler signed into law a temporary ban against physician-assisted suicide (June 4, 1990 to December 15, 1992) and the "revenge" period after Kevorkian was acquitted on the deaths of Marjorie Wantz and Sherrie Miller (May 14, 1996), until the defeat of Kevorkian's nemesis, Richard Thompson, for re-election (August 6, 1996). Perhaps the selection of all women in these periods reflected Kevorkian's natural inclinations when he was unimpeded by legal consideration. Alternatively, Kevorkian may have tried to inflame those he opposed by choosing women because of the stereotype of female helplessness.

In the "prosecution" phase (December 16, 1992 to May 14, 1996) Kevorkian was vigorously prosecuted by Thompson and others. Here, the selection criteria seemed to change drastically, with more men than women. In the last "business as usual" phase, (August 7, 1996 to February 3, 1997) Kevorkian was dealing not with Thompson, but his successor, David Gorcyca. Here he again chose a balance of men and women, although more women than men. The point of this pattern is that Kevorkian seemed to choose all women when he wanted to, and chose a balance of men and women at other times.

Another example of the extra-medical purposiveness evident in Kevorkian's behavior can be seen in the venue he chose to aid in the killing. During the first and third phases, all of the patients died in Oakland county (the home base of Prosecutor Thompson). During the second phase (when Kevorkian was in the greatest legal difficulty, especially with Thompson) Kevorkian seemed to choose patients outside of Oakland County as well. The increase with time of patients coming outside of Michigan may simply attest to the increasing national notice given to Kevorkian, rather than a specific selection agenda set by Kevorkian and his associates.

The issue of declining patient care over time is even more disturbing. Kevorkian (1992) set out a number of standards for physician-assisted suicide. Among the standards Kevorkian proclaims here and in other places are: 1) bringing in a psychiatrist, 2) minimum twenty-four hour waiting periods after the patient has made a final request, 3) consultation with a pain specialist when pain is a major factor in the patient's condition, 4) extensive counseling sessions to understand the reasons behind the patient's wish to die, and 5) an end to the process if there is any sign of ambivalence.

That Kevorkian is not sensitized or oriented toward a patient's ambivalence is exemplified in several of the early cases. In his taped session with his first suicide, Janet Adkins, Kevorkian does not explore alternative meanings beneath her statement, "She wants to get out," and seems to pressure her to say she wants to die. In a transcript of a phone call between Kevorkian and his third suicide, Marjorie Wantz, Kevorkian responds to Wantz's statement of ambivalence "I got two choices. Either stay like this or go the other way" with the response "You sound like you're in pain." A third example is the death of Hugh Gale in Macomb County, one of three counties that make up metropolitan Detroit (Macomb, Oakland, and Wayne). Gale, a seventy-two-year-old former merchant marine, was suffering from emphysema. There is no question that he asked to die, but there is clear evidence that Gale had a great deal of ambivalence after the gas mask was put on his face, asking twice that it be removed. Kevorkian's original record of the incident (on a so-called "Form H") found in a garbage bag outside his assistant's (Neal Nicol's) house, indicated that Kevorkian removed the mask in response to Gale's first request, but did not remove it in response to the second.[6]

Less clear is Kevorkian's attitude toward terminality, though this criterion is typically espoused by others. We have already discussed the fact that the majority (31) of Kevorkian's cases were not terminal. In addition, in only a small minority of the cases was there clear evidence that Kevorkian consulted with another health professional, whether a psychiatrist (7 cases), a specialist (7 cases), a pain relief specialist (2 cases) or the primary care physician (4 cases, though he tried to contact the primary care physician in 8 cases).[7]

All of these variables decline appallingly with time, with only three terminal patients dying in phase three and four, and no consultation with a treating physician or a pain specialist after the first phase. There were several cases of

---

[6] A second record (Form H) was found in Kevorkian's apartment in which the second request was whited out and replaced with an innocuous statement of the exact same length. It strains incredulity to accept the defense explanation that the original statement represented a "typo" and raises the question of why Kevorkian was not vigorously prosecuted in this case (cf. Kaplan, 1998).

[7] Very often when Kevorkian has tried to consult with a patient's doctor, he has been turned down. We do not know if this decrease is due to this rejection or because of his increasing isolation and moralistic certainty.

consultation with psychiatrists or specialists after the first phase, but the great majority of such consultation occurred during the first phase. These patterns uniformly point to an erosion of Kevorkian's compliance with the standards he had himself enunciated. The increase over time of the patients' meeting Kevorkian only once and dying within one day of their first contact and/or first face-to-face meeting with him is a further indication of his abandonment of his own standards. There has also been a change in method of death from a carbon monoxide mask (taking 7 minutes) to injection of potassium chloride along with sedatives/hypnotics in Kevorkian's "suicide machine" (taking 2 minutes).

Cheyfitz (1997) cites statements from Geoffrey Fieger, Kevorkian's attorney, to the effect that the siege situation Kevorkian has found himself in with the police has made it impractical or impossible for Kevorkian to follow his theoretical standards. One can only wonder, what other corners might be cut in the name of practicality should physician-assisted suicide become routinized.

Finally, there is no clear evidence that Kevorkian's assisted suicides are so strikingly different from typical suicide-prevention cases. Indeed, even chronically sick people differ in suicidality. Berman and Samuel (1993), for example, have shown the twenty-four completed suicides among multiple sclerosis (MS) patients were more disabled, less capable of expressing feelings and asking for help and were generally more isolated that a matched sample of twenty-two nonsuicidal MS patients.

The replacement of the suicide prevention model with that of physician-assisted suicide threatens to shift the default in our society from life to death. This problem may exist even in those extreme cases where it seems from the outside that a person really has very few options. Any consideration of legalizing physician-assisted suicide should ensure that it not be mechanized or routinized and that it remain a rare event. Time itself may allow the patient's condition to improve or decline. Much of the push toward PAS may be preemptive in this regard and thus force a decision prematurely without allowing the change in the patient's condition itself to generate new options. This tendency toward preemptive solutions itself may reflect the obsession with instant solutions characteristic of the United States, and is typical of the truncating of time in the suicidal personality. Just as the passage of time can be an ally in treating the traditional suicidal person, so it can also help to clarify and remedy what would seem to be at the moment an impossible medical condition. These data suggest there may be good reason to maintain the legal barriers to physician-assisted suicide.

APPENDIX
Table A1. Kevorkian's First Forty-Seven Patients

No.	Name	Gender	Age	Date of Death	County of Death
1	Janet Adkins	F	54	June 4, 1990	Oakland
2	Sherry Miller	F	43	Oct. 23, 1991	Oakland
3	Marjorie Wantz	F	58	Oct. 23, 1991	Oakland
4	Susan Williams	F	52	May 15, 1992	Oakland
5	Lois Hawes	F	52	Sept. 26, 1992	Oakland
6	Catherine Andreyev	F	45	Nov. 23, 1992	Oakland
7	Marguerite Tate	F	70	Dec. 15, 1992	Oakland
8	Marcella Lawrence	F	67	Dec. 15, 1992	Oakland
9	Jack Miller	M	53	Jan. 20, 1993	Wayne
10	Mary Biernat	F	74	Feb. 4, 1993	Leelanau
11	Stanley Ball	M	82	Feb. 4, 1993	Leelanau
12	Elaine Goldbaum	F	47	Feb. 8, 1993	Oakland
13	Hugh Gale	M	70	Feb. 15, 1993	Macomb
14	Jonathan Grenz	M	44	Feb. 18, 1993	Oakland
15	Martha Ruwart	F	40	Feb. 18, 1993	Oakland
16	Ronald Mansur	M	54	May 16, 1993	Wayne

APPENDIX
Table A1. (Cont'd.)

Primary Medical Condition	Terminal	Method of Death	Body Disposal Method
Alzheimer's disease	No	Lethal injection	Cremation
Multiple sclerosis	No	Carbon monoxide	Cremation
No anatomical evidence of disease at autopsy	No	Lethal injection	Cremation
Multiple sclerosis	No	Carbon monoxide	Cremation
Lung cancer	Yes	Carbon monoxide	Cremation
Breast cancer	Yes	Carbon monoxide	Cremation
ALS	Yes	Carbon monoxide	Cremation
Emphysema, Heart disease	No	Carbon monoxide	Cremation
Emphysema, Prostate cancer	Yes	Carbon monoxide	Cremation
Breast cancer	?	Carbon monoxide	Cremation
Pancreatic cancer, Blind	Yes	Carbon monoxide	Cremation
Multiple sclerosis	No	Carbon monoxide	Burial
Emphysema, Congestive heart disease	?	Carbon monoxide	Cremation
Squamous cell cancer of upper and lower airways with metastases	Yes	Carbon monoxide	Cremation
Ovarian cancer with metastases	Yes	Carbon monoxide	Cremation
Bone and lung cancer	Yes	Carbon monoxide	Burial

APPENDIX
Table A1. (Cont'd.)

No.	Name	Gender	Age	Date of Death	County of Death
17	Thomas Hyde	M	30	Aug. 4, 1993	Wayne
18	Donald O'Keefe	M	73	Sept. 9, 1993	Wayne
19	Merian Frederick	F	72	Oct. 22, 1993	Oakland
20	Ali Khalili	M	61	Nov. 22, 1993	Oakland
21	Margaret Garrish	F	71	Nov. 26, 1994	Oakland
22	John Evans	M	77	May 8, 1995	Oakland
23	Nicholas Loving	M	27	May 12, 1995	Oakland
24	Erika Garcellano	F	60	June 26, 1995	Oakland
25	Esther Cohan	F	46	Aug. 21, 1995	Oakland
26	Patricia Cashman	F	58	Nov. 8, 1995	Oakland
27	Linda Henslee	F	48	Jan. 29, 1996	Oakland
28	Austin Bastable	M	53	May 6, 1996	Oakland
29	Ruth Neuman	F	69	June 10, 1996	Oakland
30	Lona Jones	F	58	June 18, 1996	Oakland
31	Bette Hamilton	F	67	June 20, 1996	Oakland
32	Shirley Cline	F	63	July 4, 1996	Oakland
33	Rebecca Badger	F	39	July 9, 1996	Oakland
34	Elizabeth Mercz	F	59	Aug. 6, 1996	Oakland
35	Judith Curren	F	42	Aug. 15, 1996	Oakland

APPENDIX
Table A1. (Cont'd.)

Primary Medical Condition	Terminal	Method of Death	Body Disposal Method
ALS	Yes	Carbon monoxide	Cremation
Bone cancer	Yes	Carbon monoxide	Cremation
ALS	Yes	Carbon monoxide	Cremation
Multiple myeloma	Yes	Carbon monoxide	Cremation
Rheumatoid arthritis, Bilateral leg amputation, Loss of one eye	No	Carbon monoxide	Burial
Pulmonary fibrosis	Yes	Carbon monoxide	Cremation
ALS	No	Carbon monoxide	Cremation
ALS	No	Carbon monoxide	Cremation
Multiple sclerosis, Painful ulcers	No	Carbon monoxide	Cremation
Skeletal metastases of breast cancer	No	Both	Cremation
Multiple sclerosis	No	Both	Cremation
Multiple sclerosis	No	Both	Cremation
Cerebral vascular disease	No	Both	Cremation
Astrocytoma	No	Both	Cremation
Syringomyelia	No	Both	Cremation
Bowel cancer	Yes	Lethal injection	Cremation
No anatomical evidence of disease at autopsy	No	Lethal injection	Cremation
ALS	No	Both	Burial
No anatomical evidence of disease at autopsy	No	Lethal injection	Cremation

APPENDIX
Table A1. (Cont'd.)

No.	Name	Gender	Age	Date of Death	County of Death
36	Louise Siebens	F	76	Aug. 20, 1996	Oakland
37	Patricia Smith	F	40	Aug. 22, 1996	Oakland
38	Pat DiGangi	M	66	Aug. 22, 1996	Oakland
39	Loretta Peabody	F	54	Aug. 30, 1996	Ionia
40	Jack Leatherman	M	72	Sept. 2, 1996	Oakland
41	Isabel Correa	F	60	Sept. 7, 1996	Oakland
42	Richard Faw	M	71	Sept. 29, 1996	Oakland
43	Wallace Spolar	M	69	Oct. 10, 1996	Oakland
44	Nancy DeSoto	F	55	Oct. 17, 1996	Oakland
45	Barbara Collins	F	65	Oct. 23, 1996	Oakland
46	Elaine Day	F	79	Feb. 2, 1997	Oakland
47	Lisa Lansing	F	42	Feb. 2, 1997	Oakland

APPENDIX
Table A1. (Cont'd.)

Primary Medical Condition	Terminal	Method of Death	Body Disposal Method
ALS	No	Lethal injection	Burial
Multiple sclerosis	No	Lethal injection	Cremation
Multiple sclerosis	No	Lethal injection	Cremation
Multiple sclerosis	No	Lethal injection	Cremation
Pancreatic cancer	Yes	Lethal injection	Cremation
Status post spinal cord trauma	No	Carbon monoxide	Cremation
Colon cancer	No	Carbon monoxide	Cremation
Multiple sclerosis, Heart disease	No	Carbon monoxide	Cremation
ALS	No	Carbon monoxide	Cremation
Ovarian cancer	Yes	Lethal injection	Cremation
ALS	No	Lethal injection	Cremation
Chronic inflammatory bowel disease	No	Lethal injection	Burial

Table A2. Overall Demographic Characteristics

| | Yes | | No | | |
	Count	%	Count	%	Count
At least some college	28	59.6	19	40.4	47
Had children	38	80.9	9	19.1	47
Had no minor children	4	8.5	43	91.5	47
Homemaker	9	19.1	38	80.9	47
Helping type job	19	40.4	28	59.6	47
Resided in Michigan	17	36.2	30	63.8	47
Lived in house	31	66.0	15	31.9	47

Table A3. Biomedical History

| | Yes | | No | | Total |
	Count	%	Count	%	Count
History of psychosis	1	2.9	34	97.1	35
History of depression	11	36.7	19	63.3	30
History of sleep disorder	3	9.1	30	90.9	33
History of disability	40	87.0	6	13.0	46
Physically incapacitated	31	66.0	16	34.0	47
Functional physical limitation	19	47.5	21	52.5	40
History of incontinence	19	45.2	23	54.8	42
Able to go to the toilet	19	42.2	26	57.8	45
Able to walk	18	39.1	28	60.9	46
Able to drive	7	15.2	39	84.8	46
Able to work	5	10.6	42	89.4	47
Was working	2	4.3	45	95.7	47
Reported pain	34	73.9	12	26.1	46
Anatomical basis for pain	20	42.6	27	57.4	47
Patient considered terminal	14	31.1	31	68.9	45

Table A4. Psychosocial History

	Yes		No		Total
	Count	%	Count	%	Count
Lived alone	14	29.8	33	70.2	47
Lived with spouse/partner	19	40.4	28	59.6	47
Lived with children	14	29.8	33	70.2	47
Lived with other family	6	12.8	41	87.2	47
Lived with paid help	2	4.3	44	95.7	46
Periodic paid care	14	34.1	27	65.9	41
Expressed fear of being dependent	36	90.0	4	10.0	40
Non spouse life insurance beneficiary	6	50.0	6	50.0	12
Financial condition deteriorating	12	30.0	28	70.0	40
Financial/professional reversal within 5 years	6	14.3	36	85.7	42
Parent died within 5 years	9	22.5	31	77.5	40
Divorced or separated within 5 years	6	13.0	40	87.0	46
Spouse died within 5 years	2	4.3	45	95.7	47
Child died wtihin 5 years	2	4.4	43	95.6	45
Friend died within 5 years	1	3.6	27	96.4	28
Victim of crime or disaster within 5 years	1	2.5	39	97.5	40
Other trauma within 5 years	6	17.1	29	82.9	35
History of physical abuse	3	8.1	34	91.9	37
History of sexual abuse	1	2.6	37	97.4	38
History of alcoholism	2	4.3	32	68.1	47
History of substance abuse	4	11.4	31	88.6	35
History of suicide attempts	10	23.8	32	76.2	42
History of suicide in family	3	9.4	29	90.6	32

Table A5. Consultation History/Treatment Before Kevorkian

	Yes		No		Total
	Count	%	Count	%	Count
Consulted with religious figure	7	24.1	22	75.9	29
Consulted with family about patient's wishes	42	91.3	4	8.7	46
Consulted with mental health professional	9	28.1	23	71.9	32
Doctor provided insufficient pain relief	12	29.3	29	70.7	41
Rejected medical treatment	13	28.9	32	71.1	45
Patient declined pain medication	5	11.6	38	88.4	43

Table A6. Drugs Present at Treatment and Autopsy

	During Treatment					At Autopsy				
	Present		Absent		Total	Present		Absent		Total
Drugs in System	Count	%	Count	%	Count	Count	%	Count	%	Count
Antidepressants	6	12.8	41	87.2	47	3	6.4	44	93.6	47
Anti-psychotics	0	0.0	47	100.0	47	0	0.0	47	100.0	47
Antiseizure drugs	2	4.3	45	95.7	47	2	4.3	45	95.7	47
Muscle relaxers and nonpioids	10	21.3	37	78.7	47	5	10.6	42	89.4	47
Opiates	16	34.0	31	66.0	47	17	36.2	30	63.8	47
Sedatives/ hypnotics	9	19.1	38	80.9	47	24	51.1	23	48.9	47
Stimulants	1	2.1	46	97.9	47	4	8.5	43	91.5	47
Other drugs	13	27.7	34	72.3	47	2	4.3	45	95.7	47
No drugs	17	36.2	30	63.8	47	13	27.7	34	73.3	47

Table A7. Experience with Kevorkian

	Yes		No		Total
	Count	%	Count	%	Count
Patient made initial contact	27	69.2	12	30.8	39
Kevorkian was first person contacted	20	60.6	13	39.4	33
Kevorkian contacted by phone	12	34.3	23	65.7	35
Family/friend opposed to meeting Kevorkian	11	25.6	32	74.4	43
Kevorkian responded in less than 1 day	35	74.5	12	25.5	47
Time between first diagnosis and death less than 6 months	7	17.1	34	82.9	41
Time from 1st contact to death was 1 day or less	14	29.8	33	70.2	47
Time from 1st face to face until death was 1 day or less	30	63.8	17	36.2	47
Only one face to face meeting occurred	17	48.6	18	51.4	35
Consulted treating physician	4	11.8	30	88.2	34
Kevorkian tried to contact treating physician	8	30.8	18	69.2	26
Consulted specialist	7	25.0	21	75.0	28
Consulted pain relief specialist	2	7.1	26	92.9	28
Consulted psychiatrist	7	26.9	19	73.1	26

Table A8. Circumstance of Death

	Yes		No		Total
	Count	%	Count	%	Count
Location of suicide was motel	7	20.6	27	79.4	34
Someone present with patient at suicide	27	84.4	5	15.6	32
Informant was spouse	19	41.3	27	58.7	46
Oakland County medical examiners processed body	38	80.8	9	19.1	47
Homicide on death certificate	33	71.7	13	28.3	46
Suicide on death certificate	6	13.0	40	87.0	46
Cause of death was listed as carbon monoxide	32	68.1	15	31.9	47
Body was cremated	41	87.2	6	12.8	47

Table A9. Gender Differences in Kevorkian's Patients

	Total		Males		Females		Chi-Square	P
	Count	%	Count	%	Count	%		
Homemaker	9/47	19.1	0/15	0.0	9/32	28.1	5.22	.02
Helping type job	19/47	40.4	2/15	13.3	17/32	53.1	6.71	.01
Reported pain	34/46	73.9	11/15	73.3	23/31	74.2	.01	.95
Anatomical basis for pain	20/47	42.6	9/15	60.0	11/32	34.4	2.74	.10
Able to drive	39/46	84.8	10/14	71.4	29/32	90.6	2.78	.10
Able to work	5/47	10.6	4/15	26.7	1/32	3.1	5.95	.02
Was working	2/47	4.3	2/15	13.3	0/32	0.0	4.46	.03
Patient considered terminal	14/45	31.1	8/14	57.1	6/31	19.4	6.43	.01
Surviving spouse/ children	18/44	40.9	9/15	60	9/29	31	3.43	.06
Lived with spouse/partner	19/47	40.4	9/15	60.0	10/32	31.3	3.50	.06
Other trauma within 1 year	5/37	13.5	0/13	0.0	5/24	20.8	3.13	.08
Two or more conditions present	13/47	27.7	2/15	13.3	11/32	34.4	2.26	.13
Sedatives and hypnotics in system at time of death	24/47	51	5/15	33.3	19/32	59.4	2.77	.10
Kevorkian was first person contacted	20/33	60.6	2/8	25.0	18/25	72.0	5.61	.02
Time from 1st contact to death was 1 day or less	14/47	29.8	7/15	46.7	7/32	21.9	3.00	.08
Someone present with patient at suicide	27/32	84.4	6/11	54.5	21/21	100.0	11.31	.01
Informant was spouse	19/46	41.3	10/15	66.7	9/31	29.0	5.91	.02
Carbon monoxide used for suicide	27/47	57.4	12/15	80	15/32	46.9	4.58	.03
Body found in Oakland County	39/47	83.0	9/15	60.0	30/32	93.8	8.24	.01
Homicide on death certificate	33/46	71.7	7/14	50	20/32	81.3	4.69	.03
Suicide on death certificate	6/46	13.0	5/14	35.7	1/32	3.1	9.12	.01
History of suicide attempts	10/42	23.8	2/14	14.2	8/28	28.5	1.05	.31
History of depression	11/30	36.7	3/10	30.0	8/20	40.0	.29	.59

Table A10. Age Differences in Kevorkian's Patients

| | Age Categories | | | | | | | | | |
| | Total | | >50 | | 50-69 | | 70+ | | Chi-Square | P |
	Count	%	Count	%	Count	%	Count	%		
Middle class income	27/43	62.8	6/13	46.2	13/20	65.0	8/10	80.0	8.30	.08
Had children	38/47	80.9	7/13	53.8	19/22	86.4	12/12	100.0	9.30	.01
Married	17/47	36.2	2/13	15.4	11/22	50.0	4/12	33.3	4.30	.11
History of incontinence	19/42	45.2	10/13	76.9	7/19	36.8	2/10	20.0	83.00	.02
Reported pain	34/46	73.9	12/13	92.3	16/21	76.2	6/12	50.0	5.90	.05
Anatomical basis for pain	20/47	42.6	5/13	38.5	9/22	40.9	6/12	50.0	.38	.82
Lived with spouse/partner	19/47	40.4	3/13	23.1	12/22	54.5	4/12	33.3	3.70	.16
Lived with children	14/47	29.8	4/13	30.8	7/22	31.8	3/12	25.0	.18	.91
Lived with other family	6/47	12.8	4/13	30.8	2/22	9.1	0/12	0	5.80	.05
Financial condition deteriorating	12/40	30.0	6/12	50.0	6/19	31.6	0/9	0	6.10	.04
Parent died within 1 year	3/40	7.5	3/12	25.0	0/17	0	0/11	0	7.60	.02
Parent died within 5 years	9/40	22.5	6/12	50.0	2/17	11.8	1/11	9.1	7.50	.02
Financial/ professional reversal within 5 years	6/42	14.3	4/13	30.8	2/18	11.1	0/11	0	4.90	.09
Consulted with mental health professional	9/32	28.1	4/8	50.0	5/15	33.3	0/9	0	5.60	.06
Consulted with religious figure	7/29	24.1	0/8	0	6/12	50.0	1/9	11.1	7.80	.02
Rejected medical treatment	13/45	28.9	0/12	0	9/22	40.9	4/11	36.4	6.70	.03
No drugs used during treatment	17/47	36.2	1/13	7.7	9/22	40.9	7/12	58.3	7.30	.03
Stimulants in system at time of death	4/47	8.5	3/13	23.1	0/22	0	1/12	8.3	5.50	.06
Other drugs in system at time of death	2/47	4.3	2/13	15.4	0/22	0	0/12	0	5.40	.06
Time between initial diagnosis and death less than 6 months	7/41	17.1	0/12	0	3/18	16.7	4/11	36.4	5.40	.07
Informant was spouse	19/46	41.3	2/13	15.4	11/22	50.0	6/11	54.5	5.10	.08

Table A11. Marital Status Differences in Kevorkian's Patients

	Total		Not Married		Married		Chi-Square	P
	Count	%	Count	%	Count	%		
WASP ancestry	32/47	68.1	18/30	60.0	14/17	82.4	2.50	.11
Had children	38/47	80.9	21/30	70.0	17/17	100.0	6.31	.01
Helping type job	19/47	40.4	9/30	30.0	10/17	58.8	3.74	.05
Lived in house	31/46	67.4	16/29	55.2	15/17	88.2	5.33	.02
Mentally incapacitated	10/37	27.0	4/22	18.2	6/15	40.0	2.15	.14
Reported pain	34/46	73.9	23/29	79.3	11/17	64.7	1.19	.28
Anatomical basis for pain	20/47	42.6	16/30	53.3	4/17	23.5	3.94	.05
Patient considered terminal	14/45	31.1	12/29	41.4	2/16	12.5	4.01	.05
Lived alone	14/47	29.8	14/30	46.7	0/17	0.0	11.30	.01
Lived with spouse/partner	19/47	40.4	2/30	6.7	17/17	100.0	39.25	.01
Non spouse life insurance beneficiary	6/12	50.0	6/6	100.0	0/6	0.0	12.00	.01
Financial condition deteriorating	12/40	30.0	10/24	41.7	2/16	12.5	3.89	.05
Parent died within 5 years	9/40	22.5	8/26	30.8	1/14	7.1	2.91	.09
Two or more conditions present	13/47	27.7	6/30	20.0	7/17	41.2	2.43	.12
Antiseizure drugs used during treatment	2/47	4.3	0/30	0.0	2/17	4.3	3.69	.05
Informant was spouse	19/46	41.3	3/29	10.3	16/17	94.1	31.02	.01

Table A12. Socioeconomic Status Differences in Kevorkian's Patients

	Total		Lower		Middle		Upper		Chi-Square	P
	Count	%	Count	%	Count	%	Count	%		
Younger than 50	13/43	30.2	6/9	66.7	6/27	22.2	1/7	14.3	8.28	.08
Between 50 & 69	20/43	46.5	3/9	33.3	13/27	48.1	4/7	57.1	8.28	.08
70 and older	10/43	23.3	0/9	0.0	8/27	29.6	2/7	28.6	8.28	.08
At least some college education	25/43	58.1	3/9	33.3	16/27	59.3	5/7	85.7	4.48	.11
Married	17/47	36.2	2/10	20.0	10/29	34.4	5/8	40.0	4.18	.12
Lived in house	30/43	69.8	3/9	33.3	22/27	81.5	5/7	71.4	7.43	.02
History of disability	36/42	85.7	9/9	100.0	24/27	88.9	3/6	50.0	7.97	.02
History of incontinence	19/40	47.5	8/9	88.9	9/24	37.5	2/7	28.6	8.15	.02
Physically incapacitated	29/43	67.4	7/9	77.8	20/27	74.1	2/7	28.6	5.80	.06
Functional physical limitation	19/38	50.0	6/8	75.0	12/24	50.0	1/6	16.7	4.67	.10
Patient considered terminal	13/41	31.7	2/9	22.2	9/25	36.0	2/7	28.6	.62	.73
Reported pain	31/42	73.8	8/9	88.9	18/26	69.2	5/7	71.4	1.36	.51
Anatomical basis for pain	17/43	39.5	2/9	22.2	12/27	44.4	3/7	42.9	1.43	.49
Was working	2/43	4.7	0/9	0.0	0/27	0.0	2/7	28.6	10.79	.01
Periodic paid care	14/40	35.0	5/8	62.5	6/26	23.1	3/6	50.0	4.88	.09
Surviving spouse/ children	18/41	43.9	2/9	22.2	10/25	40.0	6/7	85.7	6.84	.03
Divorced or separated within 5 years	6/42	14.3	2/9	22.2	1/26	3.8	3/7	42.9	7.44	.02
Financial condition deteriorating	11/39	28.2	5/8	62.5	3/24	12.5	3/7	42.9	8.31	.02
History of substance abuse	4/34	11.8	4/8	50.0	0/20	0.0	0/6	0.0	14.73	.001
Patient declined additional medical treatment	4/40	10.0	0/9	0.0	3/25	12.0	1/6	16.7	1.41	.49
Consulted psychiatrist	6/25	24.0	0/6	0.0	4/16	25.0	2/3	66.7	4.90	.09
Anti-depressants used during treatment	6/47	12.8	3/0	30.0	3/29	10.3	0/8	0.0	4.13	.13
No other drugs used during treatment	30/47	63.8	4/10	40.0	22/29	75.9	4/8	50.0	5.02	.08
Antiseizure medication in body at time of death	2/47	4.3	0/10	0.0	0/29	0.0	2/8	25.0	10.79	.005

Table A12. (Cont'd.)

	SES Categories									
	Total		Lower		Middle		Upper		Chi-Square	P
	Count	%	Count	%	Count	%	Count	%		
Opiates in system at time of death	16/43	37.2	3/9	33.3	8/27	29.6	5/7	71.4	4.23	.12
Time from 1st contact to death was 1 day or less	12/43	27.9	0/9	0.0	8/27	29.6	4/7	57.1	6.50	.04
Time from 1st face to face until death was 1 day or less	26/43	60.5	3/9	33.3	18/27	66.7	5/7	71.4	3.56	.17
Informant was spouse	18/42	42.9	3/9	33.3	9/26	34.6	6/7	85.7	6.30	.04
Suicide on death certificate	6/42	14.3	2/9	22.2	1/26	3.8	3/7	42.9	7.44	.02
Someone present with patient at suicide	24/29	82.8	5/7	71.4	15/15	100.0	4/7	57.1	6.97	.03

Table A13. Ancestry Differences in Kevorkian's Patients

	Total		WASP		Non-WASP		Chi-Square	P
	Count	%	Count	%	Count	%		
Married	17/47	36.2	14/32	43.7	3/15	20.0	2.50	.11
History of psychosis	1/35	2.9	0/27	0.0	1/8	12.5	3.47	.06
History of sleep disorder	3/33	9.1	1/26	3.8	2/7	28.6	4.08	.04
Mentally incapacitated	10/37	27.0	9/27	33.3	1/10	10.0	2.01	.16
Functional physical limitation	19/40	47.5	15/28	53.6	4/12	33.3	1.38	.24
History of incontinence	19/42	45.2	13/29	44.8	6/13	46.2	.01	.94
Reported pain	34/46	73.9	24/32	75.0	10/14	71.4	.06	.80
Anatomical basis for pain	20/47	42.6	11/32	34.4	9/15	60.0	2.74	.10
Patient considered terminal	14/45	31.1	9/31	29.0	5/14	35.7	.20	.65
Lived alone	14/47	29.8	6/32	18.8	8/15	53.3	5.84	.02
Lived with spouse/partner	19/47	40.4	16/32	50.0	3/15	20.0	3.82	.05
Lived with paid help	2/46	4.3	0/31	0.0	2/15	13.3	4.32	.04
Spouse died within 5 years	2/47	4.3	0/32	0.0	2/15	13.3	4.46	.03
Child died within 5 years	2/45	4.4	0/30	0.0	2/15	13.3	4.19	.04
Financial/professional reversal within 1 year	4/41	9.8	1/28	3.6	3/13	23.1	3.84	.05
Consulted pain relief specialist	2/28	7.1	0/21	0.0	2/7	28.6	6.46	.01
Consulted with religious figure	7/29	24.1	4/24	16.7	3/5	60.0	4.24	.04
Kevorkian consulted with family about patient's wishes	42/46	91.3	31/32	96.9	11/14	78.6	4.10	.04
Sedatives/hypnotics used during treatment	9/47	19.1	3/32	9.4	5/15	40.0	6.19	.01
No other drugs used during treatment	30/47	63.8	17/32	53.0	13/15	86.7	4.85	.03
Kevorkian tried to contact treating physician	8/26	30.8	4/20	20.0	4/6	66.7	4.7	.03
Only one face to face meeting occurred	17/35	48.6	11/27	40.7	6/8	75.0	2.90	.09
Informant was spouse	19/46	41.3	16/32	50.0	3/14	21.4	3.28	.07
Body was cremated	41/47	87.2	30/32	93.8	11/15	73.3	3.80	.05

Table A14. Phase Differences in Kevorkian's Patients

	Total		Phase 1		Phase 2		Phase 3		Phase 4		Chi-Square	P
	Count	%	Count	%	Count	%	Count	%	Count	%		
Female	32/47	68.1	8/8	100.0	9/20	45.0	6/6	100.0	9/13	69.2	11.50	.10
Younger than 50	13/47	27.7	2/8	25.0	7/20	35.0	1/6	16.7	3/13	23.1	-	-
Between 50 and 70	22/47	46.8	5/8	62.5	6/20	30.0	5/6	83.8	6/13	46.2	-	-
Older than 70	12/47	25.5	1/8	12.5	7/20	35.0	0/6	0.0	4/13	30.8	-	-
Middle class income	27/43	62.8	3/7	42.9	10/18	55.6	4/6	66.7	10/12	83.3	6.01	.42
WASP ancestry	32/47	68.1	4/8	50.0	15/20	75.0	3/6	50.0	10/13	76.9	3.01	.39
Married	17/47	36.2	3/8	37.5	6/20	30.0	1/6	16.7	7/13	53.8	3.08	.38
History of depression	11/30	36.7	4/5	80.0	5/13	38.5	1/2	50.0	1/10	10.0	7.28	.06
Mentally incapacitated	10/37	27.0	4/7	57.1	4/16	25.0	1/4	25.0	1/10	10.0	4.73	.19
Reported pain	34/46	73.9	5/8	62.5	17/20	85.0	3/5	60.0	9/13	69.2	2.47	.48
Anatomical basis for pain	20/47	42.6	3/8	37.5	12/20	60.0	2/6	33.3	3/13	23.1	4.80	.19
Patient considered terminal	14/45	31.1	3/8	32.5	8/18	44.4	1/6	16.7	2/13	15.4	3.73	.29
Able to go to the toilet	19/45	42.2	4/7	57.1	6/20	30.0	4/5	80.0	5/13	38.5	4.86	.18
Able to walk	18/46	39.1	3/8	37.5	6/20	30.0	4/5	80.0	5/13	38.5	4.22	.24
Able to drive	7/46	15.2	0/8	0.0	3/19	15.8	0/6	0.0	4/13	30.8	4.95	.18
Able to work	5/47	10.6	0/8	0.0	1/20	5.0	0/6	0.0	4/13	30.8	7.88	.05
Was working	2/47	4.3	0/8	0.0	1/20	5.0	0/6	0.0	1/13	7.7	1.03	.80

Financial condition deteriorating	12/40	30.0									8.97	.03
Financial/professional reversal within 1 year	4/41	9.8	0/7	0.0	1/17	5.9	2/4	50.0	1/13	7.7	8.47	.04
Sedatives and hypnotics in system at time of death	24/47	51.1	4/8	50.0	6/20	30.0	6/6	100.0	8/13	61.5	9.88	.02
Consulted treating physician	4/34	11.8	4/7	57.1	0/15	0.0	0/4	0.0	0/8	0.0	17.50	.01
Consulted pain relief specialist	2/28	7.1	2/6	33.3	0/9	0.0	0/6	0.0	0/7	0.0	7.90	.05
Consulted psychiatrist	7/26	26.9	4/7	57.1	1/9	11.1	1/3	33.3	1/7	14.3	5.02	.17
Consulted specialist	7/28	25.0	5/7	71.4	0/9	0.0	1/6	16.7	1/6	16.7	11.50	.01
Family/friend opposed to meeting Kevorkian	11/43	25.6	5/8	62.5	3/19	15.8	0/5	0.0	3/11	27.5	8.42	.04
Time from 1st contact to death was 1 day or less	14/47	29.8	0/8	0.0	6/20	30.0	1/6	16.7	7/13	53.8	7.49	.06
Time from 1st face to face until death was 1 day or less	30/47	63.8	2/8	25.0	11/20	55.0	6/6	100.0	11/13	84.6	11.70	.01
Only one face to face meeting occurred	17/35	48.6	0/5	0.0	4/15	26.7	4/5	80.0	9/10	90.0	16.50	.01
Cause of death was listed as carbon monoxide	32/47	68.1	6/8	75.0	19/20	95.0	2/6	33.3	5/13	38.5	15.40	.01
Location of suicide was motel	7/34	20.6	0/8	0.0	0/18	0.0	3/3	100.0	4/5	80.0	29.10	.01
Body found in Oakland County	39/47	83.0	8/8	100.0	13/20	65.0	6/6	100.0	12/13	92.3	8.25	.04
Resided in Michigan	17/47	36.2	6/8	75.0	10/20	50.0	0/6	0.0	1/13	7.7	19.90	.01

REFERENCES

Anderson, R. N., Kochanek, K. D., & Murphy, S. L. (1997). Advanced report to final mortality statistics, 1995. *Monthly Vital Statistics Report, 45* (11, Suppl. 2). Hyattsville, MD: National Center for Health Statistics. DHHS Publication No. (PHS) 97-1120.

Berman, A. L., & Samuel, L. (1993). Suicide among people with multiple sclerosis. *Journal of Neurological Rehabilitation, 7,* 53-62.

Breitbart, W., Rosenfeld, B. D., & Passik, S. D. (1996). *American Journal of Psychiatry, 153,* 238-242.

Brown, J. H., Henteleff, P., Barakat, S., & Rowe, C. J. (1986). Is it normal for terminally ill patients to desire death? *American Journal of Psychiatry, 14,* 208-211.

Cheyfitz, K. (1997). Dr. Death, 1915. In *The suicide machine* (pp. 176-180). Detroit, MI: The Detroit Free Press.

Chochinov, H. M., Wilson, K. J., Enns, M., Mowchun, M., Lander, S., Levitt, M., & Clinch, J. J. (1995). Desire for death in the terminally ill. *American Journal of Psychiatry, 152* (8), 1186-1191.

Chynoweth, R., Tongo, J. I., & Armstrong, J. (1980). Suicide in Brisbane: A retrospective psychosocial study. *Australian and New Zealand Journal of Psychology, 14,* 37-45.

Clark, D. C. (1992). Rational suicide and people with terminal conditions or disabilities. *Issues in Law and Medicine, 8,* 147-166.

Clark, D., & Horton-Deutsch, S. (1992). Assessment in absentia: The value of the psychological autopsy method for studying antecedents of suicide and predicting future suicides. In R. W. Maris, A. L. Berman, J. T. Maltsberger, & R. I. Yufit (Eds.). *Assessment and prediction of suicide* (pp. 144-182), New York: The Guilford Press.

Conwell, Y., Caine, E. D., & Olson, K. (1990). Suicide and cancer in later life. *Hospital and Community Psychology, 41,* 1334-1339.

Detroit Free Press Staff, The (1997). *The suicide machine,* Detroit, MI: The Detroit Free Press.

Dorpat, T. L., Anderson, W. F., & Ripley, N. S. (1968). The relationship of physical illness to suicide. In H. L. Resnick (Ed.), *Suicidal behaviors: Diagnosis and management* (pp. 209-219). Boston, MA: Little Brown.

Emanuel, E. J., Fairclough, D. L., Daniels, E. R., & Clarridge, B. R. (1996). Euthanasia and physician-assisted suicide: Attitudes and experiences of oncology patients, oncologists and the public. *The Lancet, 347,* 1805-1810.

Fawcett, J. (1972). Suicidal depression and physical illness. *Journal of the American Medical Association, 219,* 1303-1306.

Ganzini, L., Johnston, W. S., McFarland, B. H., Tolle, S. W., & Lee, M. A. (1998). Attitudes of patients with amyotrophic lateral sclerosis and their care givers toward assisted suicide *The New England Journal of Medicine, 339* (14), 967-973.

Harris, E. C., & Barraclough, B. B. (1994). Suicide as an outcome for medical disorders. *Medicine, 73,* 281-296.

Horton-Deutsch, S. L., Clark, B. C., & Farrah, C. J. (1992). Chronic dyspnea and suicide in elderly men. *Hospital and Community Psychology, 43,* 1198-1203.

Kaplan, K. J. (1991). Suicide and suicide prevention: Greek versus Biblical perspectives. *Omega, 24* (3), 227-239.

Kaplan, K. J. (1998). The case of Dr. Kevorkian and Mr. Gale: A brief historical note. *Omega, 36,* 169-176.

Kaplan, K. J., & Leonhardi, M. (1997). Kevorkian, Martha Wichorek and us: A personal account. *Newslink, 23* (4), 9-10.

Kaplan, K. J., & Leonhardi, M. (1999-2000). Kevorkian, Martha Wichorek and us: A personal account. *Omega, 40* (1), 267-270 (this issue).

Kevorkian, J. (1992). A fail-safe model for justifiable medically-assisted suicide ("medicide"). *American Journal of Forensic Psychiatry, 13* (1), 7-42.

Minkoff, K., Bergman, E., Beck, A. T., & Beck, R. (1973). Hopelessness, depression, and attempted suicide. *American Journal of Psychiatry, 130,* 455-459.

Murphy, G. K. (1977). Cancer and the corner. *Journal of the American Medical Association, 237,* 786-788.

Robins, E., Gassner, S., Kayes, J., Wilkinson, R. M., & Murphy, G. E. C. (1959). The communication of suicidal intent: A study of 13 consecutive cases of successful (completed) suicides. *American Journal of Psychiatry, 115,* 724-733.

Sainsbury, P. (1955). *Suicide in London.* London, UK: Chapman and Hall.

Seneca, L. A., The younger. (1979). *Seneca.* Cambridge, MA: Harvard University Press.

Steward, I. (1960). Suicide: The influence of organic disease. *The Lancet, 2,* 919-920.

Whitlock F. A., (1978). Suicide, cancer and depression. *British Journal of Psychiatry, 132,* 269-274.

GENDER AND PHYSICIAN-ASSISTED SUICIDE: AN ANALYSIS OF THE KEVORKIAN CASES, 1990-1997*

SILVIA SARA CANETTO

JANET D. HOLLENSHEAD

Colorado State University, Fort Collins

ABSTRACT

This study examines the seventy-five suicide cases Dr. Jack Kevorkian acknowledged assisting during the period between 1990 and 1997. Although these cases represent a range of regional and occupational backgrounds, a significant majority are women. Most of these individuals had a disabling, chronic, nonterminal-stage illness. In five female cases, the medical examiner found no evidence of disease whatsoever. About half of the women were between the ages of forty-one and sixty, and another third were older adults. In contrast, men were almost as likely to be middle-aged as to be older adults. Men's conditions were somewhat less likely than women's to be chronic and nonterminal-stage. The main reasons for the hastened death mentioned by both the person and their significant others were having disabilities, being in pain, and fear of being a burden. The predominance of women among Kevorkian's assisted suicides contrasts with national trends in suicide mortality, where men are a clear majority. It is possible that individuals whose death was hastened by Kevorkian are not representative of physician-assisted suicide cases around the country, because of Kevorkian's unique approach. Alternatively, the preponderance of women among Kevorkian's assisted suicides may represent a real phenomenon. One possibility is that, in the United States, assisted suicide is particularly acceptable for women. Individual, interpersonal, social, economic, and cultural factors encouraging assisted suicide in women are examined.

*This research was supported in part by a grant from Colorado State University awarded to the first author in 1993.

In the United States, information about assisted suicide cases is generally unavailable because assisted suicide is illegal in a majority of states (Smith, 1997). Despite the legal prohibition, we know that assisted suicides do take place. Several recent surveys revealed that many physicians and nurses comply with requests for hastened death[1] (Asch, 1996; Back, Wallace, Starks, & Pearlman, 1996; Doukas, Waterhouse, Gorenflo, & Seid, 1995; Emanuel, Fairclough, Daniels, & Clarridge, 1996; Fried, Stein, O'Sullivan, Brock, & Novack, 1993; Lee, Nelson, Tilden, Ganzini, Schmidt, & Tolle, 1996; Meier, Emmons, Wallenstein, Quill, Morrison, & Cassel, 1998; Slome, Mitchell, Charlebois, Benevedes, & Abrams, 1997). In these surveys, 3.3 to 53 percent of physicians and 16 percent of nurses acknowledged granting a request for hastened death. While these surveys help estimate the scope of the phenomenon, they do not provide much information about the persons and circumstances associated with such a practice. Outside of a few publicized cases, such as Dr. Quill's patients Diane and Jane (Quill, 1991, 1996), we know very little about the characteristics of individuals who die of assisted suicide or the circumstances of their death.

An exception are the suicides assisted by Dr. Jack Kevorkian, a retired pathologist from Royal Oak, Michigan. Between 1990 and 1997, Dr. Jack Kevorkian has acknowledged hastening the deaths of seventy-five individuals. The Kevorkian cases are a uniquely rich data set. Because of his interest in promoting the cause of hastened death, Dr. Kevorkian has made public a fair amount of information about these individuals and the circumstances of their deaths.

This study examines the personal characteristics and circumstances of individuals whose deaths were hastened by Dr. Kevorkian between 1990 and 1997. One goal is to identify the characteristics of this sample. Another goal is to understand the circumstances associated with their hastened deaths, including the psychological and interpersonal dynamics preceding the death.

METHOD

Data Sources

Information regarding the seventy-five Kevorkian assisted suicides was obtained from state (primarily *The Detroit News and Free Press* and *The Denver Post*) and national newspapers (i.e., *The New York Times* and *The Washington Post*), in paper and/or electronic version, as well as books published by *Detroit Free Press* journalists. *The Detroit News and Free Press,* whose local coverage

---

[1] Some surveys asked about assisted suicide (i.e., Doukas et al., 1995; Emanuel et al., 1996; Lee et al., 1996; Meier et al., 1998; Slome et al., 1997); others about assisted suicide or euthanasia (i.e., Asch, 1996; Back et al., 1996).

includes the vicinities of the incidents, served as the primary source and usually provided the most detailed data. *The New York Times* and *The Washington Post* were examined to obtain a national perspective. In some instances the local newspaper from the deceased's town of residence was examined to fill in missing background details. Finally, *The Denver Post* was used, because of its accessibility, to verify and sometimes add to the data. For information on diseases, terminal status, and/or cause of death we consulted the medical examiners, whenever possible, as well as the electronic record of the *Euthanasia World Directory* (http://www.FinalExit.org/kevorkian.html). The list of references for our data sources are in Appendix A.

Nature of the Data

Consistent with our first goal, to identify the characteristics of persons whose deaths were hastened by Kevorkian, we collected information on demographic (i.e., gender, age, occupation, living arrangement, family relations, and state of residence) and health variables (e.g., primary physical illness and associated chronicity, terminal status, disability, and physical pain; mental disorders and history of suicidal behavior) about the deceased. Primary physical illness and terminal status, defined as a life expectancy of six months or less, were determined on the basis of the judgment of the medical examiner.

To understand the circumstances leading to the hastened death, our second goal, we analyzed the person's statements, including suicide notes, about reasons for seeking a hastened death. In addition, we examined the perceptions of family members and friends regarding the reasons for the assisted suicide; the responses of family members and friends to the person's decision to seek a hastened death, including their role in making it happen; the presence of family and/or friends at the suicide; and the time between diagnosis of the person's primary illness and death.

Because of the nature of the data, we could not always determine the source of the information. In general, we gave priority to information that clearly originated from the deceased (e.g., pre-suicide videos, letters, interviews), information that was contributed by people who knew the deceased person well (e.g., family members, friends), and information from people who had been in recent contact with the deceased (e.g., neighbors, personal physicians). We usually did not include information that came exclusively from Dr. Kevorkian or his lawyers, because of their unique stake in the cases.

Statistical Analyses

Simple comparisons used Binomial Tests, t-tests, χ^2 Goodness of Fit indicators, or χ^2 Tests of Association, as appropriate. An alpha level of .05 was used for all analyses. All significance levels are for two-tailed comparisons. Statistically significant findings are explicitly identified. Other differences may be reported but should not be interpreted as significant.

RESULTS

Between 1990 and 1997, seventy-five people were reported as having died with the assistance of Dr. Kevorkian. According to Geoffrey Fieger, Kevorkian's lawyer, this number represented a fraction of the deaths Dr. Kevorkian had been involved with (Martin & Brasier, 1996). A majority of the early cases (16 out of the first 22) were from Michigan. However, starting from 1996, Fieger claimed that many Michigan cases went unreported (Martin & Brasier, 1996). Most (69%) of these hastened deaths occurred in Oakland county—this includes 74 percent of female and 57 percent of male deaths. Death was brought about by the administration of quick acting poisons, either via inhalation (44% of cases), injection (40% of cases), or both (3% of cases). The method was unknown for the remaining 13 percent of cases. Men were more likely to die of carbon monoxide poisoning than of lethal injection (62% versus 24%). Women, on the other hand, were more likely to die of lethal injection than of carbon monoxide inhalation (46% versus 37%). In the case of two women (4%), both methods were used.

Who Were the Persons Whose Deaths Were Hastened by Dr. Kevorkian?

Personal Background

The individuals whose deaths were hastened by Dr. Kevorkian between 1990 and 1997 came from a range of locations in North America. They were from twenty-three U.S. states and two provinces of Canada. The largest number of cases ($n = 21$) were from Michigan. The second highest number were from California ($n = 11$). Illinois, New York, and Pennsylvania ranked next, with four people residing in each.

These individuals represented a relatively diverse group of occupations, ranging from skilled professionals (e.g., physician, attorney), semi-skilled professionals (e.g., teacher, executive secretary), and unskilled laborers (e.g., homemaker, farmer) (see Table 1). Fifteen percent of the deceased were homemakers, 13 percent had a background in healthcare, 11 percent had worked in education, and 8 percent had held administrative/clerical positions. At the time of death, many individuals were retired, on disability, or unemployed.

The individuals whose death was hastened by Dr. Kevorkian were, however, fairly homogenous with regard to gender, a significant majority (72%) being female ($p < .05$) (see Table 1). Nearly all were of white, European-American descent. A comparison of the annual number of female and male cases reveals distinct distributions (see Figure 1). The first eight cases, which occurred between 1990 and 1992, were all females. Dr. Kevorkian assisted the first male in 1993, a year in which the majority of his reported assisted suicides (67%) were males. In fact, in 1993 more males died with Kevorkian's assistance than in any other year during the period of our study. After 1993, there was a consistent drop in the proportion of male cases. Males constituted 40 percent of cases reported in 1995, 26 percent of cases in 1996, and 20 percent of cases in 1997. Only one assisted suicide was reported in 1994, a female. In contrast, the proportion of female deaths increased over time. There were 1.5 times as many females than males in the first twenty-five cases; 3.2 as many females in the second twenty-five cases, and 4 times as many females as males in the final twenty-five cases.

Individuals who died with the assistance of Dr. Kevorkian ranged in age from twenty-seven to eighty-nine, with an average age of fifty-eight years ($SD = 14.55$). When the data on age were coded in terms of adult (i.e., 40 or younger), middle-aged (i.e., between 41 and 60), and older adult (i.e., 61 or older) categories, the distribution was found to be significantly different than that expected due to chance ($p < .05$). Fewer cases fell into the adult category. The average age for women was fifty-eight years ($SD = 14.28$). The youngest female was twenty-seven years old and the oldest was eighty-nine, representing a span of sixty-two years. The average age for men was fifty-nine years ($SD = 15.56$), with a range of twenty-seven to eighty-two. The difference between women's and men's average age was not statistically significant. Women were most often middle-aged (50%), with fewer (39%) being older adults. On the other hand, men were almost equally as likely to be middle aged (43%) as to be older adults (48%). These trends do not represent a significant association between age and gender.

As illustrated in Table 2, women were more likely to be single, divorced, or widowed (44% of the cases) than married or in a relationship (28% of cases). Men, on the other hand, were almost as likely to be married or in a relationship as to be single, divorced, or widowed (43% versus 38%, respectively). Fifty-nine percent of the women and 76 percent of the men were reported to have children. Siblings were mentioned in about a third of all cases. At the time of their death, most men lived with family (52% of cases); a minority lived alone (10%) or in a nursing home (5%). While a majority of women also lived with family (41%), about one-fourth lived alone, and 13 percent in a nursing home. None of these trends reached statistical significance.[2]

---

[2] On April 13, 1999, Dr. Kevorkian was convicted to ten to twenty-five years in prison for second degree murder and three to seven years for delivery of a controlled substance in the euthanasia death of Thomas Youk, a fifty-two-year-old accountant who suffered from amyotrophic lateral sclerosis. Until then, through 1998, he was publicly involved in the deaths of nine more women and nine more men (including Youk). In the final count ($N = 93$) persons whose death was hastened by Dr. Kevorkian were still predominantly female (68%), mid (44%) to older adult (44%), and of European-American descent (96%).

Table 1. The Kevorkian Assisted Suicide Cases 1990-1997:
Date of Death, Sex, Age, Occupation, and Illness

Case	Date of Death	Sex	Age	Occupation	Illness
1	6/4/90	Female	54	Former teacher on disability	Alzheimer's disease
2	10/23/91	Female	58	Former elementary school teaching assistant	Unexplained and untreatable pelvic pain[a]
3	10/23/91	Female	43	Former secretary on disability	Multiple sclerosis
4	5/15/92	Female	52	Homemaker/Avon salesperson	Multiple sclerosis
5	9/26/92	Female	52	Homemaker/volunteer	Lung and brain cancer
6	11/23/92	Female	45	Schoolteacher/ real estate agent	Breast cancer
7	12/15/92	Female	70	Former computer operator/volunteer	Amyotrophic lateral sclerosis
8	12/15/92	Female	67	Retired nurse	Heart disease/emphysema
9	1/20/93	Male	53	Retired forester/ tree trimmer	Bone cancer/emphysema
10	2/4/93	Male	82	Retired farmer/county extension agent	Pancreatic cancer
11	2/4/93	Female	73	Seamstress/homemaker	Breast cancer
12	2/8/93	Female	47	Former sales clerk	Multiple sclerosis
13	2/15/93	Male	70	Retired merchant marine/ former security guard	Emphysema/congestive heart disease
14	2/18/93	Female	41	Computer programmer	Duodenal/ovarian cancer
15	2/18/93	Male	44	Former real estate agent	Throat cancer
16	5/16/93	Male	54	Real estate broker	Bone and lung cancer
17	8/4/93	Male	30	Former landscaper/ carpenter	Amyotrophic lateral sclerosis
18	9/9/93	Male	73	Retired tool & die maker	Bone cancer and amyloidosis

Table 1. (Cont'd.)

Case	Date of Death	Sex	Age	Occupation	Illness
19	10/22/93	Female	72	Homemaker/politician	Amyotrophic lateral sclerosis
20	11/22/93	Male	61	Physician/university professor	Bone cancer
21	11/26/94	Female	72	Homemaker/unable to work for years	Rheumatoid arthritis
22	5/8/95	Male	78	Retired minister	Pulmonary fibrosis
23	5/8/95	Male	27	College student/grocery clerk	Amyotrophic lateral sclerosis
24	6/26/95	Female	60	Former nursing home aide	Amyotrophic lateral sclerosis
25	8/21/95	Female	45	Executive secretary on disability	Multiple sclerosis
26	11/8/95	Female	58	Owner of travel agency/ former teacher	Breast cancer
27	1/29/96	Female	48	Data communications manager	Multiple sclerosis
28	5/6/96	Male	53	Former tool & die maker	Multiple sclerosis
29	6/10/96	Female	69	Retired school bus driver	Recent stroke/diabetes
30	6/18/96	Female	58	Nurse	Brain tumor/seizures
31	6/20/96	Female	67	Former commercial artist	Syringomyelia
32	7/4/96	Female	63	Retired high school administrator	Bowel cancer
33	7/9/96	Female	39	Former medical technician	Multiple sclerosis (autopsy indicated a misdiagnosis)[a]
34	8/6/96	Female	59	Supervisor at factory	Amyotrophic lateral sclerosis
35	8/15/96	Female	42	Former nurse	Chronic fatigue syndrome/ fibromyalgia[a]

Table 1. (Cont'd.)

Case	Date of Death	Sex	Age	Occupation	Illness
36	8/20/96	Female	76	Former typist/volunteer church secretary	Amyotrophic lateral sclerosis
37	8/22/96	Male	66	Former college professor	Multiple sclerosis
38	8/22/96	Female	40	Former nurse on disability	Multiple sclerosis
39	8/30/96	Female	54	Homemaker	Multiple sclerosis
40	9/2/96	Male	73	Retired engineer	Pancreatic cancer
41	9/7/96	Female	60	Retired factory worker	Degenerative spinal cord disorder/diabetes
42	9/29/96	Male	71	Psychiatrist	Colon cancer
43	10/10/96	Male	69	Retired teacher	Multiple sclerosis
44	10/17/96	Female	55	Retired florist/homemaker	Amyotrophic lateral sclerosis
45	10/23/96	Female	65	Retired microbiologist	Ovarian cancer
46	2/2/97	Female	42	Attorney	Crohn's disease (complained of chronic intestine pain)
47	2/2/97	Female	79	Retired law office employee	Amyotrophic lateral sclerosis
48	3/6/97	Female	59	Homemaker	Chronic arthritis/ esophagus problems
49	3/18/97	Male	41	Inspirational speaker on disabilities	Quadriplegic
50	3/24/97	Female	75	Retired librarian/ music teacher	Amyotrophic lateral sclerosis
51	4/8/97	Female	27	Graduate student	AIDS
52	5/7/97	Female	63	Grocery store worker	Amyotrophic lateral sclerosis
53	6/26/97	Female	40	Homemaker	Fibromyalgia/chronic fatigue syndrome[a]

Table 1. (Cont'd.)

Case	Date of Death	Sex	Age	Occupation	Illness
54	7/2/97	Female	54	Retired bookkeeper	Multiple sclerosis
55	7/2/97	Female	51	Retired nurse	Multiple sclerosis
56	8/13/97	Female	34	Account representative	Multiple sclerosis
57	8/27/97	Female	73	Former unemployment claim processor	Pancreatic cancer
58	8/29/97	Male	55	Civil engineer	Multiple sclerosis
59	9/3/97	Female	54	Insurance agent/ business owner	Ovarian cancer
60	9/6/97	Female	43	Homemaker	Multiple sclerosis
61	9/20/97	Male	78	Land developer/ former professor	Parkinson's disease
62	9/27/97	Female	54	Homemaker	Multiple sclerosis
63	10/3/97	Male	50	Optical technician	Amyotrophic lateral sclerosis
64	10/8/97	Female	65	Homemaker	Coronary disease (complained of chronic pain syndrome)
65	10/13/97	Female	34	Unknown	Multiple sclerosis
66	10/29/97	Male	54	Retired probation officer	Stroke/kidney problems
67	11/13/97	Female	74	Retired real estate broker	Pancreatic cancer
68	11/21/97	Female	78	Retired secretary	Multiple sclerosis
69	11/21/97	Female	84	Former actress/founder of theater group/degree in social work	Osteoporosis
70	12/3/97	Female	82	Retired teacher	Various age-related ailments[b]
71	12/11/97	Female	59	Apartment manager	Breast cancer
72	12/16/97	Female	46	Train conductor	Breast cancer

Table 1. (Cont'd.)

Case	Date of Death	Sex	Age	Occupation	Illness
73	12/16/97	Female	89	Former secretary	Strokes/paralysis
74	12/28/97	Male	53	Retired truck driver	Bladder cancer
75	12/28/97	Female	71	Former personnel supervisor	Breast cancer

[a]The coroner found no evidence of disease.

[b]According to reports, this person was the "first to say she had no overriding cause of pain or suffering" (Mishra, 1997, December 5, p. 1A). Her suicide note said that she was eighty-two years old and wanted to die (Mishra, 1997, December 4, p. 1A).

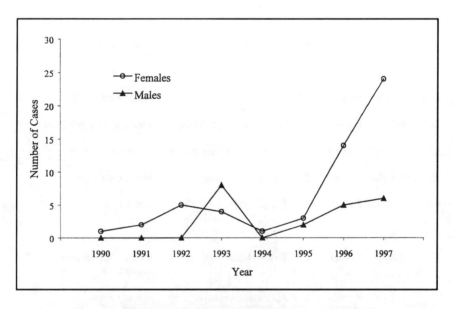

Figure 1. The Kevorkian assisted suicide cases 1990-1997:
number of female and male deaths per year.

Table 2. The Kevorkian Assisted Suicide Cases 1990-1997:
Family Structure and Living Arrangements

Characteristic	Females ($n = 54$)		Males ($n = 21$)		All ($n = 75$)	
	n	%	n	%	n	%
Relationship Status						
Married	15	(28%)	7	(33%)	22	(29%)
Unmarried but in a relationship	0	(0%)	2	(10%)	2	(3%)
Single	6	(11%)	3	(14%)	9	(12%)
Divorced	12	(22%)	4	(19%)	16	(21%)
Widowed	6	(11%)	1	(5%)	7	(9%)
Unknown	15	(28%)	4	(19%)	19	(25%)
Children						
Had children	32	(59%)	16	(76%)	48	(64%)
Did not have children	10	(19%)	3	(14%)	13	(17%)
Unknown	12	(22%)	2	(10%)	14	(19%)
Siblings						
Had siblings	19	(35%)	7	(33%)	26	(35%)
Did not have siblings	4	(7%)	0	(0%)	4	(5%)
Unknown	31	(57%)	14	(67%)	45	(60%)
Living Arrangements						
Lived with family	22	(41%)	11	(52%)	33	(44%)
Lived alone	15	(28%)	2	(10%)	17	(23%)
Nursing home	7	(13%)	1	(5%)	8	(11%)
Unknown	10	(19%)	7	(33%)	17	(23%)

Physical Health

A significant proportion of individuals (64%) whose death was hastened by
Dr. Kevorkian suffered from a chronic condition ($p < .05$) (see Table 3). While
females were more likely to have a chronic condition than males (69% versus
52%), a statistically significant relationship between gender and chronicity was
not indicated by the data. Among chronic conditions, multiple sclerosis (MS) was
the most common, having been diagnosed in 25 percent of cases (28% of females
and 19% of male cases). The second most prevalent chronic illness was amyotrophic lateral sclerosis (ALS), which was the primary diagnosis in 15 percent of
all cases. ALS afflicted 15 percent of females and 14 percent of males. Cancer

Table 3. The Kevorkian Assisted Suicide Cases 1990-1997:
Characteristics of the Person's Primary Illness

Illness Characteristics	Females (n = 54)		Males (n = 21)		All (n = 75)	
	n	%	n	%	n	%
Chronic	37	(69%)	11	(52%)	48	(64%)
Non-chronic	13	(24%)	9	(43%)	22	(29%)
Unknown	4	(7%)	1	(5%)	5	(7%)
Terminal	11	(20%)	8	(38%)	19	(25%)
Non-terminal	41	(76%)	11	(52%)	52	(69%)
Unknown	2	(4%)	2	(10%)	4	(5%)
Physical disability	38	(70%)	16	(76%)	54	(72%)
No physical disability	8	(15%)	0	(0%)	8	(1%)
Unknown	8	(15%)	5	(24%)	13	(17%)
Pain	34	(63%)	12	(57%)	46	(61%)
No pain	2	(4%)	0	(0%)	2	(3%)
Unknown	18	(33%)	9	(43%)	27	(36%)

was also a common diagnosis, affecting 29 percent of cases. This illness was somewhat more common in males (43%) than in females (24%) (see Table 1).

In a significant proportion of cases (69%), the illnesses of those assisted in suicide were not at the terminal stage ($p < .05$). Only one-quarter of illnesses were judged as terminal-stage by the medical examiner (see Table 3). Thirty-eight percent of the males and 20 percent of the females were classified as terminal ($p = ns$).

A significant proportion of individuals (72%) experienced some form of physical disability ($p < .05$) (see Table 3). This disability typically involved an inability to walk (56% of cases), incontinence (15% of cases), vision problems (12% of cases), and/or difficulties talking (9% of cases). Many individuals had more than one disability. Women and men were similar with regard to the experience of physical disability (70% versus 76%, $p = ns$).

Physical pain was mentioned in a significant proportion (61%) of cases ($p < .05$). In about a quarter of the cases it was the individuals themselves who reported being in pain. Usually (in 72% of all cases), however, pain was mentioned by family, friends, acquaintances, or physicians of the deceased. Women and men were similar with regard to the experience of pain (63% versus 57%, $p = ns$).

Mental Health

Information about the mental health of the persons whose death was hastened by Dr. Kevorkian was typically unavailable. In ten (19%) female cases and seven (34%) male cases, there was mention of current and/or past depression, emotional instability, and/or other psychological problems. For eight individuals (4 females and 4 males) there was a report of past suicidal behavior.

A striking finding in terms of mental health, is that in five cases, all female, the medical examiner found no evidence of disease. Four of these women had a history of depression, and three took high doses of mood-altering drugs. Three had a history of serious personal problems, including spousal abuse. These women were younger (the average age was 52; the median age was 42) than the average woman in the Kevorkian assisted suicide group. Most (4 out of 5) complained of illnesses that are difficult to diagnose, such as chronic fatigue syndrome. One of these women was Rebecca Badger, who at the time of her death was thirty-nine years old. She was diagnosed as having multiple sclerosis for which she took high doses of morphine and Valium. Besides her prescription drug dependence, Badger had a history of alcohol abuse and depression. Like Badger, Judith Curren was addicted to psychotropic drugs, which she obtained through her husband, a psychiatrist and her former psychotherapist. She had a history of depression, for which she underwent many ineffective interventions, including electroconvulsive therapy. Curren had filed nine complaints against her husband for domestic violence. The latest episode occurred the same month she died of lethal injection, at age forty-two. Marjorie Wantz, a fifty-eight year-old woman with a long history of mental disorders, spent her latest years trying to obtain relief for an unexplained pelvic pain. She had ten unsuccessful surgeries and was on high doses of painkillers and psychotropic medications. The oldest woman in this group was Martha Wichorek, an eighty-two-year-old widow. She suffered from various age-related disabilities (e.g., incontinence) but was healthy for her age. Prior to her death she stated she believed in assisted suicide on demand for anyone older than eighty. In her suicide note she stated she was not "stressed, oppressed or depressed," she just "want[ed] to die" (Mishra, 1997, p. 1A). A neighbor and friend of twenty-three years, however, was surprised at the news of her death, as she recently put a new roof and completed a paint job for her house.

What Were the Circumstances Surrounding their Deaths?

Personal Reasons for the Assisted Suicide

Information about the person's reasons for the assisted suicide came from a variety of documents, including suicide notes, letters, interviews, and pre-suicide videotapes. Suicide notes and/or pre-suicide videotapes were reported in forty-three of the seventy-five cases—this includes twenty-nine females and fourteen males. Pre-suicide videotapes were available only through August of 1996. Prior to this time, the farewell messages were often elaborate and rich in information. After that date, suicide notes typically included only a statement to contact Dr. Kevorkian's lawyers.

In over half of the cases (57%), no information was available concerning the person's reasons for the hastened death (see Table 4). However, when such information was provided, more than one reason was often mentioned.

The most common motive given by the individuals Dr. Kevorkian assisted in suicide was having physical disabilities (see Table 4). This explanation was mentioned by about one-fourth of all individuals. Persons who gave this reason focused on the poor quality of life and loss of dignity brought on by the

Table 4. The Kevorkian Assisted Suicide Cases 1990-1997:
Explanations For, and Reactions To the Assisted Suicide

	Females (n = 54)		Males (n = 21)		All (n = 75)	
	n	%	n	%	n	%
Reasons for the Assisted Suicide Given by the Individual[a]						
Disability	13	(24%)	6	(29%)	19	(25%)
Physical pain	9	(17%)	2	(10%)	11	(15%)
Fear of being a burden	8	(15%)	2	(10%)	10	(13%)
Right-to-die	7	(13%)	2	(10%)	9	(12%)
Unknown	30	(56%)	13	(62%)	43	(57%)
Reasons for the Assisted Suicide Given by Family/Friends[a]						
Disability	11	(20%)	5	(24%)	17	(23%)
Fear of being a burden	7	(13%)	2	(10%)	9	(12%)
Physical pain	5	(9%)	4	(19%)	9	(12%)
Right-to-die	4	(7%)	2	(10%)	6	(8%)
Depression	2	(4%)	0	(0%)	2	(3%)
Unknown	34	(63%)	13	(62%)	47	(63%)
Family/Friends Response to the Assisted Suicide Decision						
Supported the Decision	42	(78%)	15	(71%)	57	(76%)
Did Not Support the Decision	0	(0%)	0	(0%)	0	(0%)
Unaware of the Decision	4	(7%)	3	(14%)	7	(9%)
Unknown	8	(15%)	3	(14%)	11	(15%)

[a]Percentages do not sum to 100 because more than one reason for hastened death was given in many cases.

disabilities. They argued that the disabilities destroyed their will to live, their interest and pleasure in life. Some examples of this kind of explanation from women included the following statements: "I do not want to live in this condition any longer;"[3] "I can't walk, I can't write. It's hard for me to talk. I can't function as a human being;"[4] "I see life from here on as a losing battle . . . too much effort spent solving the problem of how to stay alive and no energy or time left for real living. I want out, the earliest, most human way possible;"[5] "As . . . I was nothing more than 'bed-vege,' I knew it was time to say, 'See ya'.[6] Men expressed similar feelings about their physical disabilities and their plan to die. A man complained that he was no longer able to leave the house, eat, or exercise: "there's no reason to prolong any of this. I'm just not going to get any better and time goes by so slowly that it is unbearable. Life is not life anymore."[7] Another man said his condition was "like being imprisoned in your own body—kind of like being sentenced to life imprisonment with no chance of parole—for a crime you didn't commit."[8]

The next most common reasons mentioned by individuals who hastened their death were pain (15% of cases) and fear of being a burden (13% of cases) (see Table 4). Individuals who feared being a burden anticipated, did not want to, and/or could not afford to be dependent on others. For example, a woman who only a year before had learned she had Alzheimer's disease wrote in her suicide note: "This is a decision taken in a normal state of mind. I do not choose to put my family or myself through the agony of this terrible disease."[9] A man who had Parkinson's disease wrote that he wanted to die in a dignified way rather than be "reduced to the indignities of childhood diapers; spoon-feeding; semi-death."[10] Finally, in 12 percent of the cases the plan for assisted suicide was viewed as an affirmation of the right to choose the time to die. Individuals who mentioned this reason were often members of The Hemlock Society or activists in the right-to-die movement.

[3] Susan Williams' (case 4) suicide note, cited in Betzold and Gerdes (1992, p. D12).

[4] Sherry Miller (case 3), quoted in Wilkerson (1991, p. A14).

[5] Merian Frederick's (case 19) suicide note, cited in "Kevorkian aids suicide in bid for jail" (1993, p. 8).

[6] Esther Cohan (case 25), in a letter quoted in "After latest assisted suicide, body is left near a hospital (1995, p. C19).

[7] Jonathan Grenz (case 15), in a letter cited in Ourlian (1993, p. 2B).

[8] Austin Bastable (case 28), in a videotape recorded before his death, cited in Farnsworth (1996, p. A5).

[9] Janet Adkins' (case 1) suicide note, cited in Basheda (1990, p. C7).

[10]Natverlal Thakore's (case 61) suicide note, cited in Associated Press (1997).

Reasons for Assisted Suicide:
Family and Friends Perspectives

In about a third of the cases, family members and friends also offered an opinion on the reasons for the hastened death. In this study a family member is defined as a person who had a close relationship with the deceased, whether via legal, biological, or common-law bonds, or via being an unrelated companion. Physical disability was the most commonly mentioned explanation given by significant others, followed by fear of being a burden, pain, right-to-die issues, and depression (see Table 4).

A focus on disability is illustrated by the following three examples. In a statement released after the hastened death of his forty-year-old daughter, who suffered from chronic fatigue syndrome, the father stated "there is no quality left to her life and no hope for any cure. . . . There are things in this world worse than death."[11] In this case (case 53), no evidence of disease was actually found by the medical examiner, who was quoted as saying: "Although there was information that this robust 40-year-old lady suffered from chronic fatigue syndrome, there was no evidence of anatomically demonstrable disease in her body" (Hyde, 1997). In another case, a daughter wrote to Kevorkian, shortly before her father's hastened death, that her father's "blindness and rapid deterioration from cancer" made assisted suicide "a most urgent matter for him."[12] Finally, a mother was reported as saying that ALS rendered her twenty-seven-year-old "son's life almost meaningless to him."[13]

The fear of being a burden is captured by the following three examples. A woman said of the hastened death of her friend: "She felt it was a gift to her family, sparing them of the burden of taking care of her."[14] A husband said that his wife was on the verge of requiring nursing home care and "did not want to devastate our financial picture."[15] Another woman, whose fifty-nine-year-old sister was diagnosed with breast cancer after losing her health insurance in a divorce, stated: "She wanted to live. She tried very hard to live" [but] "if you can't afford to fight it you just die."[16]

---

[11]Janis Murphy's (case 53) father, cited in Murphy and McDiarmid (1997).

[12]Stanley Ball's (case 10) daughter, cited in Ourlian (1993, p. 4A).

[13]Nicholas Loving's (case 23) mother, cited in Ourlian (1995, p. 4C).

[14]Janet Adkins' (case 1) friend, Peggy Morrison, quoted in Johnson, Greenwalt, and Hauser (1990, p. 42).

[15]Patricia Smith's (case 38) husband, cited in Associated Press (1996).

[16]Rosalind Haas' (case 71) sister, cited in Schrader (1997, p. 4B) and in Montgomery (1997), respectively.

Family and Friends' Responses to the Assisted Suicide Plan

About two-thirds of significant others (78% of women's and 71% of men's significant others) supported the decision to seek a hastened death (see Table 4). Support came in various forms: from help in planning the death (e.g., contacting Kevorkian or driving to Michigan) to participating in a pre-suicide videotaped interview with Kevorkian; from being present at the time of death to making post-mortem statements to the media indicating agreement with the hastened death decision. Some family members and/or friends were described as reluctant at first, and more supportive of the plan to seek an assisted suicide over time. In a few cases (9%), close family members stated they were unaware of their relative's plan to seek a hastened death.

Family and Friends' Presence at the Hastened Death

Family members and/or friends were known to be present at thirty-two of the seventy-five deaths (43%). This number is a conservative estimate, as the presence of family was unknown in fourteen female and in six male cases, while the presence of friends was unknown for nine females and four males. Fifty-two percent of females and 48 percent of males had one or more family members attending their death. In contrast, friends were reported as present only at female deaths (in 20% of cases).

Time from Diagnosis of Illness to Death

The time between diagnosis of the illness (which led to the request for assisted suicide) and death ranged from less than one month to more than twenty-seven years. A chi-square analysis indicated that for significantly more individuals (35%), death occurred within five years of diagnosis, as opposed to other categories (i.e., more-than-5 to 10 years, more-than-10 to 15 years, and more-than-15 years) ($p < .05$). Men were more likely to die in fewer than five years than women (48% versus 31%). However, there was no statistically significant relationship between sex-of-the-deceased and time between diagnosis and death. The time from diagnosis to death was unknown for 36 percent of the cases.

Summary of Findings

Between 1990 and 1997, seventy-five individuals were reported as having died with the assistance of Dr. Kevorkian. The individuals represent a broad range of regional and occupational backgrounds, but a majority (72%) were women of European-American descent. Most suffered from a condition that was disabling (72%), chronic (64%), and nonterminal-stage (69%). No evidence of disease whatsoever was found by the medical examiner in 10 percent of female cases. Fifty percent of the women whose death was hastened by Kevorkian were middle-aged and another 39 percent were older adults. In contrast, 43 percent of the men were middle-aged and 48 percent were older adults. In addition, men were somewhat less likely than women to have a condition that was chronic (52% versus 69%) or nonterminal stage (52% versus 76%). The main reasons for the hastened death mentioned by both the person and their significant others were having disabilities, being in pain, and fear of being a burden.

DISCUSSION

One of our most noteworthy findings, in our opinion, is that women repre-sented a majority of Kevorkian's assisted suicide cases. This finding is remark-able because in the United States women represent a minority of suicide cases (Canetto & Lester, 1995). In this country, women are less likely to kill themselves than men by a ratio of 1:4 (Canetto & Lester, 1995). While this ratio diminishes between ages forty-five and fifty-four, when women's mortality by suicide peaks, even at mid-life, women's rates of death by suicide are less than half those of men (McIntosh, 1991; McIntosh, Santos, Hubbard, & Overholser, 1994). Furthermore, the female-to-male suicide ratio increases after mid-life when women's rates drop and men's escalate. For example, in 1992, the female-to-male suicide ratio for those age sixty-five and over was 1:6 (McIntosh, Pearson, & Lebowitz, 1997). These data suggest that the gender psychology of assisted suicide is different from the gender psychology of self-inflicted death.

Several trends in the Kevorkian assisted suicides run counter to those that emerged from studies of assisted suicide in the Netherlands, a country where assisted suicide is legitimized. First, while in the current study a majority (72%) of assisted suicide cases were women, in studies conducted in the Netherlands fewer women than men died of assisted suicide (women represented 32% of assisted suicide cases in the 1990 survey and 39% of cases in the 1995 survey) van der Maas, van Delden, & Pijnenborg, 1992; van der Maas et al., 1996, respectively). However, in 1990, there were fewer women than men among those whose request for physician assisted suicide or euthanasia was refused (45% versus 55%). Also, euthanasia, a far more common death in the Nether-lands, was more prevalent among women than men (women represented 52% of euthanasia cases in the 1990 survey, and 57% of cases in the 1995 survey).

The results of this study also differ from those of surveys from the Netherlands with regard to the most common diagnosis of the deceased. Chronic illnesses were the most prevalent diagnosis (64% of cases) in the Kevorkian cases, while cancer was the most common diagnosis in the Netherlands (83% of cases in 1990; 78% of cases in 1995). Yet another difference is that only 25 percent of the persons who died with the assistance of Dr. Kevorkian were at the terminal stage, as compared to 85 percent of assisted suicide cases in the 1990 Netherlands survey. We realized there are reasons for caution in making comparisons across studies using different methodologies and with samples drawn from countries with different cultural traditions and social structures. At the same time, we believe it is valuable to examine related trends across methodologies and cultures such that similarities and differences can be documented and understood.

In the Kevorkian sample, gender differences are salient and unique within the context of related local and international data. Thus, we dedicate the rest of the discussion to an examination of gender issues in Kevorkian's assisted suicide cases.

Why Women?

In this section we consider explanations of the preponderance of women among those who died with Kevorkian's assistance. We focus on factors such as pragmatism about one's death, a diminished sense of entitlement, social, and economic disadvantage, and cultural definitions of the full life.

Because of Unique Selection Factors in Kevorkian's Cases

It is possible that individuals who died with Kevorkian's assistance are not representative of physician-assisted suicide cases in general, because of the unique circumstances of Kevorkian's practice. Because Kevorkian has not shared information about persons whose request for assisted suicide he turned down, we do not know whether his assisted suicide public record is representative of his assisted suicide applicant pool. "There's [sic] many more people that contact me than I help" he has said (Harmon, 1996, p. 1C). It is possible that disproportionately more women than men make assisted suicide requests of Kevorkian. It is also possible that there is an excess of male cases among those post-1995 assisted suicides that Kevorkian has not made public (Martin & Brasier, 1996).

A second possibility is that more women than men experience the conditions that Kevorkian considered a good fit for assisted suicide. For example, women are more likely than men to experience chronic, incurable, and debilitating diseases (Gatz, Harris, & Turk-Charles, 1995). These are the conditions that were most prevalent among the people whose death he assisted, especially women. It is interesting to note in this regard that in a 1992 article Kevorkian wrote about "justifiable medically-assisted suicide" (cited in Betzold, 1993), the model case is a woman. This fictitious woman, whom he named Wanda Enditall, is a forty-five year old afflicted with multiple sclerosis, and with a family who understands and almost unanimously supports her intent to seek a hastened death (pp. 120-121). Enditall's condition and circumstances are very similar to those of many women whose death Kevorkian actually assisted. Enditall has a chronic, debilitating, but nonterminal-stage illness, and a family who agrees with her plan to voluntarily die.

A third possibility is that Kevorkian may have viewed women as better candidates for assisted suicide than men, independent of their condition. "I only help when they really need it," he said of the people who contact him (Harmon, 1996, p. 1C). How did Kevorkian know when "they really need it?" While Fieger, Kevorkian's lawyer, has argued that Kevorkian "scrupulously" followed strict guidelines (Williams & Greenwood, 1996), a *Detroit Free Press* investigation found that he frequently ignored his own rules. For example, he consistently violated his own recommendation that "every candidate for suicide must be examined by a psychiatrist" (The Detroit Free Press Staff, 1997, p. 64).

Kevorkian's assisted suicide cases may be distinctive in other ways. Persons who sought Kevorkian's assistance in death may be unique due to the high likelihood of publicity associated with a Kevorkian assisted suicide. For example, they may have been more likely to be activists in the right-to-die movement. Several of Kevorkian's cases in fact fit this category, including Janet Adkins, Janet Good, and Austin Bastable. At the very least, those who sought Kevorkian's assistance may have been comfortable with the possibility of media exposure, and perhaps even motivated for their death to serve as a public example. For instance, Janet Adkins, Kevorkian's first assisted suicide, was quoted as saying before dying, "You just make my case known" (Ilka, 1990, p. C9).

Because Women are More Willing to Face Their Own Deaths

Kevorkian (1996) himself offered this interpretation of the gender imbalance in his assisted suicide record. Women are "stronger. . . . more practical than men," he said, "That's why I think they can face it better than men." Women "are more in tune with nature than men," while a man's "mind is boggled with a bunch of hair-splitting philosophy."

These interpretations are echoed in comments by Janet Good, an activist in the right-to-die movement, and one of Kevorkian's assisted suicides. "It's taking charge of your life" she said when asked why women (and only women at the time) were dying with Kevorkian's assistance. She was described as indignant over the suggestion that passivity, deference to male authority, and seeking approval from a father figure were important motivations for the women whose suicide was assisted by Kevorkian (Martin, 1991).[17]

Similarly, Sheila Cook, a coordinator of Compassion in Dying case-management team, talked about the "beauty . . . [of] directing the end of . . . [own's] life." Susan Dunshee, another activist in Compassion in Dying and "a believer in independence" and strength, described a woman whose assisted suicide she

---

[17]Some evidence, however, suggests that Janet Good, a woman who in many ways was daring and determined, might have been rather deferential in her relationship to Kevorkian. "As close as we are, I just can't call him Jack. . . . He is always the Doctor" she is quoted as saying (Lessenberry, 1997, p. 85). After being diagnosed with cancer, she was asked whether she would die with Kevorkian's assistance. "No! I can't. I don't feel that I can ask him! I could not live with the thought that I might be the one to put him in jail," she responded. A few months before her assisted suicide, she said: "I think it would be an honor to die with Dr. Kevorkian, if he will agree and I need it" (Lessenberry, 1997, p. 130).

witnessed: "She met me at the door holding a vacuum cleaner. . . . she was doing a final housecleaning. . . . [She even] had mouthwash on her nightstand . . . to use after she swallowed the barbiturates mixed in applesauce." According to Dunshee, this woman was "clearheaded, decisive, and in full-control" (Friedman, 1997, p. 165). Reflecting on the question of women and hastened death, another commentator, however, concluded that "for the well-organized house-wife, . . . [a hastened death] is . . . [the ultimate, final] tidy solution" (Verlander, 1997, p. 16).

Because Women are Particularly Concerned About Self-Determination in Death

Some evidence suggests that the concern about self-determination in death may be particularly relevant for women. For example, a study of judicial reasoning in cases involving termination of treatment for incompetent persons found that, in the absence of written directives, the courts were more likely to infer a preference to terminate life support when the patient was a man than when the patient was a woman (Miles & August, 1990). In these cases the courts tended to view past pro-euthanasia statements and behaviors as valid, mature, and rational only for the male patients. In addition, life supports were regarded as undignified and dehumanizing for men but not for women. According to Jecker (1994), these findings "reflect in part the historical treatment of women under the law: histori-cally, women were viewed as lacking the qualities of autonomy and rationality considered preconditions for the exercise of valid consent" (p. 676).

Data on women's attitudes about right-to-die issues are, however, mixed. Some evidence suggests that many women have embraced the cause of hastened death. For example, according to a 1996 article entitled "Who's fighting to die? A look at the Hemlock Society membership," women constitute the majority (two-thirds) of Hemlock Society members (Fox & Kamakahi, 1996). One note of caution about this conclusion is that the response rate of the Hemlock Society survey was less than 20 percent. Therefore, all one can conclude on the basis of this 1995 Hemlock Society survey is that female members were more likely than male members to respond to the survey. In any case, the current Executive Director of the Hemlock Society is a woman. Other women are, and have been visibly involved in the "fight to die" (e.g., Janet Good, Kevorkian's "assistant" and one of his assisted suicides). "Of course women are in the forefront of the right-to-die issues, because they have been struggling their whole lives to control their bodies, and in fact their destinies" said Carol King, then the executive director of the Michigan Abortion Rights Action League. "Deciding how and when to die when terminally ill or riddled with unending pain is an issue of choice" she argued (Martin, 1991).

Other evidence, however, indicates that women are more negative than men about physician's hastened deaths. For example, surveys indicate that women (as well as older persons, ethnic minorities, and the poor) are more likely to oppose assisted suicide and euthanasia than men (e.g., see the California exit polls, described in Steinfels, 1993; an analysis of older adult responses to a Gallup poll, in Seidlitz, Duberstein, Cox, & Conwell, 1995; and a study of elderly patients and their families by Koenig, Wildman-Hanlon, & Schmader, 1996). These findings have typically been interpreted as indicating that women, like other disadvantaged groups, are more worried about being forced to die than about being forced to live, because of persistent experiences with being cut off from resources (see Canetto, 1996, and Wolf, 1996a, for a gender analysis of assisted suicide issues; and *The Detroit Free Press,* 1997, for an analysis of "Black reluctance" to support assisted suicide). In addition, the visible leaders of the "right-to-die" movement have been men. In this country, Derek Humphry, a British expatriate, Jack Kevorkian, and Timothy Quill are among the best known of such figures.

Because Women's Choices for Care are Limited by Social and Economic Disadvantage

In a 1994 report on assisted suicide and euthanasia, The New York State Task Force on Life and the Law concluded that in the United States, a country where medicine is practiced in a context of serious social inequities and biases, legalized assisted suicide and euthanasia would be "profoundly dangerous" for many ill individuals. According to this group, the risk "would be most severe for those whose autonomy and well-being are already compromised by poverty, lack of access to good medical care, or membership in a stigmatized social group" (pp. vii-viii, 1994). While not specifically named as a risk group, women fit all of the characteristics identified as risk factors in the report by the New York State Task Force on Life and the Law.

Women enter mid- to late-adulthood, the time when decisions about hastened death are most likely to occur, with vastly different personal, social and economic resources than men (see Gatz et al., 1995; and Hess, 1990, for reviews). Women live about seven years longer than men. At the same time, older women are more likely than older men to suffer from disabling chronic diseases. In addition, older women are more likely to be poor, widowed, live alone, and to have limited access to medical insurance and family care. For example, women are less likely than men to be cared for at home. They also tend to stay longer in acute-care beds and are more likely to be transferred to long-term facilities for their recovery than older men. More women than men live in nursing homes. In other words, women tend to live longer than men, but in poor health, and with fewer economic and family resources to compensate for their ailments and disabilities. Thus, longevity, coupled with morbidity and diminished resources, may be viewed as a liability and a burden rather than an asset.

Because of their limited access to resources and longer lives, women are more severely handicapped by illnesses and disabilities. As a result, they may be more likely to see themselves, and/or be seen by others, as appropriate candidates for a hastened death (Canetto, 1995, 1996). Their living may be perceived as burdensome to them, their families, the medical system and society. This scenario is coming into focus in the current context of managed care medicine, where assisted suicide represents a "cost-saving measure" (Wolf, 1996b, p. 465). The idea of "tempting health care providers to persuade chronic patients to minimize costs by ending it all painlessly is no fantasy" (Kreimer, 1995, p. 841). For example, Fung (1993), in an article entitled "Dying for money: Overcoming moral hazard in terminal illnesses through compensated physician-assisted death," proposed that financial incentives be offered for choosing assisted death over life-extending interventions. He dedicated the article to his mother whose death he wished had been hastened.

Because Women Have a Diminished Sense of Entitlement

This explanation focuses on cultural definitions of femininity as self-effacement and self-sacrifice. It proposes that more women than men opted for a Kevorkian-hastened death, when ill and/or disabled, because of a socialized sense of self as undeserving, and a duty to be altruistic (Canetto, 1995; 1996; Gutmann, 1996).

Psychological studies suggest that women have less of a sense of entitlement than men (see Major, 1987, for a review). According to Gilligan's (1982) research on moral development, one of the conventions of femininity is that "virtue for women lies in self-sacrifice" (p. 132).

In Western countries, this convention is rooted in a long history of glorification of women's self-effacement and self sacrifice (see Wolf, 1996a, for a review). For example, in Greek tragedy "silence is the adornment of women," and a suicide is a widow's reasonable behavior (Loraux, p. 21). As noted by Kaplan and DeWitt (1996), Kevorkian himself acknowledged the power of the Greek legacy when, in a taped interview, he told Janet Adkins, his first assisted suicide, and her husband: "I think the world one day will thank you and Ron because what you're doing is a historical move. I don't think it's ever been done officially since the days of classical Greece" (Betzold, 1993, p. 73).

This cultural lineage has implications, as suggested by Wolf (1996a): "It means that while we debate physician assisted suicide and euthanasia rationally, we may be animated by unacknowledged images that give the practices a certain rendered logic and felt correctness" (p. 289). Self-sacrificing in women is reinforced and expected in many contexts, including in families. "The history and persistence of family patterns in this country in which women are expected to adopt self-sacrificing behavior for the sake of the family may pave the way too for the patient's request for death," concludes Wolf (1996a, p. 291).

Because of a Devaluing of Women's Lives

This explanation focuses on another aspect of social disadvantage previously addressed by The New York State Task Force on Life and the Law, that of the social value of a person's life. Several kinds of evidence show that women's lives are devalued, especially when women are ill, disabled or simply up in age.

First, women all over the world have access to substantially fewer and less quality resources than men, from food to medical care (United Nations, 1991). For example, even though in the United States women receive more medical care than men, this care is usually worse or inappropriate (Council on Ethical and Judicial Affairs, American Medical Association, 1991). In several parts of the world, women have had to fight against the duty to die—as was the custom for widows, but not for widowers, in India and Papua New Guinea. According to the Lusi of Papua New Guinea, a widow would rather be ritually killed than depend on her children, who might resent having another mouth to feed as she becomes disabled with age (Canetto & Lester, 1998).

Second, there are studies on the perception of the acceptability of suicidal behavior. These studies show that while suicide is perceived as incongruous with femininity, the decision to kill oneself is viewed as most understandable for older women. For example, according to a study by Stillion and colleagues (1989), people are most likely to agree, and least likely to sympathize, with older women's "attempting" to kill themselves. Stillion and associates suggested that older women are not seen as worthy of survival or sympathy, following a suicidal act, because they lack status, wealth, and power. They note that "the devaluing of females lives . . . may become more pronounced in old age" (p. 247).

This devaluing of women's lives is likely to play a role in assessments of the life worth preserving (Canetto, 1996). Confronted with a judgment for which there are no objective criteria, physicians are going to be influenced by societal values and personal biases about disposable lives (Kamisar, 1996). In a society where women's lives are objectively more difficult and more likely to be devalued, women are more likely than men to be seen as reasonable candidates for a hastened death. Since "there is no valid clinical method for distinguishing rational . . . [requests] from those that are motivated by sadness, demoralization, discouragement, or altruism" (Miles, 1995, p. 18), a disabled, discouraged woman who seeks hastened death may be viewed as making a practical, sensible "choice."

As noted by Kass and Lund (1996), "the problem is not primarily that physicians believe some lives more worthy or better lived than others; nearly all people hold such opinions and make such judgments. The danger comes when they *act* on these judgments," and with the authority of their profession (p. 26).

Because of Gender Biases in Societal Definitions of the Completed, Full Life

One of the issues in the debate about "rational suicide among the elderly" (Humphry, 1992, p. 125) is the idea of a completed, full life. According to some authors (e.g., Brody, 1992), a completed, full life is one that has run its "natural lifespan" (intended not necessarily as the biological maximum) and which has brought a sense of completion to the person's biographical narrative. Death after such "completed life" is viewed by some as relatively acceptable and rational. For example, Callahan (1990, 1995) argues that a tolerable death is one that occurs when one has reached a certain age, accomplished "on the whole" one's life goals and fulfilled one's moral obligations.

As noted by Bell (1992), gender-unspecified definitions of the long-enough and full-enough life are often based on a male model of the natural lifespan and full biography. As such, these definitions are biased against, and adversely affect women more than men. For example, Callahan's (1995) definition of the natural lifespan appears to be based on a male referent, as indicated by the language and examples he uses to describe the older person: "When we know someone's age, but nothing else about him, what do we know of significance? If the person is old—say, in his 70s (and certainly by his 80s)—we . . . would not expect to find him playing football or climbing trees for recreation" (p. 166). In addition, Callahan's proposal of using a single age-range as the criterion for limiting access to health care disproportionally harms women because women live longer than men. It means treating life beyond the age of seventy-three, male life expectancy, as expendable and excessive.

Similarly a biographical definition of the full life that fails to take into account differences in the biographies of men and women has the potential of encouraging premature death in women. Consider the case of a widowed or divorced homemaker whose children have left home. Should this woman become sick and disabled and request assistance in death, it is easy to imagine someone arguing that her wish for death is sensible and rational because she has completed her lifework. This kind of biography is found in several of the Kevorkian cases (e.g., Wichorek). A variation in this biography ("a physically healthy, grief-stricken 50-year-old [divorced] social worker" who lost her two children) was approved for a famous assisted suicide in the Netherlands (e.g., Chabot's case, see Hendin, 1995, p. 197).

Why Assisted Suicide?

Another important question in the gender patterns of Kevorkian's assisted suicides has to do with the mode of death. Assuming that women who died with Kevorkian's assistance had only "good" and "rational" reasons to hasten their death, why did not they simply kill themselves? Why did they choose a hastened death? Why did they go through Dr. Kevorkian? In this section we consider explanations for the choice of assisted suicide.

Because Killing Oneself by Oneself is Perceived as Masculine Behavior

According to a recent review of studies (Canetto, 1995), killing oneself is considered a masculine act in the United States. Suicide is viewed as less acceptable for females than for males. For example, in a study by Deluty (1988-89), death by suicide in females was rated as more wrong and more foolish than death by suicide in males. In another study (Lewis & Shepeard, 1992), females who killed themselves were seen as less well-adjusted than men who killed themselves, independent of the precipitant of suicide (e.g., achievement versus relationship problems). It is plausible that these negative attitudes about female suicide may discourage women from killing themselves. In addition, studies consistently find that women are less likely than men to believe that people have the right to kill themselves (e.g., Johnson, Fitch, Alston, & McIntosh, 1980; Marks, 1988-89).

Because Assisted Suicide May Be Perceived as a Feminine Death

It has been suggested that suicide is perceived as unacceptable in females because it involves taking charge of one's fate, an action which goes against conventions of femininity (Canetto, 1995). If suicidal death could be made to appear passive, deferential, and "gentle," then it might be considered acceptable for women. Perhaps physician-assisted suicide fits such criteria.

Janet Good, an activist in the right-to-die movement whose death was hastened by Dr. Kevorkian, thought so. She interpreted women's high rate of suicidal behavior and low suicide mortality as indicating that women want to kill themselves but do not want to die alone nor to "use means that are effective but violent, such as guns." According to her, assisted suicide is the perfect solution for suicidal women because it allows them to die with company and "peacefully." "Isn't that a rational position?" she asked (Martin, 1991).

So far there have been no studies on gender and the perceived acceptability of assisted suicide. There is indirect evidence, however, suggesting that a hastened death may be viewed as particularly fitting for females. One such line of evidence are the published cases of hastened death. While there have been men among those who died of hastened deaths, the model cases in news' accounts and in scholarly journals have all been women (Wolf, 1996a). Almost all of the "classic" hastened-death legal cases in the United States and Canada involved women (Downie & Sherman, 1996).

"Jean's way: A love story" was the assisted suicide book of the late 1970s. The book, written by Derek Humphry and his second wife Anne Wickett (who later killed herself), documents the assisted suicide of Humphry's first wife, Jean (Cox, 1993). In the early 1980s, the model case was Elizabeth Bouvia, a woman severely handicapped by quadriplegia and advanced cerebral palsy, who tried to legally compel a hospital to help her die of starvation (Battin, 1994). The case that energized the hastened death debate ten years ago was Debbie (Anonymous, 1988). She was euthanized by a resident who wrote up the event in a one-page anonymous article published in the *Journal of the American Medical Association.* Then came Dr. Kevorkian's string of nationally publicized female assisted-suicides. It took two years and eight female deaths before Kevorkian assisted a male in suicide. In the meantime Dr. Quill's published an article in *The New England Journal of Medicine* about assisting a patient, Diane, in suicide (1991). Some years later he wrote about Jane's assisted suicide (Quill, 1996). Louise was the person whose hastened death was featured in a 1993 *New York Times* cover article to illustrate the approach to assisted suicide of Compassion in Dying, an organization dedicated "to helping terminally ill patients end their lives" and to legalizing assisted suicide (Belkin, 1993, p. 50). In the same year, a book by the president of the Delaware Valley Hemlock Society was dedicated to seven women, Karen Anne Quinlan, Nancy Cruzan, Patti Rosier, Diane Trumbull, Janet Adkins, Sherri Miller, Marjorie Wantz, whom the author viewed as key cases in *"The struggle for death with dignity"* (Cox, 1993, p. 3). In Canada the front-page case was Sue Rodriguez, a forty-three-year-old woman afflicted with ALS who unsuccessfully attempted to change the Criminal Code concerning assisted suicide and eventually killed herself in 1994 with the help of an unknown doctor (Battin, 1994). Recently, the first person to publicly take advantage of Oregon's assisted suicide law was a woman (Hoover & Hill, 1998).[18] The use of female cases to promote hastened death may hold for the Netherlands as well. Dr. Herbert Cohen, one of the best-known Dutch practitioners of hastened death, was quoted as saying: "Have you noticed . . . that all of the cases that have broken new ground in Dutch law have been women?" (Hendin, 1994, p. 136).

What tacit assumptions about women may be influencing the consistent choice of female cases to advocate for hastened death? As discussed by Wolf (1996a), the persistence of these female images leads one to wonder whether there is something about being a female that makes female hastened deaths look right and good.

Because of Gender Dynamics in the Doctor-Patient Relationship

Several physicians have commented on the dynamics of the doctor-patient relationship and how these dynamics may play out when one of the potential cures is death (e.g., Miles, 1994; Wesley, 1993). For example, Miles (1994) reminds us that "physicians often have difficulties responding therapeutically to chronically ill or dying patients" (p. 1786). According to Miles, physicians feel frustrated and inadequate about irreversible medical problems in their patients. He reviews evidence showing that physicians undertreat pain and overlook depression. He also reports that physicians tend to underestimate the quality of life of their chronically ill patients and assume that such patients would want to forego life-prolonging interventions. He speculates that such behavior results from physicians' own dread about disabilities and death, and from the belief that their patients are as discouraged by their condition as they are. "In such emotional

---

[18]The sex of the very first person whose assisted suicide was reported by the press was not identified. The first and second assisted suicide were covered in the same article.

relationships, physicians may acquire an inflated sense of their insights into suicidal patients' feelings and proceed to unusual and improper clinical acts," including the "medical enabling of suicidal choices" continues Miles (p. 1786). In other words, according to Miles, a suicide may at least in part "arise in response to a physician's need for release from a painful clinical relationship, rather than as an independent patient's choice" (p. 1786).

Similarly, Kass and Lund (1996) reflect on issues of choice and informed consent in the physician-patient relationship. They view the goal of patient autonomy in medical decisions as difficult to attain even in the best of circumstances, such as when the patient is in relatively good health. They believe such autonomy is a fiction when the person is seriously ill. Physicians have control and authority over key information regarding prognosis, alternative treatment, and their appropriateness: "like many technical experts, they are masters at framing the options to guarantee a particular outcome" (p. 408). When the physician tells a patient about an illness with a terrible prognosis" and includes among the options the offer of a 'gentle quick release,' what will the patient likely choose, especially in the face of a spiraling hospital bill or resentful children?" (p. 408). Also, "with patients thus reduced—helpless in action and ambivalent about life" physicians and families do not need to be "consciously manipulative," note Kass and Lund. "Well-meaning and discreet suggestions, or even unconscious changes in expression, gesture, and tone of voice, can move a dependent and suggestible patient toward a choice for death" (p. 407).

When the element of gender is added to this interaction, with the female as the patient and the male as the physician, the power differential dynamics described by Miles (1994), and by Kass and Lund (1996) are likely to be exacerbated (Wolf, 1996a). The potential for unconscious projections and for acting out gender scripts of subordination and dominance is heightened. We know that women suffer from discrimination in their relationships to physicians, a majority of whom are male (Council on Ethical and Judicial Affairs, American Medical Association, 1991). This discrimination includes a failure to take women's complaints seriously, and a failure to equitably provide major diagnostic and therapeutic interventions. According to the Council on Ethical and Judicial Affairs, American Medical Association, these disparities in care may be fueled by a general perception that women's contributions to society are less than men, and that women, therefore, do not deserve high-quality and high-cost care. The evidence leads one to wonder whether male physicians may be particularly prone to validate women's requests for hastened death (see Canetto, 1995, 1996). Dr. Herbert Cohen, a Dutch practitioner of hastened death, speculated that women in general "can make an appeal to a doctor that is stronger, more existential" (Hendin, 1994, p. 136). According to Wolf (1996a), it would be remarkable if a lifetime of experiences in social structures which devalue women would not influence a physician's judgment about the quality and worth of the lives of female patients.

In the case of hastened death, having a meaningful and long-lasting relationship with the physician may actually add to the dangers (Canetto, 1996) rather than increase the safeguards for the patient, as some have argued (e.g., Battin, 1994; Quill, Cassel, & Meier, 1992). Such a personal relationship may increase the physician's feelings of frustration and embarrassment about being unable to help, and add to the physician's impulse to withdraw from the patient via enabling the acceleration of the patient's dying process. A close relationship between a physician and a patient could also amplify the psychological authority of the physician in the eyes of the patient, adding to the patient's vulnerability to the physician's expert and "caring" opinion.

Gender dynamics in the relationship between Kevorkian and his female clients were explored in a *Detroit Free Press* article back in 1991, when there had been only three female deaths (Bratt, 1991). "The fatal attraction for the women who used the Kevorkian techniques . . . is that it offered them a passive way to end their life with the approval of a paternalistic figure" wrote Bratt (p. 1A). "There may be an element of the kindly father figure granting permission," Irene Deitch, a clinical psychologist, was quoted as saying in the same article. She suggested that, while the person believes she is in control, she has actually relinquished control to Kevorkian. The presence of someone who promises a "peaceful," "dignified" and "gentle" "deliverance"—"a soft landing," as Good put it (Lessenberry, 1997, p. 82)—may mollify a person's ambivalence (Bratt, 1991, p. 9A). In a more recent article, Gutmann (1996) also addressed the fatal attraction element in Kevorkian's relationship with his female clients, and argued that "Dr. Jack" appealed to women's altruism and wish to be perfect. For example, according to Gutmann, Janet Adkins, Kevorkian's first client, and someone "who spent her life attempting to be perfect" was attracted to "the formality, the jargon, the bureaucracy" of Kevorkian's operation.

CONCLUSIONS

In a recent article on euthanasia, Battin argued that documentation is the "most important mechanism for the control of abuse" in hastened death. "Retroactive inspection" of cases allows an answer to "many quite revealing questions" such as: "Do some doctors provide assistance in suicide more frequently than others?" or "Do African-American patients 'choose' euthanasia more often than white?" she wrote (1994, p. 178). We believe that our study represents a contribution to documenting the practice of assisted suicide. To our knowledge, this is the first study to explore the gender dynamics in the choice and implementation of assisted suicide.

Our main finding is that most of the persons who died with the assistance of Dr. Kevorkian were women of European-American descent. Typically these women were suffering from a chronic, disabling but nonterminal-stage condition. Because of the nature of our data, we do not know what may account for the patterns we observed. It is possible that our findings are primarily due to unique selection biases associated with Kevorkian's practice. Alternatively, they may result from an interaction of factors specific to women, including women's courage and pragmatic attitudes about their own deaths, their diminished sense of entitlement, their reduced access to resources, a societal devaluing of women's lives, and a legacy of positive images of women's hastened deaths. Real and symbolic power issues in the relationship between male doctor and female patient probably also played a role. Clearly we need more research on what leads to a hastened death, and on why women and men make that choice.

Because many of the factors potentially involved in the decision to seek a hastened death differentially affect women and men, we believe this research should keep a clear focus on gender. In the meantime, examining these findings in light of related evidence should lead to concern that the option of hastened death may be more of a danger than an opportunity, a duty more than a choice, particularly for women. A focus on individual choice and self-determination obscures the complex, and often subtle, pressures on women to seek death. It renders invisible those interpersonal, economic, social, and cultural forces that make the collaboration of women, their families and physicians in actively ending women's lives look right and rational.

ACKNOWLEDGMENTS

The authors acknowledge the contribution of Miqelle DeMeis, Kimberly Hawley, Heather Hirschfeld, and Tammy K. Maglia, who assisted in the data collection and management. We are grateful to Kevin Ann Oltjenbruns, Ph.D., Wendy Warren, Keith Wilson, Ph.D., and David B. Wohl, Ph.D., for their review of the manuscript. Special thanks to Alicia S. Cook, Ph.D., who asked us critical questions. We also wish to recognize the staff of Colorado State University Library, Interlibrary Loan Services, for their assistance in procuring many of the out-of-state newspaper articles; Valerie J. Assetto, Ph.D., and Steve P. Mumme, Ph.D., Department of Political Sciences, Colorado State University, for many of the in-state newspaper references; and Madalyn Kelly, Ph.D., Department of Psychology, Northern Territory University, Darwin, Australia, for the Australian references. Finally, we thank Ljubisa J. Dragovic, M.D., and Werner U. Spitz, M.D., Michigan Medical Examiners for Oakland and Macomb County respectively, for providing the data on diseases, terminal status, and/or cause of death. Earlier versions of this article were presented at the meeting of the American Association of Suicidology, Phoenix, Arizona, May 1995; at the meeting of the 26th International Congress of Psychology, Montréal, Québec, Canada, August 1996; and at a colloquium given at Northern Territory University, Darwin, Northern Territory, Australia, March 1997.

APPENDIX A
Data Sources

Abramowitz, M. (1992, December 17). Kevorkian aids in two more suicides. *The Washington Post*, p. A2.

After latest assisted suicide, body is left near a hospital (1995, August 22). *The New York Times*, p. C19.

An ill woman kills herself with help from Kevorkian. (1996, June 22). *The New York Times*, p. 9A.

Anstett, P., & Cheyfitz, K. (1996, September 9). Police judgment debated. *The Detroit News Home Page* [On-line].

Anstett, P., Crumm, D., & Cheyfitz, K. (1996, September 13). Disease not found after 3 suicides. *The Detroit News Home Page [On-line]*.

Associated Press. (1991, October 24). Doctor assists in two more suicides in Michigan. *The New York Times*, pp. A1, B9.

Associated Press. (1991, October 24). Suicide doctor assists in 2 more deaths. *The Washington Post*, p. A31.

Associated Press. (1992, November 24). Doctor in Michigan assists in a 6th suicide. *The Washington Post*, p. A10.

Associated Press. (1992, December 16). Two commit suicide, aided by Michigan doctor. *The New York Times*, p. A22.

Associated Press. (1993, February 9). Kevorkian aids in two more suicides: Total is at 15. *The New York Times*, p. A6.

Associated Press. (1993, February 16). Kevorkian helps invalid kill himself with gas. *The Denver Post*, p. B2.

Associated Press. (1993, February 19). Kevorkian assists two more suicides: Approaching law spurs speedup. *The Denver Post*, p. A3.

Associated Press. (1993, September 11). Officials debate how to handle suicide doctor. *The Detroit Free Press*, p. 7A.

Associated Press. (1993, October 23). Kevorkian helps woman die, aiding suicide for 19th time. *The Washington Post*, p. A2.

Associated Press. (1994, November 27). Kevorkian present at death ruled homicide in Michigan. *The Washington Post*, p. A12.

Associated Press. (1995, May 14). Latest death in Kevorkian's presence ruled homicide. *The Washington Post*, p. A17.

Associated Press. (1995, June 27). Kevorkian attends a death at his new clinic. *The Washington Post*, p. A3.

Associated Press. (1996, June 12). Kevorkian attends the suicide of stroke-ridden N.J. woman. *The Washington Post*, p. A22.

Associated Press. (1996, August 8). Jack Kevorkian at 34th suicide. *The Detroit News*, p. 1A.

Associated Press. (1996, August 20). In Detroit, sides clash over suicide. *The New York Times*, p. A11.

Associated Press. (1996, August 23). Kevorkian brings 2 more bodies to Michigan hospital. *The Washington Post*, p. A4.

Associated Press. (1996, August 27). In Oakland County: Suicide of Kevorkian's 37th patient was a family decision. *The Detroit News* [On-line].

Associated Press. (1996, September 4). Latest person to die in Kevorkian's presence had pancreatic cancer. *The Detroit News* [On-line].

Associated Press. (1997, August 30). Kevorkian attends death of Colorado man at Farmington Hills motel. *The Detroit News* [On-line].

Associated Press. (1997, September 6). Coroner: Janet Good would have lived more than 6 months. *The Detroit News* [On-line].

Associated Press. (1997, September 21). Canadian man leaves letter saying he committed suicide with Kevorkian's help. *The Detroit News* [On-line].

Associated Press. (1997, October 4). Note found near body mentions Kevorkian. *The Detroit Free Press,* p. 11A.

Associated Press. (1997, October 9). Kevorkian patient's death called homicide. *Kentucky Post.* p. 3K.

Associated Press. (1997, October 17). Kevorkian ends meeting with woman when police arrive. *The Detroit News* [On-line].

Associated Press. (1997, November 22). Kevorkian aids West Palm woman in death. *Palm Beach Post,* p. 3A.

Associated Press. (1997, November 23). Residents recall women in assisted suicide case. *The New York Times* [On-line].

Associated Press. (1997, December 13). Kevorkian supporter assists California woman's suicide. *The Detroit News* [On-line].

Bakri, L. (1997, December 29). Kevorkian deaths anger lawmakers. *The Detroit News* [On-line].

Bakri, L., DeHaven, J., & French, R. (1997, March 20). Pennsylvania man may be Kevorkian's latest. *The Detroit News* [On-line].

Basheda, V. (1990, June 6). Suicide woman's quiet death sets off debate. *The Detroit News and Free Press,* pp. C7-C8.

Bebow, J., & Trent, K. (1994, November 27). Kevorkian assists at suicide of woman, 72. *The Detroit News and Free Press,* pp. 1A, 14A.

Belkin, L. (1990, June 6). Doctor tells of first death using his suicide device. *The New York Times,* p. A1.

Bell, D. (1997, December 31). Suicide patient mentally unwell niece says he had history of problems. *The Detroit Free Press,* p. 1A.

Bennet, J. (1995, May 9). Kevorkian is in attendance at suicide for the 22d time. *The New York Times,* p. B15.

Betzold, M. (1993). *Appointment with Doctor Death.* Troy, MI: Momentum Books.

Betzold, M. (1995, May 13). 23rd suicide brings calls for jailing. *The Detroit Free Press,* pp. 1A, 6A.

Betzold, M. & Gerdes, W. (1992, May 16). Kevorkian attends another suicide. *The Detroit News and Free Press,* pp. D12-D14.

Body in auto is reported to be Kevorkian's 26th assisted suicide. (1995, November 9). *The New York Times,* p. A17.

Body found in Romulus motel; Fieger represents family. (1997, May 7). *The Detroit News* [On-line].

Bowler, T. (1993, February 5). Pain was too great for 'happy Irishman.' *The Detroit News,* p. 4A.

Bowles, S., DeSimons, B., & Sweeney, A. (1992, September 27). Kevorkian assists in suicide no. 5. *The Detroit News and Free Press,* p. 1A.

Brand-Williams, O., & Hurt, C. (1996, September 30). Psychiatrist 41st to die in Kevorkian's presence. *The Detroit News* [On-line].

Bratt, H., & Hernandez, R. (1992, November 24). React: Woman's angry friend lashes at Dr. Death. *The Detroit News,* pp. 1A, 9A.

Cole, K. (1994, November 28). Lawmaker says legalization of assisted suicide needed now. *The Detroit News,* pp. 1B, 4B.

Costello, N. (1995, May 13). Monday victim 'made gift of his death,' widow says. *The Detroit News,* pp. 1A, 3A.

Coyne, T. (1996, September 8). Kevorkian client takes life after police delay suicide. *The Detroit News,* p. A10.

Chefitz, K., & Anstett, P. (1996, September 20). Kevorkian video suggests deception. *The Detroit News* [On-line].

Daughterry, J. (1996, August 21). Judith Curren's last days were a blur of drugs and pain. *The Detroit News,* p. 5C.

DeHaven, J. (1996, June 12). Kevorkian changes strategy. *The Detroit News,* pp. 1C, 5C.

DeHaven, J. (1996, August 21). Cops question suicide victim's spouse. *The Detroit News,* pp. 1C, 5C.

DeHaven, J. (1996, September 9). Women recalls mother's final battle. *The Detroit News* [On-line].

DeHaven, J. (1996, October 25). Hospital workers say police didn't assault Kevorkian. *The Detroit News* [On-line].

DeHaven, J., & Harmon, B. (1996, September 4). In Birmingham: Police puzzled over where assisted suicide occurred. *The Detroit News* [On-line].

DeHaven, J. & Harmon, B. (1997, February 5). Funeral home most used by Kevorkian is called in again. *The Detroit News* [On-line].

De La Cruz, D. (1997, November 15). Suicide victim's neighbor says 'no one knew she was sick.' *The Detroit news* [On-line].

Detroit Free Press Staff (1997). *The suicide machine.* Detroit Free Press.

Doctor assists 2 more suicides in Michigan. (1992, December 16). *The New York Times,* p. 14A.

Doctor in Michigan helps a 6th person to commit suicide. (1992, November 24). *The New York Times,* p. A10L.

Douglas, I. (1990, June 6). Doctor assists woman's suicide. *The Detroit News and Free Press,* p. 1A.

Dubrowski, J. (1993, September 11). Dr. Death defies law, deal again. *The Rocky Mountain News,* p. 36A.

Ensslin, J. (1997, October 1). Woman's death linked to Kevorkian Arapaho resident found in motel room; note describes agony multiple sclerosis. *The Rocky Mountain News,* p. 5A.

Farnsworth, C. (1996, May 9). Tape recalls a Canadian's gratitude to Kevorkian. *The New York Times,* p. A5.

Fornoff, R., & Arellano, A. (1993, May 17). In Detroit, suicide doctor challenges new state law. *The Detroit Free Press,* pp. 1A, 4A.

Fracassa, H. (1997, March 20). In Macomb County: No charges expected in death of Nebraskan. *The Detroit News* [On-line].

Garrett, C. (1996, January 30). Kevorkian assists in 27th suicide. *The Detroit News,* pp. 1A, 4A.

Garrett, C. (1997, April 10). Kevorkian, woman talked about suicide, lawyer says. *The Detroit News* [On-line].

Goldberg, R. (1997, December 28). Kevorkian questioned after delivering body to medical examiner's office. *The Detroit Free Press* [On-line].

Grant, D., & Bakri, L. (1997, December 4). Kevorkian associate aids Detroit suicide. *The Detroit News* [On-line].

Green, J. (1992, May 16). Illness just killed her spirit, neighbors say. *Oakland Press,* pp. A1, A8.

Greenwood, T., & Daugherty, J. (1996, October 11). Texas man is Kevorkian's 42nd suicide. *The Detroit News* [On-line].

Harmon, B. (1996, June 20). Don't bring bodies here, Pontiac tells Kevorkian. *The Detroit Free Press*, p. 1C.

Harmon, B. (1996, July 11). Catholics see latest suicide as slap in face. *The Detroit News*, p. 1D.

Harmon, B. (1996, August 23). Kevorkian assists 2 deaths in one day. *The Detroit News*, pp. 1A, 10A.

Harmon, B., & Garrett, C. (1997, May 8). In Romulus: Cops find body after media call. *The Detroit News* [On-line].

Harmon, B., Josar, D., & Heinlein, G. (1996, May 9). Canadian man's suicide impacts Kevorkian case. *The Detroit News*, pp. 1A, 9A.

Harmon, B. (1997, August 14). Kevorkian assists 54th suicide. *The Detroit News* [On-line].

Harmon, B. (1997, August 28). Coroner: No sign of cancer in Good. *The Detroit News* [On-line].

Harmon, B. (1997, November 23). Autopsies challenge new Kevorkian suicides. *The Detroit News* [On-line].

Helms, M. (1996, September 3). Kevorkian present at suicide No. 39 *The Detroit Free Press* [On-line].

Helms, M. (1997, September 4). Kevorkian returns to a hotel for latest suicide. *The Detroit Free Press* [On-line].

Helms, M. & Castine, J., & Laitner, B. (1997, October 9). *The Detroit Free Press*, p. 2B.

Hettena, S. (1997, November 22). Attorney: Kevorkian present at two deaths. *The Detroit News* [On-line].

Hughes, J. (1997, July 2). Fieger announces deaths of two multiple sclerosis patients. *The Detroit News* [On-line].

Hyde, J. (1997, June 28). Kevorkian linked to Nevada woman's death in Southfield. *The Detroit News* [On-line].

Ilka, D. (1990, June 5). Doctor assists woman's suicide. *The Detroit Free Press,* p. C9.

Ilka, D. (1995, November 15). Kevorkian issue puts medical examiner to test. *The Detroit Free Press*, pp. 1D, 5D.

Ilka, D., & Larabee, J. (1995, November 9). Officials attack Kevorkian-again. *The Detroit News*, pp. C1, C4.

Ingersoll, B., Powers, R., & Martindale, M. (1993, May 17). Kevorkian role in latest death unclear; legal tangle deepens. *The Detroit News*, pp. 1A, 6A.

Irwin, J. (1997, November 23). Attorney says Kevorkian was present at two deaths. *The Detroit Free Press* [On-line].

Johnson, B., Greenwalt, J., & Hauser, S. (1990, June 25). A vital woman chooses death. *People Weekly*, 40-43.

Josar, D. (1996, October 1). Sparks fly at suicide hearing; 41st death is ruled homicide. *The Detroit News* [On-line].

Kevorkian aids in two more suicides; total is at 15. (1993, February 9). *The New York Times*, p. A6.

Kevorkian aids in suicide; Prosecutor ousted in vote (1996, August 8). *The Washington Post*, p. A11.

Kevorkian aids suicide in bid for jail. (1993, October 23). *The New York Times*, p. 8.

Kevorkian assists 33rd suicide. (1996, July 10). *ERGO! News Bulletin* [On-line].

Kevorkian assists in death of 39-year-old woman. (1996, July 11). *The Washington Post*, p. A11.

Kevorkian attends 27th suicide. (1996, January 30). *The Washington Post*, p. A3.

Kevorkian attends 36th suicide. (1996, August 21). *DeathNet* [On-line].

Kevorkian attends another Michigan Death. (1996, January 30). *The New York Times*, p. C23.

Kevorkian attends death, opens clinic. (1995, June 27). *The Coloradoan*, p. A2.

Kevorkian attends suicide of 58-year-old cancer patient. (1995, November 9). *The Washington Post*, p. A12.

Kevorkian attends suicide of minister despite rulings. (1995, May 9). *The Washington Post*, p. A16.

Kevorkian brings two more bodies to Michigan Hospital. (1996, August 23). *The Washington Post*, p. A4.

Kevorkian challenges motive in offer of aid. (1994, November 29). *The New York Times*, p. A16.

Kevorkian held briefly after 2nd suicide in a day. (1996, August 23). *The New York Times*, p. A15.

Kevorkian helps a New Jersey woman die. (1996, June 12). *The New York Times*, p. A9.

Kevorkian helps man with cancer kill self. (1996, September 2). *The Coloradoan*, p. A2.

Kevorkian helps Tennessee cancer patient to die. (1996, September 2). *DeathNet* [On-line].

Kevorkian is at suicide (1995, August 22). *The Washington Post*, p. A7.

Kevorkian leaves body of woman at hospital. (1996, October 18). *The New York Times*, p. A12.

Kevorkian linked to another suicide. (1997, September 8). *Miami Herald* [On-line].

Kevorkian present at 31st suicide. (1996, June 21). *CNN Home Page* [On-line].

Kevorkian's toll. (1997, August 14). *The Washington Post*, p. A9.

King, R. (1997, November 23). Area woman cheery as she readied to die. *Palm Beach Post*, p. 1A.

Kostelni, N. (1997, September 5). PA woman sought out Kevorkian after three years of being in pain. *New Jersey Inquirer* [On-line].

Krodel, B., & Murphy, B. (1997, April 10). Fourth suicide found 27-year-old woman suffered from AIDS. *The Detroit Free Press* [On-line].

Larabee, J., McClear, J., & Powers, R. (1995, May 9). Kevorkian at 22nd suicide. *The Detroit News*, pp. 1A, 3A.

Lessenberry, J. (1995, November 12). Dr. Kevorkian resumes use of machine. *The New York Times*, p. 25.

Lessenberry, J. (1996, September 8). Kevorkian helps 40th suicide, day after police tried to intervene. *The New York Times*, p. 38.

Lessenberry, J. (1996, September 21). Video may lead to case against Kevorkian. *The New York Times*, p. 6.

Lopez, M., & Brand-Williams, O. (1996, October 24). Fieger says Royal Oaks cops bruised Kevorkian after his 44th attended suicide. *The Detroit News* [On-line].

Lopez, M., & Garrett, C. (1997, December 17). California woman, 89, dies with Kevorkian at her side. *The Detroit News* [On-line].

Martin, J. (1996, July 6). Kevorkian is present at 32nd suicide. *The Detroit Free Press*, p. 3A.

Martin, J. (1996, September 4). Fieger scorns Kevorkian's critics. *The Detroit News* [On-line].

Martindale, M. (1991, October 25). Strangers linked in death by Kevorkian. *The Detroit News*, pp. A1, A3.

Martindale, M., & Ourlian, R. (1991, November 3). Kevorkian suicide patient was on Halcion. *The Detroit News*, pp. 1A, 9A.

Martindale, M. (1993, November 23). Kevorkian quiet after 20th death. *The Detroit News*, pp. 1A, 4A.

Matthews, L., & McKay, D. (1995, August 22). Kevorkian attends 25th suicide since '90. *The Detroit Free Press*, pp. B1, B3.

McClear, J. A. (1990, December 14). Suicide Doc clear of murder. *The Detroit News*, p. 1A.

McClear, J. A., Martindale, M., & Ourlian, R. (1992, November 24). Kevorkian: Medicide is 'acceptable'. *The Detroit News*, pp. 1A, 9A.

McHugh, J. (1996, September 16). Post Mortem. *People Weekly, 46,* 52-55.

Meredith, R. (1997, November 15). Kevorkian helps woman die in a Roman Catholic Church. *The New York Times* [On-line].

Michalak, J. (1992, May 24). Mum witnesses hold up probe. *Daily Tribune,* pp. 1A, 6A.

Mishra, R. (1997, December 4). State going after Kevorkian new doctor involved in the latest suicide. *The Detroit Free Press* [On-line].

Mishra, R. (1997, December 5). Latest suicide breaks pattern Kevorkian colleague aids woman's death. *The Detroit Free Press* [On-line].

Montgomery, T. (1997, December 13). O.C. life ends in assisted suicide. *The OC Register* [On-line].

Murphy, B. (1997, February 4). Kevorkian is mum on latest 2 corpses. *The Detroit Free Press* [On-line].

Murphy, B. (1997, August 15). Expert rules hotel death a homicide. *The Detroit Free Press*, p. 4B.

Murphy, B. (1997, December 13). Kevorkian apprentice helps 2nd woman die; another homicide investigation begins. *The Detroit Free Press*, p. 3A.

Murphy, B., & Helms, M. (1997, September 9). Fieger denies woman was mentally unfit. *The Detroit Free Press* [On-line].

Murphy, B., & Jonas, I. (1997, March 26). Secrecy surrounds recent suicides; Fieger quiet. *The Detroit Free Press* [On-line].

Murphy, B., & McDiarmid, H. (1997, June 28). A decision in D.C.—A death in Southfield woman's body found in hotel on day of ruling. *The Detroit Free Press* [On-line].

Murphy, B., McKee, K., & Siegel, S. (1997, February 4). 2 corpses found; Kevorkian is mum both ruled dead of drug injection. *The Detroit Free Press* [On-line].

Murphy, B., & Niemiec, D. (1997, March 20). Pennsylvania man travels to Livonia to kill himself. *The Detroit Free Press* [On-line].

Murphy, B., Montemurri, P., & Abraham, M. (1997, November 14). Kevorkian aids suicide at church lawyer Fieger denies act was slap at Catholic Foes. *The Detroit Free Press*, p. 1A.

Musial, R. (1995, May 13). Family supported victim's decision; his life 'was torture'. *The Detroit Free Press*, p. 6A.

National News Briefs; Kevorkian lawyer gives rational for a suicide. (1997, March 8). *The New York Times*, p. 11.

Nayolor, J., & Pardo, S. (1997, October 1). Colorado woman with MS ends life; police investigate link to Kevorkian. *The Detroit News* [On-line].

News Services. (1997, February 4). Women's bodies are left at Michigan facilities, one in Kevorkian's van. *The Washington Post*, p. A2.

News Services. (1997, November 15). Kevorkian patient had kept quiet about ill N.Y. neighbors describe her as kind, friendly. *The Detroit News*, pp. 1A, 4A.

North, K., Cheyfitz, K., & Martin, J. (1996, October 18). Indiana community mourns latest suicide. *The Detroit News* [On-line].

Nortin, J. (1997, March 8). Woman wracked by crippling arthritis flew to Michigan to die. *The Detroit News* [On-line].

Obituaries. (1997, September). *The Gazette* [On-line]. Available: Gazette.com.

O'Keeffe, M. (1997, May 8). Kevorkian helps Arvadan kill herself husband accompanies paralyzed victim of multiple sclerosis, 63, to Detroit-Area motel. *The Rocky Mountain News*, p. 4A.

Ourlian, R. (1992, December 16). Ailing, but ready: 'I led a good life.' *The Detroit News and Free Press*, p. 11C.

Ourlian, R. (1993, January 21). Kevorkian strikes in Wayne county: Prosecutor hasn't decided about charges. *The Detroit News*, pp. 1B, 2B.

Ourlian, R. (1993, February 5). Kevorkian goes up north; town shaken by two suicides. *The Detroit News*, pp. 1A, 4A.

Ourlian, R. (1993, February 19). Area doctors take a stand: Wayne County Medical Society opposes new law banning assisted suicides. *The Detroit News*, p. 1B.

Ourlian, R. (1993, February 19). Kevorkian helps two more persons die. *The Detroit News*, pp. 1B, 2B.

Ourlian, (1993, August 5). Kevorkian assists in suicide on Belle Isle. *The Detroit News*, pp. 1A, 6A.

Ourlian, R. (1995, May 14). Angry mother praises Kevorkian, criticizes physicians: 'No doctor would help us'. *The Detroit News*, p. 4C.

Ourlian, R., & Martindale, M. (1993, February 9). Kevorkian assists in 12th suicide. *The Detroit News*, pp. 1B, 6B.

Ourlian, R., Martindale, M., & Bratt, H. M. (1992, May 17). Suicide rehearsal: 'I want to die'. *The Detroit News and Free Press*, p. 1A.

Ourlian, R., & Williams, C. (1993, May 18). Police lack evidence on Kevorkian. *The Detroit News*, pp. 1A, 6A.

Pardo, S. (1997, October 15). Latest death could be rebuke from Kevorkian. *The Detroit News* [On-line].

Powers, R. (1992, December 16). Her wait ends—death fulfills dream. *The Detroit News*, p. 11C.

Prosecutor of Kevorkian loses re-election bid. (1996, August 8). *The New York Times*, p. A23.

Reuters. (1997, June 27). Kevorkian lawyer hired in death case. *The New York Times*, p. 10 [On-line].

Reuters. (1997, October 4). National News Briefs: Kevorkian patient found dead at hotel. *The New York Times*, p. 16 [On-line].

Reuters. (1997, October 10). National News Brief: Patient of Kevorkian is found dead in a motel. *The New York Times*, p. 19 [On-line].

Reyes, B. (1997, October 4). Body found in Livonia motel, with note to call Fieger. *The Detroit News* [On-line].

Schabath, G., & Ourlian, R. (1993, February 16). Kevorkian critics wanted assisted-suicide ban now. *The Detroit News*, pp. 1B, 4B.

Schrader, E. (1997, December 13). O.C. woman's suicide is reported. *Los Angeles Times* [On-line].

Sekhar, A., & Durfee, D. (1997, July 3). 2 women with MS found dead; Kevorkian is mum. *The Detroit News* [On-line].

Seymour, L., & Ourlian, R. (1995, June 27). 'Mercy clinic' has its first suicide. *The Detroit News*, p. A1.

Sheinwald, R. (1997, March 8). Fieger says woman found in Romulus committed suicide. *The Detroit News* [On-line].

Shepardson, D. (1997, October 31). Kevorkian helps stroke victim die. *The Detroit News* [On-line].

Storey, K., & Bakri, L. (1997, November 14). Suicide victim dies in church: Kevorkian assists, drops off N.Y. woman at hospital, Fieger says. *The Detroit News* [On-line].

Storey, K., & Lama, B. (1997, September 4). Kevorkian assists suicide of PA woman. *The Detroit Free Press* [On-line].

Stout, D. (1997, August 28). Janet Good, 73; Advocated the right to die. *The New York Times*, p. 19 [On-line].

Terry, D. (1993, August 5). Kevorkian aids in suicide, no. 17, near police station. *The New York Times*, p. A8.

Terry, D., (1993, August 5). Kevorkian assists in suicide of 30-year-old ALS sufferer. *The Denver Post*, p. A2.

Terry, D. (1993, November 23). While out on bail, Kevorkian attends a doctor's suicide. *The New York Times*, pp. A1, A12.

The suicide regime. (1998, January 14). *The Detroit News Home Page* [On-line].

Two commit suicide, aided by Michigan doctor. (1992, December 16). *The New York Times,* p. A22.

Walsh, E. (1993, November 23). Physician, 61, dies with Kevorkian's assistance. *The Washington Post,* p. A1.

Walsh, E. (1996, August 24). No legal action is anticipated as Kevorkian suicides multiply. *The Washington Post,* p. A2.

Wife wanted to die. (1997, October 10). *Kentucky Post,* p. 15A.

Wilkerson, I. (1991, January 9). Talk of a search for relief and suicide. *The New York Times,* p. A14.

Wilkerson, I. (1991, October 25). Opponents weigh action against doctor who aided suicides. *The New York Times,* p. A10.

Wilkerson, I. (1993, May 17). In apparent defiance, doctor is present at another suicide. *The New York Times,* pp. A1, A9.

Williams, C. (1996, June 21). Kevorkian ready to set up mobile site for deaths, offer organ donations. *The Detroit News,* p. 9A.

Williams, C. (1996, June 20). Kevorkian strikes again: Assisted suicide toll at 30. *The Detroit News* [On-line].

Williams, C., & Greenwood, T. (1996, June 12). Kevorkian present at death of N.J. woman. *The Detroit News Home Page* [On-line].

Williams, C., & Lopez, M. (1996, June 21). Kevorkian at 2nd death in two days. *The Detroit News* p. 1A.

Williams, C., & Lopez, M. (1996, June 21). Ohio woman Kevorkian 31st death. *The Detroit News* [On-line].

Wylie, G., McClure, S., & Williams, M. (1990, June 6). Prosecutors want to stop doctor who helped suicide. *The Detroit News and Free Press,* p. 1A.

Young, A. (1997, August 28). Kevorkian helped Good die-Doctor there with family, daughter says. *The Detroit Free Press* [On-line].

Zeman, D. (1993, August 28). Kevorkian video shows death wish. *The Detroit News and Free Press,* pp. 1A, 10A.

Zeman, D. (1993, September 11). Kevorkian's bond may be shaky. *The Detroit News and Free Press,* p. 3A.

Zeman, D. (1993, October 23). Kevorkian acts again, risks jail. *The Detroit News and Free Press,* pp. 3A, 12A.

Zeman, D. (1993, October 23). Kevorkian helps another suicide. *The Denver Post,* p. A3.

REFERENCES

After latest assisted suicide, body is left near a hospital (1995, August 22). *The New York Times,* p. C19.

American Medical Association, Council on Ethical and Judicial Affairs (1992). Decisions near the end of life. *Journal of the American Medical Association, 267,* 2229-2233.

Anonymous (1988). It's over, Debbie. *Journal of the American Medical Association, 259,* 272.

Asch, D. A. (1996). The role of critical care nurses in euthanasia and assisted suicide. *The New England Journal of Medicine, 334,* 1374-1379.

Associated Press (1996, August 27). In Oakland County: Suicide of Kevorkian's 37th patient was a family decision. *The Detroit News* [On-line].

Associated Press. (1997, September 21). Canadian man leaves letter saying he committed suicide with Kevorkian's help. *The Detroit News* [On-line].

Back, A. L., Wallace, J. I., Starks, H. E., & Pearlman, R. A. (1996). Physician-assisted suicide and euthanasia in Washington State: Patient requests and physician response. *Journal of the American Medical Association, 275,* 919-925.

Basheda, V. (1990, June 6). Suicide woman's quiet death sets off debate. *The Detroit News and Free Press,* pp. C7-C8.

Battin, M. P. (1994). *The least worst death: Essays in bioethics on the end of life.* New York: Oxford University Press.

Belkin, L. (1993, November 14). There's no simple suicide. *The New York Times Magazine,* pp. 48-55, 63-64, 74-75.

Bell, N. B. (1992). If age becomes a standard for rationing health care . . . In H. B. Holmes & L. L. Purdy (Eds.), *Feminist perspectives in medical ethics* (pp. 82-90). Bloomington, IN: Indiana University Press.

Betzold, M. (1993). *Appointment with Doctor Death.* Troy, MI: Momentum Books.

Betzold, M., & Gerdes, W. (1992, May 16). Kevorkian attends another suicide. *The Detroit News and Free Press.* pp. D12-D14.

Bratt, H. M. (1991, October 25). Passive way to end life lures women. *The Detroit Free Press,* 1A, 9A.

Brody, H. (1992). Assisted death—A compassionate response to a medical failure. *The New England Journal of Medicine, 327,* 1384-1388.

Callahan, D. (1990). *What kind of life.* New York: Simon E. Schuster.

Callahan, D. (1995). *Setting limits: Medical goals in an aging society.* New York: Simon and Schuster.

Canetto, S. S. (1995). Elderly women and suicidal behavior. In S. S. Canetto & D. Lester (Eds.), *Women and suicidal behavior* (pp. 215-233). New York: Springer.

Canetto, S. S. (1996, August). *Suicide, assisted suicide and euthanasia among women.* 26th International Congress of Psychology, Montréal, Québec, Canada.

Canetto, S. S., & Lester, D. (1995). The epidemiology of women's suicidal behavior. In S. S. Canetto & D. Lester (Eds.), *Women and suicidal behavior* (pp. 35-57). New York: Springer.

Canetto, S. S., & Lester, D. (1998). Gender, culture and suicidal behavior. *Transcultural Psychiatry, 35,* 163-191.

Council on Ethical and Judicial Affairs, American Medical Association (1991). Gender disparities in clinical decision making. *Journal of the American Medical Association, 266,* 559-562.

Cox, D. W. (1993). *Hemlock's cup: The struggle for death with dignity.* Buffalo, NY: Prometheus Books.

Deluty, R. H. (1988-89). Physical illness, psychiatric illness, and the acceptability of suicide. *Omega—Journal of Death and Dying, 19,* 79-91.

Detroit Free Press Staff (1997). *The suicide machine.* Detroit, MI: Detroit Free Press.

Doukas, D. J., Waterhouse, D., Gorenflo, D. W., & Seid, J. (1995). Attitudes and behaviors on physician-assisted death: A study of Michigan oncologists. *Journal of Clinical Oncology, 13,* 1055-1061.

Downey, J., & Sherwin, S. (1996). A feminist exploration of issue around assisted death. *Saint Louis University Public Law Review, 15* (2), 303-330.

Emanuel, E. J., Fairclough, D. L., Daniels, E. R., & Clarridge, B. R. (1996). Euthanasia and physician-assisted suicide: Attitudes and experiences of oncology patients, oncologists, and the public. *Lancet, 347,* 1805-1810.

Farnsworth, C. (1996, May 9). Tape recalls a Canadian's gratitude to Kevorkian. *The New York Times,* p. A5.

Fox, E., & Kamakahi, J. J. (1996). Who is fighting to die? A look at the Hemlock Society membership. *TimeLines, The Hemlock Society, USA 68,* 1-10.

Fried, T. R., Stein, M. S., O'Sullivan, P. S., Brock, D. W., & Novack, D. H. (1993). Limits of patient autonomy: Physician attitudes and practices regarding life-sustaining treatments and euthanasia. *Archives of Internal Medicine, 153,* 722-728.

Friedman, D. (1997, February). One last choice, *Vogue,* 158-165.

Fung, K. K. (1993). Dying for money: Overcoming moral hazard in terminal illnesses through compensated physician-assisted death. *American Journal of Economics and Sociology, 52*(3), 275-288.

Gatz, M., Harris, J. R., & Turk-Charles, S. (1995). The meaning of health for older women. In A. L. Stanton & S. J. Gallant (Eds.), *The psychology of women's health* (pp. 491-529). Washington, DC: American Psychological Association.

Gilligan, C. (1982). *In a different voice: Psychological theory and women's development,* Cambridge, MA: Harvard University Press.

Gutmann, S. (1996, June 26). Death and the maiden. *The New Republic* [On-line].

Harmon, B. (1996, June 20). Don't bring bodies here, Pontiac tells Kevorkian. *The Detroit Free Press,* p. 1C.

Hendin, H. (1994). Seduced by death: Doctors, patients, and the Dutch cure. *Issues in Law and Medicine, 10* (2), 123-168.

Hendin, H. (1995). Assisted suicide, euthanasia, and suicide prevention: The implication of the Dutch experience. *Suicide and Life-Threatening Behavior, 25,* 193-204.

Hess, B. H. (1990). The demographic parameters of gender and aging. *Generations, 14,* 12-16.

Hoover, E., & Hill, G. K. (1998, March 26). Women on tape says she looks forward to relief, *The Oregonian* [On-line].

Humphry, D. (1992). Rational suicide among the elderly. *Suicide and Life-Threatening Behavior, 22,* 125-129.

Hyde, J. (1997, June 28). Kevorkian linked to Nevada woman's death in Southfield. *The Detroit News* [On-line].

Ilka, D. (1990, June 5). Doctor assists woman's suicide. *The Detroit Free Press,* p. C9.

Jecker, N. S. (1994). Physician-assisted death in the Netherlands and the United States: Ethical and cultural aspects of health policy development. *Journal of the American Geriatrics Society, 42,* 672-678.

Johnson, B., Greenwalt, J., & Hauser, S. (1990, June 25). A vital woman chooses death. *People Weekly,* 40-43.

Johnson, D., Fitch, S. D., Alston, J. P., & McIntosh, W. A. (1980). Acceptance of conditional suicide and euthanasia among older Americans. *Suicide and Life-Threatening Behavior, 10,* 157-166.

Kamisar, Y. (1996). The reasons so many people support physician-assisted suicide—And why these reasons are not convincing. *Issues in Law and Medicine, 12* (2), 113-131.

Kaplan, K. J., & DeWitt, J. (1996). Kevorkian's list: Gender bias or what? *Newslink, 22* (3), pp. 1-14.

Kass, L. R., & Lund, N. (1996). Physician-assisted suicide, medical ethics and the future of the medical profession. *Duquesne Law Review, 35* (1), 395-425.

Kevorkian, J. (1996, July). Speech before the National Press Club. *The Kevorkian File, DeathNet* [On-line].

Koenig, H. G., Wildman-Hanlon, D., & Schmader, K. (1996). Attitudes of elderly patients and their families toward physician-assisted suicide. *Archives of Internal Medicine, 156,* 2240-2248.

Kreimer, S. F. (1995). Does pro-choice mean pro-Kevorkian? An essay on *Roe, Casey,* and the right to die. *American University Law Review, 44,* 803-854.

Lee, M. A., Nelson, H. D., Tilden, V. P., Ganzini, L., Schmidt, T. A., & Tolle, S. W. (1996). Legalizing assisted suicide—Views of physicians in Oregon, *New England Journal of Medicine, 334,* 310-315.

Lessenberry, J. (1997, April). Death and the matron. *Esquire,* pp. 80-85, 131.

Lewis, R. J., & Shepeard, G. (1992). Inferred characteristics of successful suicides as function of gender and context. *Suicide and Life-Threatening Behavior, 22,* 187-196.

Loraux, N. (1987). *Tragic ways of killing a woman.* Cambridge, MA: Harvard University Press.

Major, B. (1987). Gender, justice, and the psychology of entitlement. In P. Shaver & C. Hendrick (Eds.), *Sex and gender* (pp. 124-148). Newbury Park, CA: Sage.

Marks, A. (1988-89). Structural parameters of sex, race, age, and education and their influence on attitudes toward suicide. *Omega—Journal of Death and Dying, 19,* 327-336.

Martin, A. (1991, November 4). Would it have made a difference if they were men? Feminists deplore second-guessing. *The Detroit Free Press* [On-line].

Martin, J., & Brasier, L. L. (1996, September 12). Fieger sees people going quietly. *The Detroit News* [On-line].

McIntosh, J. L. (1991). Middle-age suicide: A literature review and epidemiological study. *Death Studies, 15,* 21-37.

McIntosh, J. L., Pearson, J. L., & Lebowitz, B. D. (1997). Mental disorders of elderly men. In J. I. Kosberg & L. W. Kaye (Eds.), *Elderly men: Special problems and professional challenges* (pp. 193-215). New York: Springer.

McIntosh, J. L., Santos, J. F., Hubbard, R. W., & Overholser, J. C. (1994). *Elder suicide: Research, theory and treatment.* Washington, DC: American Psychological Association.

Meier, D. E., Emmons, C.-A., Wallenstein, S., Quill, T., Morrison, R. S., & Cassel, C. K. (1998). A national survey of physician-assisted suicide and euthanasia in the United States. *The New England Journal of Medicine, 338,* 1193-1201.

Miles, S. H. (1994). Physicians and their patients' suicides. *Journal of the American Medical Association, 271,* 1786-1788.

Miles, S. H. (1995). Physician assisted suicide and the profession's gyrocompass. *Hastings Center Report, 25*(3), 17-19.

Miles, S. H., & August, A. (1990). Courts, gender and the "right to die." *Law, Medicine, and Health Care, 18,* 85-95.

Mishra, R. (1997, December 4). State going after Kevorkian new doctor involved in the latest suicide. *The Detroit Free Press* [On-line].

Mishra, R. (1997, December 5). Latest suicide breaks pattern Kevorkian colleague aids woman's death. *The Detroit Free Press* [On-line].

Montgomery, T. (1997, December 13). O.C. life ends in assisted suicide. *The OC Register* [On-line].

Murphy, B., & McDiarmid, H. (1997, June 28). A decision in D.C.—A death in Southfield woman's body found in hotel on day of ruling. *The Detroit Free Press* [On-line].

Ourlian, R. (1993, February 5). Kevorkian goes up North; town shaken by two suicides. *The Detroit News,* pp. 1A, 4A.

Ourlian, R. (1993, February 19). Kevorkian helps 2 more persons die. *The Detroit News,* pp. 1B, 2B.

Ourlian, R. (1995, May 14). Angry mother praises Kevorkian, criticizes physicians: 'No doctor would help us'. *The Detroit News,* p. 4C.

Quill, T. E. (1991). Death and dignity: A case of individualized decision making. *The New England Journal of Medicine, 324,* 691-694.

Quill, T. E. (1996). *A midwife through the dying process: Stories of healing and hard choices at the end of life.* Baltimore, MD: The Johns Hopkins University Press.

Quill, T. E., Cassel, C. K., & Meier, D. E. (1992). Care of the hopelessly ill: Proposed clinical criteria for physician-assisted suicide. *The New England Journal of Medicine, 327,* 1380-1383.

Schrader, E. (1997, December 13). O.C. woman's suicide is reported. *Los Angeles Times* [On-line].

Seidlitz, L., Duberstein, P. R., Cox, C., & Conwell, Y. (1995). Attitudes of older people toward suicide and assisted suicide: An analysis of Gallup poll findings. *Journal of the American Geriatrics Society, 43,* 993-998.

Slome, L. R., Mitchell, T. F., Charlebois, E., Benevedes, J. M., & Abrams, D. I. (1997). Physician-assisted suicide and patients with human immunodeficiency virus disease. *The New England Journal of Medicine, 336,* 417-421.

Smith, W. J. (1997). Death wars. *National Review, 49* (13), 36-37.

Steinfels, P. (1993, February 14). Help for the helping hand in death. *The New York Times,* The Week in Review, pp. 1, 6.

Stillion, J. M., White, H., Edwards, P. J., & McDowell, E. E. (1989). Ageism and sexism in suicide attitudes. *Death Studies, 13,* 247-261.

The New York State Task Force on Life and the Law (1994). *When death is sought: Assisted suicide and euthanasia in the medical context.* New York: Author.

United Nations (1991). *Women: Challenges to the year 2000.* New York: Author.

van der Maas, P. J., van Delden, J. J. M., & Pijnenborg, L. (1992). Euthanasia and other medical decisions concerning the end of life: An investigation performed upon the request of the commission of inquiry into the medical practice concerning euthanasia [Special issue]. *Health Policy, 22* (1-2), 1-262.

van der Maas, P. J., van der Wal, G., Haverkate, I., De Graaff, C. L. M., Kester, J. G. C., Onwuteaka-Philpsen, B. D., van der Heide, A., Bosma, J. M., & Willems, D. L. (1996).

Euthanasia, physician-assisted suicide, and other medical practices involving the end of life in the Netherlands, 1990-1995. *The New England Journal of Medicine, 335,* 1699-1705.

Verlander, H. (1997, February 15). Women and the final solution. *The Canberra Times,* p. 16.

Wesley, P. (1993). Dying safely. *Issues in Law and Medicine, 8* (4), 467-485.

Wilkerson, I. (1991, January 9). Talk of a search for relief and suicide. *The New York Times,* p. A14.

Williams, C., & Greenwood, T. (1996, June 12). Kevorkian present at death of N.J. woman. *The Detroit News Home Page* [On-line].

Wolf, S. M. (1996a). Gender, feminism, and death: Physician-assisted suicide and euthanasia. In S. M. Wolf (Ed.), *Feminism and bioethics: Beyond reproduction* (pp. 282-317). New York: Oxford University Press.

Wolf, S. M. (1996b). Physician-assisted suicide in the context of managed care. *Duquesne Law Review, 35* (1), 455-479.

AN UPDATE ON THE KEVORKIAN-REDING 93 PHYSICIAN-ASSISTED DEATHS IN MICHIGAN: IS KEVORKIAN A SAVIOR, SERIAL-KILLER OR SUICIDAL MARTYR?

KALMAN, J. KAPLAN, PH.D.
Wayne State University and
Michael Reese Hospital and Medical Center

JYLL C. O'DELL, M.A.
John Jay College of Justice

LJUBISA J. DRAGOVIC, M.D.
Wayne State University Medical School
and Oakland County Medical Examiner's Office

M. CATHERINE McKEON, R.N.

EMILY BENTLEY

KAJA L. TELMET

Wayne State University

ABSTRACT

This report presents an update of the Kevorkian-Reding physician-assisted (or physician-aided) deaths to include the ninety-three publicly acknowledged cases as of November 25, 1998. These deaths are divided into ten distinct time phases. The following trends emerge. Over two-thirds of the decedents are women, the ratio of females to males varying widely with phase. The proportion of women seems to be highest when Kevorkian is free to act as he wants and lowest when he seems to be acting under legal or political restraints. Based on autopsy results, only 29.0 percent of the cases are terminal, this percentage being higher among men (37.9%) than among women (25.4%). However, 66.7% of the decedents were disabled, no significant difference emerging between men and women. Further, five out of the six decedents showing no apparent anatomical sign of disease at autopsy were women. Over 80 percent of the physician-assisted deaths are cremated, approximately twice as high a proportion as that emerging for suicides in Michigan and four times as high as cremations occurring with regard to overall deaths. Finally, death by carbon monoxide decreases dramatically with time phase while the use of the contraption dubbed the "suicide machine" increases, suggesting an increasing routinization over time. Finally, during the ninth and tenth phases, Kevorkian's aims and his own suicidality emerge more clearly, involving 1) harvesting of organs and 2) threat of starving himself in prison if he is convicted. Phase 10 can be seen as an escalation from assisted-death[1] to overt euthanasia, repeating the same need for a demonstration (Thomas Youk) that was first exhibited in Phase 1 (Janet Adkins).

Two previous articles in this special issue have focused specifically on data emerging from the physician-assisted deaths conducted in Michigan by Dr. Kevorkian and his associates. The first article (Kaplan, Lachenmeier, Harrow, O'Dell, Uziel, Schneiderhan, & Cheyfitz, 1999-2000) treated detailed data emerging from a quasi-psychological autopsy study conducted in conjunction with the Detroit Free Press which was obtained from friends and relatives of the first forty-seven of Kevorkian's publicly acknowledged deaths up to February 2, 1997. The second article (Canetto & Hollenshead, 1999-2000) dealt with information obtained largely from secondary sources (e.g., newspaper reports) regarding the first seventy-five Kevorkian-Reding deaths ending on December 28, 1997. These two reports present quite similar findings with regard to a predominance of women over men and an erosion of written safeguards over time.

Of special interest in the Kaplan, Lachenmeier, Harrow, O'Dell, Uziel, Schneiderhan, and Cheyfitz (1999-2000) article is the analysis of differences between four phases (Honeymoon, Prosecution, Revenge, and Business as Usual) defined by events occurring in the larger socio-political context in Michigan. The reader will remember that these phases were marked by three demarcation points:

1. December 15, 1992: Michigan Governor John Engler signs into law a temporary ban on physician assisted suicides.
2. May 14, 1996: Kevorkian is acquitted on murder charges in the deaths of Marjorie Wantz and Sherrie Miller, the last charges pending against him at that time.
3. August 6, 1996: Richard Thompson, Oakland County Prosecutor, who charged Kevorkian in those deaths is defeated in his bid for re-election in the Republican primary.

---

[1] All deaths investigated in Oakland County have been classified as euthanasia.

The present report presents initial data on the ninety-three publicly acknowledged and identified Kevorkian-Reding induced deaths as of November 25, 1998.[2] These are presented in Table 1.

The present report suggests seven additional significant socio-political points of demarcation:

4. February 6, 1997: Ionia County prosecutor Raymond Voet announces he will try to close a loophole which has allowed Kevorkian to assist suicides without violating the terms of his $10,000 personal bond. This occurs while Kevorkian was awaiting trial in Ionia for the assisted suicide of Loretta Peabody.

5. June 13, 1997: Circuit Court Judge Charles Miel declares a mistrial in the Ionia trial of Kevorkian because of his attorney Geoffrey Fieger's conduct in the courtroom, leaving it exceedingly unlikely that Kevorkian will ever again be tried on this case.

6. October 22, 1997: Announcing the second stage of his plan, Kevorkian gives his "organ harvesting" speech. This involves the harvesting of human organs for transplantation from the people he has helped kill themselves (Detroit Free Press, Oct. 23, 1997).

7. December 31, 1997: Kevorkian gives his "martyr" speech in which he compares himself to other historical martyrs. He predicts that he will be convicted by the state and he announces his intentions to starve himself to death. This would implicate the state by assisting him in his own suicide (Detroit Free Press, Jan. 1, 1998; Oakland Press, Jan. 1, 1998).

8. April 16, 1998: Kevorkian's attorney, Geoffrey Fieger, announces his candidacy for governor of Michigan against Republican incumbent John Engler who is another long-time nemesis of Kevorkian. On August 4, 1998, Fieger unexpectedly wins the Democratic primary in Michigan and becomes the Democratic candidate in the November 3 election against Engler. Proposal B to legalize physician-assisted suicide in Michigan is put on the November ballot. A Michigan state statute to ban assisted suicide in Michigan goes into effect on September pending the results on Proposal B in the November election.

9. November 3, 1998: Fieger is defeated for governor of Michigan by a margin of over two to one. Simultaneously, Proposal B calling for the legalization of physician-assisted suicide in Michigan (which Kevorkian opposes as being "too restrictive") is defeated by a ratio of almost three to one.

---

[2] Kevorkian has claimed over 130 physician-aided deaths but only 93 have been publicly identified as of this time. Once again, the names of the decedents are public record and have been published previously (The Detroit Free Press Staff, 1997).

Table 1. A Listing of the 93 Publicly Acknowledged Physician-Assisted
Deaths of Kevorkian and Reding (as of November 25, 1998)

	Name	Date of Death	Gender	Age	Diagnosis	Terminal
1	Janet Adkins	06/04/90	F	54	Alzheimer's disease	N
2	Sherry Miller	10/23/91	F	43	MS	N
3	Marjorie Wantz	10/23/91	F	58	No anatomical evidence of disease at autopsy	N
4	Susan Williams	05/15/92	F	52	MS	N
5	Lois F. Hawes	09/26/92	F	52	Lung cancer	Y
6	Catherine Andreyev	11/23/92	F	46	Breast cancer	Y
7	Marguerite Tate	12/15/92	F	70	ALS	Y
8	Marcella Lawrence	12/15/92	F	67	Emphysema; heart disease, arthritis	N
9	Jack E. Miller	01/20/93	M	53	Emphysema, prostate cancer	Y
10	Mary Biernat	02/04/93	F	73	Breast cancer	Y
11	Stanley Ball	02/04/93	M	82	Pancreatic cancer, blindness	Y
12	Elaine Goldbaum	02/08/93	F	47	MS	N
13	Hugh E. Gale, Sr.	02/15/93	M	70	Emphysema, congestive heart disease	N
14	Jonathan Grenz	02/18/93	M	44	Squamous cell cancer of upper and lower airways with metastases	Y
15	Martha Ruwart	02/18/93	F	41	Ovarian cancer with metastases	Y
16	Ronald Mansur	05/16/93	M	54	Bone and lung cancer	Y
17	Thomas Hyde, Jr.	08/04/93	M	30	ALS	Y
18	Donald O'Keefe	09/09/93	M	73	Bone cancer	Y
19	Merian Frederick	10/22/93	F	72	ALS	Y
20	Ali Khalili	11/22/93	M	61	Multiple myeloma	Y
21	Margaret Garrish	11/26/94	F	72	Rheumatoid arthritis, bilateral leg amputations, loss of one eye	N
22	John Evans	05/08/95	M	78	Pulmonary fibrosis	Y
23	Nicholas Loving	05/12/95	M	27	ALS	N
24	Erika Garcellano	06/26/95	F	60	ALS	N
25	Esther Cohan	08/21/95	F	45	MS, painful ulcers	N
26	Patricia Cashman	11/08/95	F	58	Skeletal metastases of breast cancer	N
27	Linda Henslee	01/29/96	F	48	MS	N
28	Austin Bastable	05/06/96	M	53	MS	N
29	Ruth Neuman	06/10/96	F	69	Cerebrovascular disease	N
30	Lona Jones	06/18/96	F	58	Astrocytoma	N
31	Bette Lou Hamilton	06/20/96	F	67	Syringemyelia	N
32	Shirley Cline	07/04/96	F	63	Bowel cancer	Y

Table 1. (Cont'd.)

	Name	Date of Death	Gender	Age	Diagnosis	Terminal
33	Rebecca Badger	07/09/96	F	39	No anatomical evidence of disease at autopsy	N
34	Elizabeth Mercz	08/06/96	F	59	ALS	N
35	Judith A. Curren	08/15/96	F	42	No anatomical evidence of disease at autopsy	N
36	Louise Siebens	08/20/96	F	76	ALS	N
37	Patricia Smith	08/22/96	F	40	MS	N
38	Pat DiGangi	08/22/96	M	66	MS	N
39	Loretta Peabody	08/30/96	F	54	MS	N
40	Jack Leatherman	09/02/96	M	73	Pancreatic cancer	Y
41	Isabel Correa	09/07/96	F	60	Status post spinal cord trauma	N
42	Richard Faw	09/29/96	M	71	Colon cancer	N
43	Wallace J. Spolar	10/10/96	M	70	MS, heart disease	N
44	Nancy de Soto	10/17/96	F	55	ALS	N
45	Barbara A. Collins	10/23/96	F	65	Ovarian cancer	Y
46	Elaine Louise Day	02/02/97	F	79	ALS	N
47	Lisa Lansing	02/02/97	F	42	Chronic inflammatory bowel disease	N
48	Helen P. Livengood	03/06/97	F	59	Rheumatoid arthritis pain, crippling esophagus problems	N
49	Albert Miley	03/19/97	M	41	Quadriplegia	N
50	Janette Knowles	03/24/97	F	75	Heart disease, emphysema	N
51	Heidi Aseltine	04/09/97	F	27	HIV	N
52	Delouise Bacher	05/07/97	F	63	MS	N
53	Janis Murphy	06/26/97	F	40	No anatomical evidence of disease at autopsy	N
54	Lynne Lennox	07/02/97	F	54	MS	N
55	Dorinda Scheipsmeier	07/02/97	F	51	MS	Y
56	Karen Shoffstal	08/13/97	F	34	MS	N
57	Janet Good	08/26/97	F	73	Microscopic evidence of residual pancreatic cancer at surgical resection margins	N
58	Thomas Summerlee	08/29/97	M	55	MS	N
59	Carol Fox	09/03/97	F	54	Ovarian cancer	Y
60	Deborah Sickels	09/07/97	F	43	MS	N
61	Natverlal Thakore	09/20/97	M	78	Parkinson's disease	N
62	Kari Miller	09/29/97	F	54	MS	Y
63	John Zdanowicz	10/03/97	M	50	ALS	N
64	Lois Carol Hawkins Caswell	10/08/97	F	65	Arteriosclerotic cardiovascular disease	N

Table 1. (Cont'd.)

	Name	Date of Death	Gender	Age	Diagnosis	Terminal
65	Annette Blackman	10/13/97	F	34	MS	Y
66	John O'Hara	10/30/97	M	54	Stroke, gout, kidney problems, heart and lung disease	N
67	Nadejdea Callimachi (Foldes)	11/13/97	F	72	Pancreatic cancer	Y
68	Naomi Sachs	11/21/97	F	84	Osteoporosis, heart disease, dementia	N
69	Bernice Gross	11/21/97	F	78	MS	N
70	Martha Wichorek	12/03/97	F	82	No anatomical evidence of disease at autopsy	N
71	Rosalind Haas	12/11/97	F	59	Breast and lung cancer	N
72	Margaret Weilhart	12/16/97	F	89	Stroke, paralysis, blindness	N
73	Cheri Tremble	12/16/97	F	46	Breast cancer	Y
74	Franz-Johann Long	12/27/97	M	53	Urinary bladder cancer	N
75	Mary Langford	12/27/97	F	73	Metastatic breast cancer	N
76	Nancy Ruth Rush	01/07/98	F	81	Lung cancer	Y
77	Carrie Hunter	01/18/98	M	35	HIV	N
78	Jeremy Allen	02/04/98	M	52	Kidney cancer	N
79	Muriel Clement	02/23/98	F	76	Parkinson's disease	N
80	Roosevelt Dawson	02/26/98	M	21	Quadriplegia	N
81	Patricia Graham	03/05/98	F	61	Heart disease	N
82	William Connaughton	03/05/98	M	42	No anatomical evidence of disease at autopsy	N
83	Waldo Herman	03/13/98	M	66	Lung cancer, heart disease	Y
84	Mary Judith Kanner	03/26/98	F	67	Huntington's disease	N
85	Shala Semino	04/08/98	F	47	ALS	N
86	Dixie Colleen Wilson	04/13/98	F	74	ALS	N
87	Jack Schenburn	04/16/98	M	89	Prostate cancer	Y
88	Priscilla Hiles	04/16/98	F	73	Chronic arthritis, sciatica, degenerative disk disease, asthma	N
89	Lucille Alderman	04/24/98	F	86	Heart disease/ osteoarthritis	N
90	Matthew Johnson	05/07/98	M	26	Quadriplegia	N
91	Emma Kassa	05/19/98	F	68	Lung cancer	Y
92	Joseph Tushkowski	06/07/98	M	45	Quadriplegia	N
93	Thomas Youk	09/17/98	M	52	ALS	N

10. November 25, 1998: Kevorkian is charged with first degree murder in the euthanasia death of Thomas Youk and released on personal bond given his assurances he will not participate in any doctor-assisted deaths. Kevorkian is subsequently convicted on March 26, 1999 of second degree murder and delivery of a controlled substance and is sentenced to ten to twenty-five years in prison on April 14, 1999.

All-in-all, the present report divides the ninety-three assisted suicides into ten distinct phases, the first four of which have been discussed previously:

Phase 1: The First Honeymoon: June 4, 1990 to December 15, 1992. In this phase, Kevorkian is unrestricted by any legal ban.

Phase 2: The First Prosecution: December 16, 1992 to May 14, 1996. In this phase, Kevorkian is facing murder charges on five of his cases, four of which have been initiated by Oakland County Prosecutor Richard Thompson (Wantz, Miller, Frederick, & Khalili). The fifth has been initiated in Wayne County with regard to the death of Thomas Hyde.

Phase 3: Revenge: May 15, 1996 to August 6, 1996. In this phase, Kevorkian has been acquitted on the existing charges filed against him and is free to take revenge on Thompson who is involved in running for re-election as prosecutor.

Phase 4: Business as Usual: August 7, 1996 to February 6, 1997. In this phase, Kevorkian has seemingly freed himself from prosecution in Oakland County as Thompson has been defeated for re-election.

Phase 5: The Second Prosecution: February 7, 1997 to June 13, 1997. In this phase, Kevorkian is facing a second prosecution in Ionia County for the death of Loretta Peabody.

Phase 6: The Second Honeymoon: June 14, 1997 to October 22, 1997. In this period, Kevorkian is free again from legal prosecution because the Ionia case has ended in a mistrial.

Phase 7: The Mission-Statement: October 23, 1997 to December 31, 1997. In this phase, Kevorkian embarks on his mission to harvest organs for transplantation from the people he has helped to kill themselves.

Phase 8: The Martyr-Statement: January 1, 1998 to April 16, 1998. In this phase, Kevorkian proclaims himself a martyr, and announces his intentions to starve himself to death in prison. If as Kevorkian expects, he is convicted by the state, it would "implicate the state in his suicide."

Phase 9: Constrained by Politics: April 17, 1998 to November 3, 1998. In this phase, Kevorkian is constrained during the race for governor of Michigan by his former attorney, Geoffrey Fieger's aspirations. In addition the ballot contains Proposal B, a proposal to legalize physician-assisted suicide in Michigan, that Kevorkian says he opposes as being too restrictive. During this period he attempts for the first time to harvest organs from a patient, removing the kidneys from Joseph Tushkowski on June 7, 1998. On September 1, a state statute banning participation in physician-assisted suicide goes into effect. After this, Kevorkian seemingly remains quiet. In reality, Kevorkian performs his first admitted euthanasia on Thomas Youk on September 17, 1998 which he does not report till after the election.

Phase 10: Free to Escalate: November 4, 1998 to November 25, 1998. Fieger and Proposal B are overwhelmingly defeated in the November 3 election. On November 4, Kevorkian offers a tape to CBS ("60 Minutes") of his act of euthanizing Thomas Youk on September 17, 1998 which had been unreported up to this point. On November 22, Kevorkian appears on "60 Minutes" with this tape, daring prosecutors to charge him and stating that in two weeks, if he is not charged, he will interpret this as allowing him to euthanize patients in distress. If he goes to prison, he will starve himself to death there. He also announces he has a new attorney. On November 25, Kevorkian is charged with first degree murder in the death of Thomas Youk which initiates a third prosecution phase. He is released on personal bond on his promise not to participate in any physician-assisted deaths. He is subsequently convicted of second degree murder and is currently in prison.

METHOD

The data on the complete set of ninety-three publicly acknowledged physician-assisted deaths as of November 25, 1998 should be regarded as preliminary. The psychological autopsy data collected on Cases one through forty-seven has not yet been done on cases forty-eight through ninety-three. Interviews have not yet been conducted on friends, family, or relevant medical personnel for these later cases. Thus we must rely only on the published autopsy findings of the respective medical examiners (Drs. Dragovic, Virani, and Pacris in Oakland County; Drs. Kanluen and Somerset in Wayne County; Dr. Spitz in Macomb County; and Dr. Houghton in Leelanau County). No autopsy was performed on the body of Loretta Peabody (Case #39) of Ionia County.

A. Independent Variables

Gender

Sixty-three women and thirty men.

Phase

The present report divides the ninety-three assisted deaths into ten distinct phases. The 93rd death of Thomas Youk has been placed in Phase 10 even though it technically occurred in Phase 9. This is because it was announced in Phase 10, and represents a dramatic escalation in Kevorkian's rhetoric from assisted suicide to euthanasia (again see Footnote 1).

Phase 1: The First Honeymoon: June 4, 1990 to December 15, 1992
Phase 2: The First Prosecution: December 16, 1992 to May 14, 1996

Phase 3: Revenge: May 15, 1996 to August 6, 1996

Phase 4: Business as Usual: August 7, 1996 to February 6, 1997

Phase 5: The Second Prosecution: February 7, 1997 to June 13, 1997

Phase 6: The Second Honeymoon: June 14, 1997 to October 22, 1997

Phase 7: The Mission-Statement: October 23, 1997 to December 31, 1997

Phase 8: The Martyr-Statement: January 1, 1998 to April 16, 1998

Phase 9: Constrained by Politics: April 17, 1998 to November 3, 1998

Phase 10: Free to Escalate: November 4, 1998 to November 25, 1998

B. Dependent Variables

The following variables were obtained from the death certificates.

Age

Age at time of death as obtained from death certificate

Years of Education

Years of education as obtained from death certificate.

Gender

Gender as obtained from death certificate.

Race

Race (Caucasian, African-American, Hispanic, or Asian) as obtained from death certificate.

Marital Status

Married or unmarried (single, divorced, or widowed) at time of death as obtained from death certificate.

County of Death

County (Oakland, Wayne, Macomb, Leelanau, or Ionia at time of death as obtained from death certificate.

Cause of Death

(By method: poisoning by carbon monoxide, poisoning by intravenous injection or poisoning by both methods) as obtained from death certificate when possible.

Disposability of the Body

Method of disposal (burial/entombment or cremation) as obtained from death certificate.

The following variables were obtained from the estimates of the respective medical examiners: Drs. Dragovic, Virani, and Pacris in Oakland County; Drs. Kanluen and Somerset in Wayne County; Dr. Spitz in Macomb County; and Dr. Houghton in Leelanau County.

Terminality

Terminality is defined at autopsy as a projection of six months or less to live as determined by the respective medical examiner.

Anatomical Basis for Pain

Anatomical basis for pain is defined by the medical examiners at autopsy as having an apparent anatomical basis for pain. No psychological autopsy data to estimate patient-experienced pain was available for the entire sample at this time.[3]

Anatomical Sign of Disease

Anatomical sign of disease is defined at autopsy by the medical examiners as an apparent anatomical sign of disease, either on gross or microscopic examination.

Disability

Disability is defined at autopsy by the medical examiner as being unable to function adequately, either physically or mentally. Again, no psychological autopsy data to estimate patient-experienced disability was available for the entire sample at this time.

C. Analyses

Analyses of variance are conducted on continuous variables and chi-squares on nominal variables.

RESULTS

A. Overall Effects

Phase

As can be seen in Table 2, eight of the deaths occurred in Phase 1 (the first honeymoon), 20 in Phase 2 (the first prosecution), six in Phase 3 (revenge), 13 in

---

[3] The report by Kaplan, Lachenmeier, Harrow, O'Dell, Uziel, Schneiderhan, and Cheyfitz (1999-2000) did report psychological autopsy reports of patient-experienced pain and disability for the first 47 decedents. We hope to extend the autopsy study to the entire sample of 93 decedents.

Phase 4 (business as usual), five in Phase 5 (the second prosecution), 13 in Phase 6 (the second honeymoon), 10 in Phase 7(the mission), 13 in Phase 8 (the martyr), four in Phase 9 (the politician), and one in Phase 10. The death in Phase 10 (Thomas Youk) was actually performed on September 17, 1998. However, it was not announced till Phase 10 and differed from the others in being proclaimed by Kevorkian a "euthanasia" rather than a "physician-assisted suicide." We thus place this death in Phase 10 as it seems to initiate a major escalation in the Kevorkian campaign.

Age

The average age of the ninety-three decedents was 58.3 years. Nine (9.7%) were under age forty, eighteen (19.4% were between forty and forty-nine, twenty-three (24.7%) were between fifty and fifty-nine, seventeen (18.3%) were between sixty and sixty-nine, and twenty-six (28%) were ages seventy and above.

Years of Education

The average number of years of education of the ninety-three decedents was 14.5 years (i.e., 2.5 years past high school).

Gender

Sixty-three of the ninety-three physician assisted deaths (67.7%) were women and thirty (32.3%) were men.

Race

The overwhelming majority (89, or 95.7%) of the ninety-three decedents were Caucasian, two were African-American, one was Hispanic, and one was Asian.

Marital Status

Only twenty-nine of the ninety-three decedents (31.2%) were married at the time of their death while the remaining sixty-four (68.8%) were single, divorced, or widowed. Of these, fifteen (16.1%) were single, another fifteen (16.1%) were widowed, and the remaining thirty-four (36.6%) were divorced.

County of Death

Almost three-fourths of the ninety-three deaths (69, or 74.2%) occurred in Oakland County, a county directly north-west of Detroit. Of the remaining twenty-four, sixteen occurred in Wayne County (including Detroit), five in Macomb County (directly north-east of Detroit), two in Leelanau County, and one in Ionia County, both counties in other parts of Michigan.

Table 2. Phase Effects

	Phase 1	Phase 2	Phase 3	Phase 4	Phase 5
Number of Deaths	8	20	6	13	5
Average Age	55.2	57.2	59.2	60.9	52.8
Average Years of Education	13.9	15.8	13.3	15.0	13.8
% Females	100% (8)	45% (9)	100% (6)	69.2% (9)	80% (4)
% Married	37.5% (3)	30% (6)	16.7% (1)	46.2% (6)	40% (2)
% Caucasian	100.0% (8)	100% (20)	100% (6)	92.3% (12)	100% (5)
% Died in Oakland County	100% (8)	65% (13)	100% (6)	92.3% (12)	0% (0)
% Died from Carbon Monoxide	75% (6)	100% (20)	33.3% (2)	38.5% (5)	0% (0)
% Cremated	100% (8)	85% (17)	83.3% (5)	76.9% (10)	40% (2)
% Terminal	37.5% (3)	55% (11)	16.7% (1)	15.4% (2)	0% (0)
% with Anatomical Basis for Pain	37.5% (3)	60.0% (12)	33.3% (2)	23.1% (3)	20.0% (1)
% with Anatomical Sign of Disease	87.5% (7)	100% (20)	83.3% (5)	92.3% (12)	100% (5)
% Disabled	62.5% (5)	80.0% (16)	33.3% (2)	61.5% (8)	80.0% (4)

Phase 6	Phase 7	Phase 8	Phase 9	Phase 10			Total
13	10	13	4	1	F, Chi-Square	p	93
52.7	69.1	59.5	56.2	52.0	.91	.52	58.3
14.9	13.9	14.0	12.2	16.0	.38	.94	14.5
76.9% (10)	80% (8)	53.8% (7)	50% (2)	0% (0)	16.77	.05	67.7% (63)
46.2% (6)	10% (1)	15.4% (2)	25% (1)	100% (1)	9.53	.39	31.2% (29)
92% (12)	100% (10)	84.6% (11)	100% (4)	100% (1)	24.92	.58	95.7% (89)
53.8% (7)	60% (6)	92.5% (12)	100% (4)	100% (1)	30.19	.001	74.2% (69)
15.4% (2)	10% (1)	0% (0)	0% (0)	0% (0)	72.13	.001	38.7% (36)
69.2% (9)	100% (10)	76% (10)	80% (4)	100% (0)	20.79	.29	80.6% (75)
30.8% (4)	20% (2)	23.1% (3)	25% (1)	0% (0)	11.57	.24	29.0% (27)
36.2% (4)	60.0% (6)	38.5% (5)	75.0% (3)	0% (0)	10.40	.32	41.9% (39)
92.3% (12)	90% (9)	92.3% (12)	100% (4)	100% (1)	3.90	.91	93.5% (87)
69.2% (9)	50.0% (5)	61.5% (8)	100% (4)	100% (1)	9.16	.42	66.7% (62)

Cause of Death (By Method)

Thirty-six of the ninety-three decedents (38.7%) died of carbon monoxide inhalation, while fifty-six (60.2%) died of lethal injection. In one death, a combination of both methods was detected, the significance of which remains unclear.

Disposability of Body

Seventy-five of the ninety-three decedents were cremated (80.6%), almost four times the cremation rate for deaths in Michigan in 1995 (23.6%) and twice the cremation rate for suicides (40%) in this same year. Of the remaining eighteen, fifteen were buried and three were entombed.

Terminality

Only twenty-seven of these ninety-three decedents were terminal (29%) while sixty-six were not terminal (71.0%).

Anatomical Basis for Pain

Only thirty-nine of the ninety-three decedents (41.9%) were judged by the medical examiners at autopsy to have an anatomical basis for pain while fifty-four (58.1%) were not so judged.

Anatomical Sign of Disease

No apparent anatomical sign of disease emerged in 6.7 percent (6 of the 90) of the autopsies for which information was available (Marjorie Wantz, Rebecca Badger, Judith Curren, Janice Murphy, Martha Wichorek, and William Connaughton).[4,5]

Disability

Two-thirds of the decedents (62 of 93) were judged by the medical examiners to be disabled at the time of their death.

---

[4] No autopsies were conducted on Mary Biernat, Stanley Ball, and Loretta Peabody. Austin Bastable was autopsied in Toronto, by the Coroner of the Province of Ontario, Canada, in the presence of Dr. Dragovic.

[5] Autopsy on Janet Good, Kevorkian's long-time assistant, revealed microscopic evidence of residual pancreatic cancer near the surgical resection margin, by Dr. Virani. Dr. Spitz performed the second autopsy on the remains of Janet Good upon private request and found no evidence or residual cancer for the simple reason that Dr. Virani had retained the tissue samples containing microscopic cancer for evidentiary purposes.

B. Gender Effects

Gender and Age

The average age of the male decedents was lower (55.5) than that of the female decedents (59.6). The age difference between men and women is not significant ($F = 1.19$, n.s.).

Gender and Years of Education

There was no significant difference in the average years of education between male decedents (Mean = 15.4) and female decedents (Mean = 14.1, $t = .88$, n.s.). However the standard deviation in this score was much higher for men ($sd = 7.73$) than for women ($sd = 1.94$, $t = 8.50$, $p < .005$).

Gender and Marital Status

Only 36.7 percent of the male decedents and 30.2 percent of the female decedents were married at the time of their deaths. This difference is not significant (Chi-Square = .39, n.s.).

Gender and Race

A greater proportion of female decedents were Caucasian (98.4%) than were male decedents (90%, Chi-Square = 6.93, $p < .08$), though the overwhelming majority for both genders was Caucasian.

Gender and County of Death

Sixty-six point seven percent of the male decedents and 77.8 percent of the female decedents ended their lives in Oakland County. This difference was not significant (Chi-Square = 1.48, n.s.).

Gender and Cause of Death (By Method)

Forty-three point three percent of the male decedents and 36.5 percent of the female decedents died of carbon monoxide poisoning. Fifty-six point seven percent of the men and 61.9 percent of the women died from lethal injections. One woman (Betty Hamilton) was poisoned by a combination of both methods. No significant gender difference emerged (Chi-Square = .67, n.s.).

Gender and Disposability of Body

Eighty-three point three percent of the male decedents and 84.1 percent of the female decedents were cremated. This was four times as great as the proportion for deaths in Michigan in 1995 and twice as great as the proportion of cremations for suicides in Michigan in this same year. No significant differences emerged between men and women (Chi-Square = .01, n.s.).

Gender and Terminality

More male decedents (11 out of 30, or 36.7%) were terminal than were female decedents (16 out of 63, or 25.4%). This difference was not significant (Chi-Square = 1.25, n.s.) in contrast to the significant gender difference in terminality reported on the first forty-seven decedents (57.1% of the male decedents among the first 47 cases judged as terminal as opposed to 19.4 percent of the female decedents, Chi-Square = 6.43, $p < .05$; Kaplan, Lachenmeier, Harrow, O'Dell, Uziel, Schneiderhan, & Cheyfitz, 1999-2000).

Gender and Anatomical Basis for Pain

Only 43.3 percent of the male decedents (13 out of 30) and 41.1 percent of the female decedents (26 out of 63) were judged by the medical examiners to have an anatomical basis for pain. This difference was not significant (Chi-Square = .04, n.s.), failing to replicate the pattern of gender differences in anatomical basis for pain (60% of male decedents as compared to 34.4% of female decedents) occurring in the first forty-seven suicides (Kaplan, Lachenmeier, Harrow, O'Dell, Uziel, Schneiderhan, & Cheyfitz, 1999-2000).

Gender and Anatomical Sign of Disease

Five out of the six decedents who showed no apparent anatomical sign of disease at autopsy were women (5 out of 61 women, or 8.2%) as opposed to (1 out of 28 men, or 3.6%). This difference was not significant (Chi-Square = .71, n.s.).

Gender and Disability

Seventy percent (21 out of 30) of the male decedents were judged by the medical examiners to be disabled at the time of death as opposed to 65.1 percent (41 out of 63) of the female decedents. This difference was not significant (Chi-Square = .22, n.s.).

C. Phase Effects

Analyses regarding phases are summarized in Table 2.

Phase and Age

No significant phase effect emerged for average age of death ($F = .91$, n.s.), average age ranging between the mid fifties and low sixties in each time period.

Phase and Years of Education

No significant phase effect emerged with regard to average years of education of the decedent ($F = .38$, n.s.).

Phase and Gender

The ratio of female to male decedents definitely varied with phase, the percentage of women being highest (100%) in Phases 1 (first honeymoon) and 3 (revenge) and low (40 or 50%) in Phases 2 (first prosecution), 8 (the martyr statement), and 9 (constrained by politics), and nonexistent in Phase 10 (free to escalate) (Chi-Square = 16.77, $p < .05$).

Phase and Marital Status

The percentage of decedents who were married at the time of their death was not significantly affected by phase (Chi-Square = 9.53, n.s.).

Phase and Race

The racial composition of the decedents did not systematically vary with phase, being overwhelming Caucasian throughout (Chi-Square = 24.92, n.s.).

Phase and County of Death

The percentage of deaths occurring in Oakland County did vary significantly with phase, being 100 percent in Phases 1 (first honeymoon), 3 (revenge), 9 (constrained by politics), and 10 (free to escalate), and 0 percent in Phase 5 (the second prosecution) (Chi-Square = 30.19, $p < .001$).

Phase and Cause of Death (By Method)

There was a dramatic effect of phase on method of death. The use of carbon monoxide decreases over time, being highest in the first two phases (75% and 100% respectively) and nonexistent in the last three phases (Chi-Square = 72.13, $p < .001$).

Phase and Disposability of Body

There was no significant phase effect on the method of disposability of body ($F = 20.79$, n.s.), a very high proportion of cremations (over 75%) occurring in all phases with the singular exception of Phase 5 (the second prosecution), where the percentage of cremations is only 40 percent.

Phase and Terminality

No significant overall phase effect emerged with regard to percentages of decedents that were regarded as terminal (Chi-Square = 11.57, n.s.). However, it is important to note that the only percentage reaching or exceeding 50 percent occurred during Phase 2 (first prosecution). The percentage of terminal cases was higher among the first forty-seven decedents (38.3%) than among the subsequent forty-six decedents (21.8%). Gender of the decedent plays an important role here, however. While the percentage of terminality among female decedents remains relatively constant from the first forty-seven cases (8 out of 32 or 25%) to the latter forty-six cases (7 out of 32 or 21.9%), this percentage drastically drops for male decedents. Specifically, the terminality rate of male decedents drops from 60 percent (9 out of 15) among the first forty-seven cases to 13.3 percent (only 2 out of 15) among the latter forty-six cases.

Phase and Anatomical Basis for Pain

No significant phase effect emerged with regard to anatomical basis for pain (Chi-Square = 10.40, n.s.). The only percentages exceeding 50 percent occurred in Phase 2—first prosecution (60%), Phase 7—mission-statement (60%), and Phase 9—constrained by politics (75%). There is no apparent difference in the percentage of decedents displaying anatomical basis for pain between the first forty-seven cases (42.6%) and the subsequent forty-six (37.9%). However, these percentages dramatically interact with gender. The percentage of male decedents displaying anatomical basis for pain decreases from 60 percent (9 out of 15) among the first forty-seven cases to 26.7 percent (4 out of 15) among the subsequent forty-six. The percentage of female decedents displaying anatomical basis for pain, in contrast, increases from 34.4 percent (11 out of 32) among the first forty-seven cases to 48.4 percent (15 out of 31) among the subsequent forty-six.

Phase and Anatomical Sign of Disease

No significant phase effect occurs with regard to apparent anatomical sign of disease in the decedents (Chi-Square = 3.90, n.s.).

Phase and Disability

There is no significant phase effect with regard to disability (Chi-Square = 9.16, n.s.), the percentage of decedents who were disabled at the time of death being over 50 percent at all phases with the single exception of Phase 3—revenge (33.3%), and actually being 100 percent for Phase 9–constrained by politics, and Phase 10—free to escalate.

DISCUSSION

The present report has extended the research on the Kevorkian-Reding physician-assisted deaths to all ninety-three publicly acknowledged cases as of November 25, 1998. Among the trends are: 1) Over two-thirds of the deaths involve women, 2) A small minority of the cases are judged terminal by the respective medical examiners, though the preponderance of men versus women in this category is less than that emerging in the analyses of the first forty-seven cases (Kaplan, Lachenmeier, Harrow, O'Dell, Uziel, Schneiderhan, & Cheyfitz, 1999-2000). Indeed, the rate of terminality drops by 75 percent among male decedents among the latter forty-six cases while it remains constant among female decedents from the first forty-seven to the latter forty-six cases. 3) A similar pattern emerges with regard to anatomical basis for pain. The percentage of women with anatomical pain increases from the first forty-seven to the latter forty-six cases (from 34.4% to 48.4%). The percentage of men with anatomical basis for pain, in contrast, decreases from 60 percent to 26.7 percent. Clearly, the Kevorkian-Reding team seems to be picking less seriously ill men over time while the female decedents seem to stay the same or become somewhat more seriously ill. At the same time, autopsies reveal no anatomical sign of disease in six cases, five of which are women. Three of these cases occur among the first forty-seven decedents and three among the latter forty-six decedents.

Expansion of our phase analyses from four to ten phases tends to confirm our earlier conclusion that the Kevorkian-Reding pattern often seems influenced by legal and political considerations extrinsic to the specific medical conditions of the patients. Consider several patterns: 4) The gender ratio of women to men varies wildly from one phase to another, being lowest when Kevorkian seems to have something to lose (Phase 2—the first prosecution and Phase 9—constrained by politics) and highest when he is unencumbered by such considerations (Phase 1—the first honeymoon, and Phase 3—revenge). 5) The method of death reverses over time, with carbon monoxide almost the exclusive method in the early phases, and the suicide machine almost the exclusive method in the later phases. This transformation seems to reveal a routinization of the process over time, the suicide machine being quicker (taking less than 2 minutes) than carbon monoxide (taking over 10 minutes). 6) The county of death varies systematically with political and legal considerations involving Kevorkian and fulfilling his own agenda quite extraneous to the patient's interest. In periods where Kevorkian seems out to get his perceived nemeses, Richard Thompson or John Engler (Phase 1—honeymoon, Phase 3—revenge, or Phase 9—constrained by politics) all the deaths occur in Oakland County. In other periods (after Thompson has been defeated, for example), the deaths seem to be scattered across counties (Phase 5—the second prosecution, Phase 6—the second honeymoon, and Phase 7—the mission statement).

Several disturbing specific examples come to mind. Consider Kevorkian's first case, Janet Adkins (June 4, 1990), Kevorkian is clearly looking for a candidate for his first assisted suicide, advertising his services in this regard in the Detroit News and Oakland Press and being written up in Newsweek. Although Kevorkian pays lip service to hoping Adkins will choose to delay her death, it is clear he is looking for a subject for his project. Indeed, Kevorkian calls Adkins a heroine in the classical Greek style when she agrees to go through with her death even though she in all probability has many quality years ahead (see Kaplan, Lachenmeier, Harrow, O'Dell, Uziel, Schneiderhan, & Cheyfitz, 1999-2000).

Another example occurs in the nationally televised tape of the death of Thomas Youk. It is clear that Kevorkian is looking for a candidate for his first euthanasia which he intends to announce the day after the November 3 Michigan election results are in involving Fieger's race for governor and Proposal B for the legislation of physician-assisted suicide.[6] In his initial meeting with Youk on September 17, 1998 Kevorkian seems to be urging him to take his time in fixing a date for his death. First, Kevorkian suggests Youk take four weeks, then three weeks, then two weeks, then finally insists on a one-week waiting period, which is abrogated when Youk's family contacts Kevorkian regarding Youk's rising anxiety and desire to die sooner. Nevertheless, there is something disingenuous about this dialogue. While Kevorkian will offer Youk four weeks, it is significant that he will not offer him eight weeks or indeed any amount of time which would put Youk's death after Kevorkian's November 4 target date. One has the feeling that if Youk wanted more time, Kevorkian would drop him as a candidate and try to find someone else to euthanize to fit into his own time frame—to publicize euthanasia as soon as the coast is clear.

The underlying aims and psychodynamics of Kevorkian himself reveal themselves at the end of Phases 9 and 10. Echoing his speeches of October 22, 1997 (his "organ harvesting" speech) and December 31, 1997 (his "suicidal martyr" speech), Kevorkian attempts to harvest the kidneys from Patient 92 (Joseph Tushkowski) and actively euthanizes Patient 93 (Thomas Youk). In the latter case, Kevorkian announces his intention on November 22, 1998 either to go on euthanizing patients if he is not charged with a crime, or to commit suicide as a martyr (by starving himself to death in prison) if he is.

Kevorkian's obsession with death reveals itself in the two prongs of the choice he is offering the prosecutors-killing others or killing himself. Although many of his choices seem quite rational, closer examination indicates that they are in the service of his obsession with death. A suicidal wish may be rationally planned out and still be in the service of an underlying compulsion. It is recommended that Kevorkian be treated from a medical rather than a legal framework, being placed under treatment to avoid doing harm to either himself or to others. We suggest treating him as a would-be suicidal martyr rather than as a savior or a serial killer. Clearly a suicide-preventive approach should be used with Kevorkian himself rather than one of assisting him in his suicide.

ACKNOWLEDGMENTS

The authors would like to offer their gratitude to the medical examiners of Oakland County (Drs. L. J. Dragovic, Kanu Virani, and Bernardino Pacris), Wayne County (Drs. Sawait Kanluen and J. Scott Somerset), Macomb County

---

[6] This making of a euthanasia "snuff tape" recapitulates Kevorkian's search for a subject (Janet Adkins) in the very beginning of his "assisted-suicide" campaign. Dr. Dragovic has maintained throughout that the term "physician-assisted suicide" is a misnomer, the deaths arranged, orchestrated and completed by another. In this article, we employ the term physician-assisted (or physician-aided) deaths.

(Dr. Werner U. Spitz), and Leelanau County (Dr. Matthew Houghton). We would also like to acknowledge the help of Adrianna Giovanini, Frank Ripullo II, Brian Tabaka, and Randy Estes.

REFERENCES

Canetto, S., & Hollenshead, J. (1999-2000). Gender and physician-assisted suicide: An analysis of the Kevorkian cases: 1990-1997. *Omega, 40* (1), 165-208 (this issue).

Detroit Free Press (1998). *Kevorkian dares legislators to ban assisted suicide* [Website edition only].

Detroit Free Press. October 23, 1997. *Kevorkian to harvest patients' organs.* p. 1A.

Detroit Free Press Staff, The (1997). *The suicide machine.* Detroit: The Detroit Free Press.

Kaplan, K. J., Lachenmeier, F., Harrow, M., O'Dell, J., Uziel, O., Schneiderhan, M., & Cheyfitz, K. (1999-2000). Psychological versus biomedical risk factors in Kevorkian's first 47 physician-assisted suicides. *Omega, 40* (1) 109-163 (this issue).

Newsweek. March 8, 1993. *Kevorkian's death wish.* pp. 46, 48.

Oakland Press. January 1, 1998. *Kevorkian offers to become a martyr.* pp. A1, A15.

DISPENSING DEATH, DESIRING DEATH: AN EXPLORATION OF MEDICAL ROLES AND PATIENT MOTIVATION DURING THE PERIOD OF LEGALIZED EUTHANASIA IN AUSTRALIA

ANNETTE STREET
LaTrobe University

DAVID W. KISSANE
University of Melbourne

ABSTRACT

A qualitative case study was conducted to explore the clinical decision making processes that underpinned the practice of euthanasia under the Rights of the Terminally Ill (ROTI) Act. The key informant for this research was Philip Nitschke, the general practitioner responsible for the legal cases of euthanasia. His information was supported by extensive document analysis based on the public texts created by patients in the form of letters and documentaries. Further collaborating sources were those texts generated by the media, rights groups, politicians, the coroner's court, and the literature on euthanasia and assisted suicide. A key study finding was that the ROTI legislation did not adequately provide for the specific medical situation in the Northern Territory, Australia. The medical roles, as proscribed by the legislation, carried many inherent assumptions about the health care context and the availability of appropriately qualified medical staff committed to providing euthanasia. These assumptions translated into difficulties in establishing clinical practices for the provision of euthanasia. A further finding concerned the motivations of those who requested euthanasia. This article addresses the medical roles and the motivations of those seeking euthanasia.

The fact that euthanasia has been illegal in most places in the industrialized world means that little research has been done on the clinical experiences of euthanasia and physician assisted suicide (PAS). The nine-month period of legalized euthanasia in the Northern Territory of Australia under the Rights of Terminally Ill (ROTI) Act, made it possible to remedy this situation. This article draws on some of the research findings of a qualitative case study (Kissane, Street, & Nitschke, 1998) which examined the clinical decision making processes underpinning the practice of euthanasia under the ROTI Act. Evidence from interviews, letters written by people seeking euthanasia, medical reports, coroner's records, and media reports provided the basis for an analysis of the motivations and knowledge that informed the decisions taken by these people and the associated medical practitioners.

Studies exploring the motivations that lead to a desire for euthanasia have highlighted the prominent role of depression in its development (Brown, Henteleff, Barakat, & Rowe, 1986; Chochinov et al. 1995). One study of Australian patients with cancer identified that hopelessness, depression, anxiety, being unmarried and having a poor prognosis significantly predicted a desire for death (Owen, Tennant, Levi, & Jones, 1994). In the same study, the perceptions of the staff members caring for these patients suggested that the patient was isolated or given up and that the quality of life was poor. It is noteworthy that interest in euthanasia was greater in patients with a good prognosis, but as prognosis deteriorated, a significant increase in rejection of euthanasia occurred (Owen, Tennant, Levi, & Jones, 1992). Predictors of a desire for euthanasia in a U.S. cohort of patients with AIDS were depression, quality of social support, fear of burden, and the recent death of a friend (Breitbart, Rosenfeld, & Passik, 1996). Pathway analysis undertaken in the studies of Chochinov et al. (1995) and Breitbart, Rosenfeld, and Passik (1996) both suggested that depression was the final common pathway, separately influenced in turn by perceptions of support, pain or other symptoms interfering with quality of life. Little evidence is available from the cases of people whose death was medically assisted. The Rimmelink report on the situation in the Netherlands is therefore a very important source of information on the topic (van der Maas et al. 1996). In the Netherlands, "loss of dignity" was the reason provided by 57 percent of cases, 46 percent cited intolerable pain, 46 percent stated they didn't want an "unworthy dying," 33 percent didn't want to be dependent on others, with 23 percent claiming to be "tired of life" (people were able to choose more than one answer, hence the percentages). A comparison of these empirically identified motivational factors with those seeking euthanasia in Darwin is warranted.

It became obvious that the processes and the context in which the decisions of the patients and medical practitioners were made, affected the motivations of those who requested euthanasia. It was also apparent that the expectations of the legislators concerning the functioning of the medical roles were unrealistic and problematic in practice. Nor was enough clear guidance available on central issues such as the structure of relationships with palliative care and the local hospitals, bereavement support, or professional education and debriefing. This article highlights some of the issues for those medical practitioners dispensing death and the motivations of those desiring death.

BACKGROUND

Most research on euthanasia and physician assisted suicide (PAS) has focused on ethical and moral discussion or on surveys of community and professional attitudes (Baume & O'Malley, 1994; Kuhse, Singer, Baume, Clark, & Rickard, 1997). Central to these debates has been the need to define the key terms of euthanasia and assisted suicide. It is not our intention in this article to deconstruct the terms and the associated meanings. We make a clear distinction between the provision of palliative treatments that will provide comfort but at the same time may hasten death, and those legally sanctioned, deliberate acts designed to induce death.

Community attitudes continue to be influenced by the widespread fear of opiate induced death (Ashby, 1995) or of suffering from unrelieved symptoms (Callahan, 1993). Similarly, bio-ethicists use moral equivalence arguments to equate clinical decisions about the withdrawal of futile treatment, to the giving of a lethal injection. Right to die groups have engaged both in political debates and provided practical advice to people on the safest ways to kill themselves (Humphry, 1991). Recent articles have argued for the roles of various health professionals in the assessment and gatekeeping processes (Ganzini, Fenn, & Lee, 1996; Sanson, Dickens, Melita, Nixon, Rowe, Tudor, & Tyrrell, 1998). The media debate has centered on the extreme view from proponents and opponents of euthanasia/PAS and sensationalized human-interest stories (O'Connor, 1998). Absent from any of these approaches to euthanasia is research which examines the critiques the actual clinical practices and structures which inform, facilitate, and limit the practice of euthanasia/PAS in society. The work of Herbert Hendin (1994) stands apart in this regard. He utilized a case study approach to articulate the clinical decision making around euthanasia in the Netherlands and to place it in its context, tracing the effects of individual cases on those involved and ultimately on the clinical decision making. His use of cases to illustrate practices, clinical decisions, and health systems influenced the approach our research has taken.

CONTEXT: PALLIATIVE CARE SERVICES IN AUSTRALIA

Historically, palliative care in Australia has developed independently of mainstream health services with localized hospice and home care programs predominating. The push to integrate palliative care and to improve access and equity has resulted in government initiatives to support better integration between hospitals, hospices, residential care, home care, and day centers. Although many health services across Australia have an identified palliative care program there is significant variation in the service delivery models being pursued and the quality of palliative care that is delivered (Commonwealth Department of Health and Family Services, 1998).

In Australia more than 80 percent of patients referred to palliative care services have cancer, yet only 43 percent of all cancer patients are referred to palliative care services (National Cancer Control Initiative, 1998). The patterns of service delivery are uneven across the eight states and territories with rural and remote areas being under-serviced.

THE PASSAGE AND REPEAL OF THE ROTI ACT

On May 25, 1995, the Northern Territory Parliament in Australia passed the Rights of the Terminally Ill Act 1995 (ROTI Act) which was enacted on July 1, 1996 and repealed on March 25, 1997 (Northern Territory Government, 1995). The fact that the ROTI Act was in operation for only nine months bears witness to the specific relationship between the national (called Commonwealth) Parliament and the Northern Territory (NT), where the Commonwealth can act as a house of review for the NT and repeal its Acts when these can be shown to be in conflict with the views of the nation.

The ROTI Act had been introduced into the NT parliament by Marshall Perron, the Chief Minister, who had seen his mother die a painful death from breast cancer. At that time the NT had no radiotherapy services for cancer patients and the palliative care service was in its infancy.

When the Act came into operation, most media interest was directed at the political process and the sensational stories of five of the seven people who officially sought to use the Act. These five people participated in televised interviews and also published letters and statements in the press. Their relatives also contributed to the media debates. Thus there is considerable amount of material in the public domain detailing the desires and experiences of these people.

The roles of the medical practitioners involved in the processes were generally ignored with the exception of the role of Dr. Philip Nitschke, the doctor who conducted the euthanasia. He actively sought constant media attention to attract the support of specialists and psychiatrists to fulfill the requirements of the Act and to "help the cause."

Comparison with the material available in media reports of Oregon, where legalized euthanasia has recently been available, suggests that the Northern Territory is not unique. Medical roles are socially constructed. The creation of new legalized roles for doctors and psychiatrists requires careful attention to the socio-political context and to the expectations of the roles in practice. The assessment role is crucial because it requires the medical practitioner to pass judgment that people requesting assistance to die are of sound mind, are terminally ill, and have been offered the appropriate treatments or palliation. The capacity to make accurate prognostications in situations where the end result is final has been soundly challenged. The capacity to determine whether the person has masked depression is particularly formidable in the course of a short psychiatric assessment.

STUDY METHOD

The key informant for this case study was Dr. Philip Nitschke, the doctor who performed the legal deaths under the ROTI Act. Eighteen hours of in-depth audiotaped interviews were conducted at his residence in Darwin. Further follow-up discussions ensued to clarify and confirm details around the clinical decision making processes that underpinned the practice of euthanasia. This information was supported by extensive document analysis based on the public texts created by patients in the form of letters and televised documentaries. Further collaborating sources were those texts generated by the media, right groups, politicians, the coroner's court and the literature on euthanasia, and assisted suicide.

The sample for this study was the seven people who officially sought to use the legislation to die. Comprehensive individual case studies on each were developed. The first two patients requested euthanasia, but died before the Act became law, four died under the Act and one following its repeal. Ages ranged from fifty-two to seventy years; four were female; two were married, the rest were single or divorced. Four revealed some symptoms of depression. Cancer was the only form of illness and most presented at advanced stages (Kissane et al., 1998).

The university's ethics committee approval was obtained for the study and Nitschke gave informed consent as the key informant. Although some patients and doctors went on the public record, their identity has been kept confidential in our reporting of this study. Nitschke reviewed transcripts of the taped interviews for validation.

A qualitative content analysis across all the cases traced commonalities and contradictions in the data. As euthanasia is a contentious public health issue a discursive analysis charted the different ideological positions inherent in the debates on euthanasia/PAS and enabled an exploration of the subsequent effects on people's lives. This article focuses on the content analysis; the discursive analysis will be published elsewhere. In writing this article we are interpreting the material through our own sets of professional lens, namely as a feminist medical sociologist researching nursing practice, palliative care, and mental health: and as a consultation-liaison psychiatrist who is also a professor of palliative medicine. We have distinct theoretical discourses that have framed and shaped the questions asked of the data and the interpretations which have been bought forth. Our interests in this study were specifically in the medical assessments, the options provided, and the care given, including the availability and quality of palliative care. We were also concerned to identify the support available to the patients, to family members, to the staff involved, and understand the way the legislative structures facilitated and hindered the practice of euthanasia under the Act. The analytical questions we asked of the textual material in this article were also informed by the literature available on the topic of the medical assessment roles in end of life decisionmaking and the responses of people suffering from life threatening illnesses. This analysis is therefore our scholarly, interpreted construction of the events. Nitschke interprets the same material through his own perspective as a euthanasia lobbyist and practitioner. Thus he argues a different reading of these processes, practices, and events.

FINDINGS

Dispensing Death:
The Medical Roles in Decision Making (See Table 1)

It is instructive to examine the way the gatekeeping assessment roles functioned and to understand the contributing socio-political factors. The roles of the various medical practitioners were proscribed under law but the socio-political situation meant that these guidelines were not able to be strictly adhered to. The ROTI Act made specific provisions for the roles of those medical personnel involved with patients requesting euthanasia. These provisions contained inherent assumptions about the availability of relevantly qualified staff prepared to support the Act. This would have been possible in a large urban environment with many specialists and psychiatrists available, but created problems in the Northern Territory with its small population scattered over a large area.

Under the ROTI Act a terminally ill patient who was experiencing pain, suffering, and/or distress to an extent deemed unacceptable, could request their medical practitioner to assist them to end their life. Their doctor needed to be satisfied on reasonable grounds that it was a terminal illness that would meet the provisions of the Act.

The Certifying Medical Practitioner

The intention of the law was that the person's usual medical practitioner would be the one who would assist the person to die after having coordinated the assessment process. In the same way the arguments for similar legislation in Oregon were based on the assumption that legalizing this process would provide support for people to negotiate assisted suicide privately with their medical practitioner.

The patients in this study were unable to continue dealing with their own medical practitioner. Nitschke was the only Australian doctor who volunteered to

Table 1. The Medical Roles in Decision Making

Case No.	Age	Gender	Marital Status	Cancer Diagnosis	Certifying GP	Certifying Specialist	Certifying Psychiatrist	Mode of Death
1	68	Female	Divorced	Caecum	Nitschke	—	Psychiatric Registrar	Suicide
2	64	Male	Single	Stomach	Nitschke	—	—	Natural
3	66	Male	Married	Prostate	Nitschke	General surgeon	Interstate psychiatrist	Euthanasia
4	52	Female	Married	Mycosis fungoides	Nitschke	Orthopedic surgeon	Interstate psychiatrist	Euthanasia
5	69	Male	Single	Stomach	Nitschke	General surgeon	NT psychiatrist	Euthanasia
6	70	Female	Divorced	Breast	Nitschke	General surgeon	NT psychiatrist	Euthanasia
7	56	Female	Single	Carcinoid	Nitschke	General surgeon	NT psychiatrist	Sedation

conduct euthanasia and for this reason it is instructive to understand his background. He had been a political activist who had devoted time, expertise, and personal resources to a number of social causes over the period of his adult life. He qualified with a Ph.D in physics, a qualification which was to assist him when he developed his deliverance machine (a computer program which connected to an intravenous line to deliver the euthanasia drugs) and later the more controversial work on a computer program to calibrate the drugs necessary for suicide based on brain wave signals. His current search for an easily concocted suicide pill also demonstrates this interest in science. He did not practice science upon graduation, as he immediately became involved in aboriginal land rights, living with an isolated aboriginal community. He began medical training in the 1980s and on completion moved to Darwin. His medical practice was a sole-operated after-hours service, which was largely used by drug dependent patients. His experiences with these people led him to agitate for a methadone program. Prior to his involvement with euthanasia, Nitschke had not been involved with the care of terminally ill people and was not part of the medical and palliative care networks in the NT.

His belief in the rights of the individual to determine the course of their life and death led him to become involved in euthanasia. He not only pioneered the clinical processes for euthanasia, but at the same time was the key political figure involved in opposing the repeal of the Act in the national parliament. His political activity required constant travel interstate, particularly to the national capital, Canberra. Absences from Darwin, allied with the fact that he was not the GP of the people requesting assistance to die, meant that he was not often the primary medical caregiver, but the person who organized the death. He was under constant pressure from the press, from patients and their families, from politicians and from the Voluntary Euthanasia Society to meet their needs. His account of this period is of a frenetic time.

While the Act was operational, he began to establish links with some palliative care nurses and a psychiatrist willing to assess patients under the Act. However the necessary secrecy which surrounded the process, and the fact that no hospitals would allow euthanasia to occur on their premises, necessitated the use of motels and homes. When palliative care nursing services were involved with patients who sought to use the ROTI Act, they communicated with Nitschke. There was no access to other members of the multidisciplinary team who may have been able to contribute to the dying process and provide support to family members. Palliative care programs provide bereavement follow up and the option of counseling for families after the death of their family member. There was no such structure or community support process in place for those seeking assistance to die. The need for this kind of supportive service warrants exploration and consideration of which agency/professional group is best placed to provide this.

The Second Opinion

A second medical practitioner, who was a resident of the Northern Territory, was required to examine the patient and confirm the existence and terminal nature of the illness, including provision of an opinion on prognosis. The Regulations required that this practitioner hold a qualification in a medical specialty related to this terminal illness, recognized by fellowship of a specialist college in Australia. This provision assumed that there were sufficient specialists resident in the Northern Territory whose specialty related to the particular medical condition and who were prepared to assist in euthanasia.

During the operation of the Act, a key activity for Nitschke was the recruitment of other medical personnel willing to assess patients under the Act by providing an informed opinion. All the deaths proposed or concluded under this legislation were from cancer. At the time of the legislation there was only one oncologist in the Territory and he declined to be involved. A general practitioner with some experience in palliative care assisted in the care of the first person to receive euthanasia, but then left for another state and was not replaced. As a result, Nitschke needed to assess cancer specialists from interstate and there were the usual differences in opinion by medical staff as to the terminal nature of the patient's illnesses. Eventually, general surgeons and an orthopaedic surgeon made assessments of the patient's treatment and prognosis as part of compliance with the Act that the specialist be from the Northern Territory.

The Psychiatric Assessment

Finally, the ROTI Act required that a psychiatrist examine the patient and confirm that he or she was not suffering from a treatable clinical depression in respect of the illness. There was a concern that many seeking euthanasia would in fact be suffering from a depressive illness or may have impaired judgment from a brain disease such that they are no longer legally responsible for themselves nor able to make a valid request for euthanasia.

Studies of death and dying which have explored attitudes to death , suicide, and euthanasia in cancer patients (Owens et al., 1992) hospice patients (Chochinov et al., 1995) and AIDS sufferers (Chochinov et al., 1995) suggest that the presence of depression may involve a treatable clinical state in which the psychiatrist could play a valid role, while alerting carers to factors such as poor social support, family difficulties, fear of burden, and other fears about death and dying which may permit remediable changes to be introduced. It can be argued that there may therefore be a substantial gatekeeping role for a psychiatrist, yet in an interesting study of confidence in making psychiatric diagnoses in the dying, Ganzini et al., (1996) reported that only 6 percent of Oregon's psychiatrists believed that they could competently make this diagnosis from a single consultation with a relevant patient. This strikingly low figure reveals the complexity of the problem in accurately appraising all relevant personal and environmental factors when a patient may not want to disclose information for fear of the consequences of doing so. Nitschke reported that all the patients found the psychiatric assessment the most stressful part of the process. Their fears about the power of the psychiatrist in the process militated against the development of a therapeutic alliance necessary for a thorough assessment. During the latter stages of his involvement with the Act Nitschke formed an alliance with a sympathetic psychiatrist who was prepared to evaluate patients.

Desire Death: The Patient's Decision for Euthanasia (See Table 2)

Central to the practice of euthanasia is the patients' decision making process and their reasons for choosing euthanasia. Motivation for euthanasia/PAS has been inferred from studies conducted on suicide and hospice patients. The information concerning PAS in Oregon is being collected through a survey with fifty-three items. The Oregon-based society Compassion in Dying (Preston & Mero, 1996) has provided assistance to people who wanted to kill themselves under very similar assessment criteria to the Death and Dignity legislation. Three hundred people were assessed with forty-six qualifying for assistance under the guidelines and processes. The main reason provided was "unbearable suffering" described in physical, emotional, or spiritual terms. The sample in this Australian study was much smaller, but it was evident that there were some similarities and differences in the motivations that propelled people to take such a final step.

Naming: The Power of Language

Language is powerful. It structures the way we think and understand our world. Words carry meanings, sometimes subtle, sometimes implied. Words can have a powerful effect on thoughts and feelings. The words which surround a prognosis of a person with a progressive illness carry messages of finality and loss of hope; words such as *incurable, no more active treatment, transfer to hospice, and terminal care.* For these patients there were a number of instances of the power of such language, often echoed three times because of the necessary medical opinions to meet the requirements of the Act. Thus, at least three times, people were told "there is nothing more that can be done for you." Euthanasia is a very final solution and doctors need to be quite sure and emphatic that their prognosis is correct (Marker & Smith, 1996). In the normal course of events, when a dying person is told that there is no more medical treatment that can prolong their life, they are also offered strategies to make the remainder of their lives as meaningful and comfortable as possible. There is less finality and more hope than is required in a process leading to euthanasia (Chevlen, 1996). Hearing that there is nothing more that can be done over and over can lead the person to feel hopeless and their loved ones both hopeless and helpless to assist.

Table 2. The Patient's Decision for Euthanasia

Case No.	Fear	Burden	Social Isolation	Suffering	Futility	Depressive Symptoms	Loss of Dignity
1	Yes	—	Yes	Yes	Yes	Suicidal	Yes
2	—	—	Yes	Yes	Yes	No	—
3	Yes	Yes	—	Yes	—	Suicidal	Yes
4	—	—	—	Yes	Yes	Yes, on antidepressants	Yes
5	—	—	Yes	Yes	—	No	—
6	Yes	Concerned	—	Yes	—	No	—
	—	—	Partial	Yes	Yes	Yes	Yes

The husband of Case 4 told the psychiatrist that his wife asked him each morning to do away with her. This persistence of her despair led him to become a strong advocate on her behalf. In this way he supported her not only in the physical actions needed to carry out euthanasia but also her belief that her life now was meaningless and death was the only answer.

"Truth telling" has been a central tenet of palliative care. However little research has been done concerning the versions of truth which are told, how the hearer interprets the "truth" and whether other circumstances occur that subsequently change the patient's understanding of what they have been told (Street, 1998). In the latter category there are instances of patient's feeling better because they received palliation and consider that the original "worst scenario" prognosis is not longer the case. Likewise there are many instances where patients report that they are not told the truth about their prognosis. Case 4 considered that the doctors were lying to her when they were offering her further treatment options. Similarly, Case 3 accused palliative care doctors of lying about his condition and "experimenting" with his treatment.

Anticipatory Distress and Fear

Euthanasia is argued on the ground that pain and suffering can be unbearable for some people and that society or medicine should provide a way for these people to end their life with dignity. This attitude was exemplified by this statement contained in the letter to the press written by Case 4:

> I believe the euthanasia is the greatest thing for people who are sick with no chance of getting better. It's a wonderful idea and it stops people from suffering when they don't need to. No one wants to die if they don't have to, but I know I have had no hesitation in asking for this. No one should suffer when they don't have to (letter to press).

Analogies are often made to veterinary practice where humans end the suffering of animals in pain; or to battle when soldiers will sometimes acquiesce to a badly wounded comrade and assist them to die rather than leave them to be tortured by soldiers from the opposing forces (Allen, 1998). Case 3 wrote: "If I were to keep a pet animal in the same condition I am in, I would be prosecuted" and Cases 1 and 4 made similar association between their situations and the case for putting a dog out of its misery.

Others were more afraid of their capacity to bear the symptoms, which inevitably accompanied their disease, a form of anticipatory distress. This was most evident in the first woman who asked for euthanasia. She was not terminal at the time, nor experiencing pain or symptoms. Her fear of symptomatic distress was a motivating factor in her request and subsequent suicide.

In a similar vein, Case 6 had some symptoms but her main reason for requesting euthanasia was anticipatory distress and frustration that, despite palliative care, she was unable to regain her capacity to do things she had done in the past. She had been very upset when her sister died a sad and painful death from breast cancer, suffering the indignity of double incontinence. Despite her recognition that each death is different, she remained fearful she would suffer a similar death. Case 3 expressed distress at the memory of friends whom he saw die "bloody horribly," dreading he would experience a similar fate. It was apparent from these cases that anticipatory distress had very real consequences for how they were feeling about themselves as they progressively deteriorated.

Burden and Family Concerns

Dr. Joanne Lynne, Director of the Centre to Improve Care of the Dying, describes the problem of fear of dependence or burden in an interview as:

> Fragile, old and dying people want to please their families and doctors, not to be a burden . . . and they don't know what to do at the end, especially amid the choices of modern medicine. They can easily be swayed by children who might say, "'How?' when these old people say they want to die, rather than, 'How can I help you, Mom? I love you and want you to live'" (Webb, 1997, p. 394).

Concern with being a burden on others was evident in all the stories in different ways. For some, their state of social isolation meant that they would be a burden to strangers, for others their love for family or friends led them to declare their sense of burden.

> My own pain is made worse by watching my wife suffering as she cares for me; cleaning up after my "accidents" in the middle of the night, and watching my body fade away (letter to press).

Similarly Case 6 did not want to be the burden to her children that she perceived her dying sister was.

Families live through intense and complex emotional experiences in which they struggle with ambivalent feelings about the worth of their sick family member. When conflict and difference of opinion occur, this ambivalence can be especially difficult to contain. Carers struggle to cope with the demands of caring for the sick relative—the constant physical neediness, irritability and anger, the inescapable routines and the broken sleep. Such family concerns were evident in these cases.

Social Isolation

Loneliness and social isolation increased as the quality of life deteriorated and this contributed to any sense of futility and despair. Cases 2 and 5 were men who were socially isolated and their deterioration was made more poignant by their loneliness. Case 7 became steadily unhappy with her quality of life. She had been an avid reader and letter writer but stopped both activities when her symptoms meant she was unable to concentrate. Letter writing had been an important means of maintaining contact with many nursing colleagues. She withdrew more socially, ceased going to the supermarket, to the theatre, and visiting people.

Futility

Those seeking assistance to die expressed a sense of futility. This was typified in the statement made by Case 2:

> I'm just existing, I can't see the point anymore I've seen my time. I'm ready
> for the sweet long sleep (McLaughlin, 1996).

Futility is bound up with a lack of purpose in pursuing life under the changed conditions brought about by debilitating illness and the inevitability of death. For Case 4 this purposelessness was related to the fact that she saw her future in hospital when women of her age (52) were healthy and vigorous:

> It's so hopeless. I'll never get out of hospital again. You want to get something to help but you can't (patient transcript recorded in psychiatric medical record).

Futility was also connected with a concern about the loss of "usefulness," an inability to "do anything," a sense of suffering. This was typified by descriptions such as:

> . . . he found himself getting increasingly weak . . . he used to sit on the back
> porch . . . he was two steps away from the toilet, two steps away from the

> bucket in case he vomited, two steps away from anything. And he just sat
> there (Nitschke transcript—Case 2).

Usefulness was not only understood by men in terms of their physical capacity.
Loss of sexual capacity was also a concern for the third case as he was no longer
able to "be a man" for his wife.

> I was sent back to Darwin hoping that the removal of my testicles and
> consequent loss of testosterone production would stop the cancer progressing.
> Unfortunately, this also made me impotent (letter to press).

Bodily Disintegration

The women in the study were less concerned about being useful and more
worried about facing the effects of bodily disintegration on themselves and
others—the loss of the fragrant attractive body to one that was disfigured, smelly,
and incontinent. The two women who suffered these conditions cut themselves
off from social intercourse as their symptoms and body odors increased.

The *fear* of bodily disfigurement and the attendant distaste concerning incontinence or fungating wounds were motivating factors for two other women in
their requests for euthanasia. Case 1 had always been proudly attractive and raged
against the ravages that cancer can bring to the body. Their perception of the
dignity of self and body was paramount in these instances.

Suffering

Unrelieved pain is cited as a strong motivator for euthanasia (Harrold, 1998;
van der Maas et al., 1996), though it is not often the major reason for the request
(Campbell, 1996). Likewise pain was not at issue in these cases. Physical
symptoms were a source of suffering for patients, particularly when poorly or
incompletely relieved. For some the symptoms were relentless and unbearable.
They were described as:

> It's bad news, because I scratch day and night. My hands and feet blister. Yes,
> I want to go. I know it's the right time. I can't take anymore (patient transcript
> recorded in psychiatric medical record)

> As it is he was living on milk, basically milk. And that was the problem really,
> he had a degree of vomiting and the like, it wasn't his real problem . . . He
> couldn't eat. He couldn't enjoy his food. He was sick to death of eating yogurt
> (Nitschke transcript—Case 2).

Case 3 wrote about the feeling of indignity he experienced as he lost control
over his bodily functions:

Morphine causes constipation—laxatives taken work erratically, often resulting in loss of bowel control in the middle of the night. I have to have a rubber
sheet on my bed, like a child who is not yet toilet-trained (Letter to press—
Case 3).

Emotional Distress and Depression

For some cases depressive symptoms were evident even though they were
formerly adjudged to be of sound mind when they made their decision to ask for
assistance to die. Case 3 described his suicidal feelings as:

Other drugs given to enhance the pain-relieving effects of the morphine have
caused me to feel suicidal to the point that I would have blown my head off
if I had had a gun.

Case 1 had already attempted suicide before she made contact and asked for
euthanasia. During the waiting time she offered to be interviewed on a television
program, a process which opened up some painful memories and set her again on
the path to her eventual suicide. The psychiatric assessment of Case 4 noted that
she had reduced reactivity to her surroundings, lowered mood, expressed hopelessness, a resignation about her future, and a desire to die.

A past history of depression earlier in life raises concern for vulnerability and
the risk of reduced coping. But recognition of clinical depression is the key
challenge. The person's sadness, despair, and demoralization may be accepted as
a normal response to their medical condition. These pleas of distress will be
understood differently by different people, depending on their training, role, and
specialization. A compassionate carer may hear grounds for euthanasia where the
consultation-liaison psychiatrist recognizes anhedonia, worthlessness, helplessness, hopelessness, and suicidal ideation, signifying a clinical depression.

DISCUSSION

The limitations of our work involve the small sample derived from the Darwin
experience, but it does represent the complete cohort of those who actively sought
euthanasia. Given this, our study of the roles and motivations of those involved
makes a worthwhile contribution about the clinical realities of such an experience, one from which we can learn.

The socio-political environment of the NT at the time, and its constitutional
relationship to the national parliament, meant that there was no formal evaluation
of the type of medical roles which developed, nor of the structures and processes
necessary to facilitate euthanasia. The development of a "euthanasia" doctor did
not reflect the spirit of the ROTI Act. In the Act the intention was for GPs to
conduct the practice of euthanasia as part of their care for the person. This
scenario assumes that Territorians have an ongoing relationship with a general

practitioner. Yet changes in the health system mean that fewer people have a long-term relationship with a family GP.

According to the Australian Medical Association spokesperson in the NT, Dr. Chris Wake, there were very few GPs who were willing to actively assist with suicide. This set up a situation where a doctor, such as Nitschke, who was committed to euthanasia, developed specific skills in the provision of this service, but did not provide overall medical management for these patients.

Whether or not the assessment and gatekeeping role can function effectively and safely is called into question by this Darwin experience. The negative message delivered in telling someone they are suitable for euthanasia merits reflection. There needs to be a mechanism through which any difference of opinion over prognosis can be resolved. Moreover, any psychiatric involvement must permit counseling and treatment of depression, rather than the role being constructed as an assessment hurdle, which is perceived as adversarial by the patient.

The motivations of these patients have become more evident with the opportunity to examine their cases in detail from a number of data sources and perspectives, to read the writings of those who died and the medical reports on their assessment and treatment. The medical personnel who were making the assessment decisions were functioning during a time of public debate and dissent over the issue. The media and parliamentary debates meant that there was intense public scrutiny and pressure on medical staff to make decisions quickly, perhaps without the chance of including a comprehensive clinical overview.

The reasons given by these patients for desiring death highlight the power of language in the doctor-patient relationship. A doctor may either affirm ongoing care of the patient or reinforce a sense of hopelessness. Yet patients require honesty about their condition and feel let down by medical staff who are unable to tell them the "truth."

Fear of what might happen in the future also emerged as a major reason for requesting death. A well-functioning and comprehensive palliative care service may provide patients with the opportunity to address these fears, many of which may prove to be unfounded. Similarly, concerns about being a burden are often resolved by a family meeting, which can reaffirm the worth of the family member. Volunteer programs via community-based palliative care counter loneliness and social isolation.

Empirical studies of desire for death have highlighted the pathway that develops in which untreated symptoms, loss of meaning and pleasure, worthlessness and hopelessness fuel the development of a clinical depression (Chochinov et al., 1995). Suicidal ideation grows directly from such negative cognitive states. We can see in the motivations of these patients this futility, despair, worthlessness, concern about body image, suffering, and depression. We have written elsewhere about the lack of effort to treat the depression (Kissane et al., 1998). Recognition of depression in the medically ill remains a serious clinical challenge for patients such as reviewed in this series.

Palliative care in Australia has benefited financially from the repeal of the ROTI Act as the government made further funds available to facilitate access, equity, and quality. Palliative care services are currently not meeting the needs of all Australians, and much further development is still needed. Access to palliative care should be an undeniable social right, one that could well predate any community consideration of euthanasia or physician-assisted suicide. Greater consultation with experts in all areas of end of life care is essential if a coordinated service is to be provided. A clearer focus on the assessment processes and supports required to deliver quality care is also necessary. One of the clear lessons from these deaths in Darwin is the community's challenge to develop comprehensive palliative care services, an issue that applies to many countries of the world.

REFERENCES

Allen, F. (1998). Euthanasia: Why torture dying people when we have sick animals put down? *Australian Psychologist, 33* (1), 12-15.

Ashby, M. (1995). Hard cases, causation and care of the dying. *Journal of Law and Medicine, 3*, 152-160.

Baume, P., & O'Malley, E. (1994). Euthanasia—Attitudes and practices of medical practitioners. *Medical Journal of Australia, 161* (2), 137.

Breitbart, W., Rosenfeld, B., & Passik, S. (1996). Interests in physician-assisted suicide among ambulatory HIV-infected patients. *American Journal of Psychiatry, 153*, 238-242.

Brown, J., Henteleff, P., Barakat, S., & Rowe, C. (1986). Is it normal for terminally ill patients to desire death? *American Journal of Psychiatry, 143*, 208-211.

Callahan, D. (1993). *The troubled dream of life: Living with mortality.* New York: Simon and Schuster.

Campbell, C. (1996). Suffering, compassion and dignity in dying. *Duquesne Law Review, 35* (1), 109-124.

Chevlen, E. (1996). The limits of prognostication. *Duquesne Law Review, 35* (1), 337-354.

Chochinov, H., Wilson, K., Enns, M., Mowchun, N., Lander, S., Levitt, M., & Clinch, J. (1995). Desire for death in the terminally ill. *American Journal of psychiatry, 152*, 1185-1191.

Commonwealth Department of Health and Family Services. (1998). *A background for a national strategy for palliative care in Australia.* Canberra, Commonwealth Department of Health and Family Services.

Ganzini, L., Fenn, D., & Lee, M. (1996). Attitudes of Oregon psychiatrists toward physician-assisted suicide. *American Journal of Psychiatry, 153*, 1469-1475.

Harrold, J. (1998). Pain, symptoms and suffering: Possibilities and barriers. In J. Harrold & J. Lynn (Eds.), *A Good Dying* (pp. 37-40). New York: The Haworth Press.

Hendin, H. (1994). Seduced by death: Doctors, patients, and the Dutch cure. *Issues in Law & Medicine, 10* (2), 123-168.

Humphry, D. (1991). *Final exit: The practicalities of self-deliverance and assisted suicide for the dying.* Oregon: The Hemlock Society.

Kissane, D. W., Street, A., & Nitschke, P. (1998). Seven deaths in Darwin: Case studies under the Rights of the Terminally Ill Act, Northern Territory, Australia. *The Lancet, 352* (9134), 1097-1102.

Kuhse, H., Singer, P., Baume, P., Clark, M., & Rickard, M. (1997). End-of-life decisions in Australian medical practice. *Medical Journal of Australia, 166* (17 February), 191-196.

Marker, R., & Smith, W. (1996). The art of verbal engineering. *Duquesne Law Review, 35* (1), 81-107.

McLaughlin, M. (1996). *The road to nowhere.* Four Corners, television program, Sydney, Australian Broadcasting Commission.

National Cancer Control Initiative (1998). *Cancer control towards 2002.* Melbourne, Commonwealth Department of Health and Family Services.

Northern Territory Government (1995). *Rights of the Terminally Ill Act 1995.* Northern Territory of Australia, Darwin: Government Publisher.

O'Connor, M. (1998). Palliative care and the euthanasia debate in Australia. *European Journal of Palliative Care, 5* (1), 27-31.

Owen, C., Tennant, C., Levi, J., & Jones, M. (1992). Suicide and euthanasia: Patient attitudes in the context of cancer. *Psycho-Oncology, 1,* 79-88.

Owen, C., Tennant, C., Levi, J., & Jones, M. (1994). Cancer patients' attitudes to final events in life: Wish for death, attitudes to cessation of treatment, suicide and euthanasia. *Psycho-Oncology, 3,* 1-9.

Preston, T., & Mero, R. (1996). Observations concerning terminally ill patients who choose suicide. *Journal of Pharmaceutical Care in Pain and Symptom Control, 4* (1-2), 183-192.

Sanson, A., Dickens, E., Melita, B., Nixon, M., Rowe, J., Tudor, A., & Tyrrell, M. (1998). Psychological perspectives on euthanasia and the terminally ill: An Australian psychological society discussion paper. *Australian Psychologists, 33* (1), 1-11.

Street, A. (1998). Competing discourses with/in palliative care. In J. Parker & S. Aranda (Eds.), *Palliative care: Explorations and challenges* (pp. 68-81). Sydney: MacLennan & Petty.

van der Maas, P., van der Wal, G., Haverkate, I., de Graaff, C., Kester, J., Onwuteaka-Philipsen, B., van der Heide, A., Bosma, J., & Willems, D. (1996). Euthanasia, physician assisted suicide, and other medical practices involving the end of life in the Netherlands. *New England Journal of Medicine, 335,* 1706-1711.

Webb, M. (1997). *The good death.* New York: Bantam Books.

"DISPENSING DEATH, DESIRING DEATH" BY ANNETTE STREET AND DAVID KISSANE: A COMMENTARY

PHILIP NITSCHKE, MBBs, PH.D.
Winnellie, Northern Territory, Australia

Dorothy Nelkin, writing in *The Lancet* (1996), recently drew attention to the practice of publishing material of a politically or socially sensitive nature in respectable journals to provide legitimacy for ideologically-based positions. The contentious question of voluntary euthanasia attracts people with strong ideologically-driven positions who seek legitimacy through the publication of research data. Because such material is then used to support or attack particular views on this issue, one is obliged to examine with great care any article which claims to present objective evidence supporting one or another side in this ongoing argument.

The article, "Desiring Death, Dispensing Death" by Annette Street and David Kissane (this issue) provides an example of this phenomenon. The authors present two main conclusions. They believe that patients are driven to seek euthanasia legislation because of what the authors describe as "negative cognitive states." They also conclude that access to good palliative care would negate any need for such legislation. The evidence presented to support these conclusions is drawn predominately from material gathered in extensive interviews between the authors and myself. I was the only person to have known and treated all of the patients who were eventually able to use the Northern Territory's Rights of the Terminally Ill Act. Unfortunately, the material reported in the article reflects only some of the views and information provided to the authors. Available material that conflicts directly with some of the material and conclusions presented has in some cases been omitted. In a previous collaborative work published as a result of this exercise, no such conclusions were drawn (Kissane, Street, & Nitschke, 1998).

To pursue the argument that "negative cognitive states" are a necessary precursor for a patient to seek access to voluntary euthanasia legislation, it is necessary to emphasize all those aspects of patients' histories that support such a thesis. Strengths displayed by individual patients have been minimized and downplayed. In particular, the common trait displayed by all patients, and overlooked completely in Street and Kissane's analysis, was the repeated statement that they all wished to remain in control of what was left in their lives. This particular characteristic meant that all seven of the patients clashed with the medical profession throughout their illness, and their statements often reflect this hostility.

Patient 3, the first person to make use of the law, had good evidence that his palliative care doctor had lied about his condition. His wife worked in the pathology laboratories at Darwin Hospital and discovered test results that had been withheld. In his public statement released after his death, the patient names the doctor concerned and accuses the medical profession of "experimentation" as they refused to be directed by him, insisting on providing further treatment even after he had made it clear this was not wanted. His feelings are summarized in the final paragraph:

> What right has anyone . . . to demand that I behave according to their rules until some omniscient doctor decides that I must have had enough and goes ahead and increases my morphine until I die? If you disagree with voluntary euthanasia, then don't use it, but don't deny me the right to use it if and when I want to (Dent, 1996).

Patient 4 had a similarly difficult time with the medical profession. In November 1996 her treating oncologist from South Australia estimated that her cancer, mycosis fungoides, had "clearly begun to run a more aggressive course," and he stated that "her prognosis is poor and is only measured in weeks" (Russell, 1996). On traveling to the Northern Territory she found that no specialist doctor was prepared to provide the necessary statement to confirm the accuracy of her diagnosis and prognosis. The Territory's only oncologist refused to cooperate and later gave evidence to a Senate inquiry indicating that he would never facilitate the use of such legislation:

> I was very intimately involved in (this patient's) care. I was not involved in her assisted suicide. That was for a conscience reason on my personal behalf, and I made that clear to them (Selva-Nayagam, 1997).

Faced with such an impasse, she took the unprecedented step of holding a national press conference, and publicly begged for a specialist Territory doctor to come forward and provide her with the assessment she needed. Only one doctor, an orthopedic surgeon, responded, and he indicated that he had done this because he was ashamed at the cowardice and insensitivity displayed by other members of the medical profession (Baddeley, 1997). Patient 4 then made use of the legislation and died on January 2, 1997. In a statement released after her death, she referred to the problems she had experienced with doctors who had attempted to stop her from using the law:

> I hope that anyone else wishing to use this Act does not have to go through such a long battle to find a doctor to help them. . . . I am pleased that the Northern Territory has such a law, even though it was so difficult for me to use, as at least now I can legally and honestly end my life. I hope this law survives and is able to help others like me, who have found that the suffering has become too great. It should not be overturned, but given a chance to work in the way it was intended. I want people to see just how important this law was to me now that I'm at the end of my life (Mills, 1997).

In some cases, hostility from doctors led patients wishing to use the law to feel obliged to provide an explanation to their doctors after their death. Patient 6 was obstructed by her doctors in NSW, and found it necessary to seek assistance from her five adult children to arrange for her stretcher transfer to Darwin. After her death, her daughter wrote to the involved doctor and tried to explain why it was so important for her mother to maintain control and to go against her doctor's wishes.

> Mom never wavered in her determination to end her life in this way. She said she wasn't frightened of dying, but that she was sad to be leaving her family and friends. She said that she knew there wasn't much life left in her and she didn't want to die a little bit at a time. I know that you wish you could have given Mom all that she needed to help her to die peacefully and naturally, but that wasn't possible for her. We, her family, are satisfied that this is what she truly wanted and are happy to have been able to help her carry out her final wish (James, 1997).

Similar statements were made by the other patients who sought to use the legislation. Street and Kissane's suggestion that the pursuit of such legislation is the result of a "negative cognitive overlay" misses the most significant unifying characteristic of this group: their endeavor to maintain control over their lives until the end. To suggest that fears of bodily disintegration, family concerns, suffering, or social isolation were dominant driving forces behind the use of this law is to misrepresent the actual situation. The evidence presented by Street and Kissane to support such claims includes serious errors. Case 7 is used as an example of "social isolation." In fact, this patient was surrounded by a network of nursing friends who rostered their time so that she was never left alone throughout the last months of her life. Her partner of many years closed his business and moved so that he could be constantly with her. In a statement to the Australian Senate he wrote:

For almost two months her former workmates instituted a roster to enable their fellow workmate in need to stay in the environment she loved so much to pass on with peace in her own home. These people's love and practical devotion to their fellow worker and friend cannot be measured on earth. They sacrificed their own time and family time to care as true friends (Collins, 1997).

This is the patient described by Street and Kissane as "socially isolated" as evidenced by the fact that she "ceased going to the supermarket, to the theatre, and visiting people."

Like the other seven, this patient made statements indicating that she appreciated being able to remain in control. She wrote:

I have reached a point where I feel that at some stage soon, I would like to end my suffering and use the Northern Territory's Rights of the Terminally Ill legislation . . . (I) have the relief of knowing that at this stage at least, I can go ahead and end my suffering at any time. . . . I will die soon, but please let me and those other terminally ill people in my position, decide when (Wild, 1997).

I treated and got to know all of the people who attempted to use the Territory voluntary euthanasia law. They were an unusual group of patients with the particular strengths needed to overcome the considerable obstacles placed in their way as they sought to access the world's first operational euthanasia legislation. In this process, the patients often found themselves in conflict with the medical profession who fought throughout this period, through their various professional organizations, to make the law inoperative. Patients found themselves pitted against doctors as they struggled for what they clearly believed was their right. The Street and Kissane article continues to promote this orthodox medical view and, as such, misses the most important lessons that could have been learned from this unique social experiment.

This debate over the issue will intensify as we move deeper into the new century. A willingness on the part of the medical profession to see patients seeking voluntary euthanasia as autonomous individuals with valid rational concerns is essential. Unfortunately, the article by Street and Kissane will not assist such resolution.

REFERENCES

Baddeley, S. (1997). Recorded telephone conversation (15 December) with P. Nitschke. Darwin.

Collins, B. (1997). *Proceedings* (2 September) Senate of Australia. Hansard.

Dent, R. (1996). Open letter to Federal Parliamentarians (21 September). Darwin.

James, L. (1997). Private communication to D. Haskins (3 March). Mt. Warrigal.

Kissane, D., Street, A., & Nitschke, P. (1998). Seven deaths in Darwin. *The Lancet, 352,* 1097-1102.

Mills, J. (1997). Final statement (2 January). Darwin.

Nelkin, D. (1998). Scientific journals and public disputes. *The Lancet, 325,* Supplement 2.

Russell, J. (1996). Statement of prognosis of Ms. J. Mills (19 November). Darwin.

Selva-Nayagam, S. (1997). Senate of Australia (24 January). Legal and Constitutional Legislation Committee Hearings, Hansard.

Wild, E. (1997). Letter to Australian Senators (17 March), Darwin.

OF EUPHEMISMS AND EUTHANASIA: THE LANGUAGE GAMES OF THE NAZI DOCTORS AND SOME IMPLICATIONS FOR THE MODERN EUTHANASIA MOVEMENT

C. BEN MITCHELL, PH.D.
Trinity International University, Deerfield, Illinois

ABSTRACT

Euphemisms are place-holders for important concepts. They may disguise a practice which one might abhor if it were given another name. In Nazi Germany during World War II, euphemisms were used to desensitize physicians and society to the horrors of a program of euthanasia. This article examines some of the euphemisms used by the Nazi physicians to redefine medicalized killing, compares the Nazi language games with those of contemporary proponents of medicalized killing, and concludes that the consistent application of euphemisms for medicalized killing significantly weakens arguments against assisted killing.

We should watch the way we talk. Human society can be described as a long conversation about what matters. In this conversation, the language we use to describe our social practices not only reveals our attitudes and virtues, it shapes them (Winslow, 1994, p. 1).

Nowhere is the revelatory and shaping function of words more evident than in the contemporary debate about physician-assisted suicide and euthanasia. Nearly everyone is aware of the role metaphors play in healthcare. For instance, Susan Sontag (1978) has written of the "punitive" uses of "illness as metaphor." A blistering commentary on medical education, Samuel Shem's (1978) *The House of God*, allows non-physicians to peek behind the veil and see the use of pejorative metaphors used by medical residents. In *The House of God*, a patient "who has lost—often through age—what goes into being a human being," was labeled a GOMER (Get Out of My Emergency Room). More recently, Edmund Pellegrino (1994) has written on the perils of metaphors in healthcare reform in his essay, "Words *Can* Hurt You: Some Reflections On the Metaphors of Managed Care." Indeed, words can hurt you.

Words can also help you. That is, the proper choice of words can ennoble the healthcare profession. Winslow (1994) has said, "To call health care a ministry is to emphasize faithful service, devotion, and compassion" (p. 5). Words can elevate the patient from "room 3, CABG procedure" to "Mary Smith, wife, mother, community leader" or from "*the* patient" to "*my* patient."

In addition to metaphors, euphemisms shape the way we think about healthcare, physicians, and patients. According to linguists Keith Allan and Kate Burridge (1991), "a euphemism is used as an alternative to a dispreferred expression, in order to avoid possible loss of face: either one's own face or, through giving offense, that of the audience, or of some third party" (p. 11). Through the use of euphemism and dysphemism, language may be used as either a shield or a weapon.

> To speak euphemistically is to use language like a shield against the feared, the disliked, the unpleasant; euphemisms are motivated by the desire not to be offensive, and so they have positive connotations; in the least euphemisms seek to avoid too many negative connotations. They are used to upgrade the denotation (as a shield against scorn); they are used deceptively to conceal the unpleasant aspects of the denotation (as a shield against anger); and they are used to display in-group identity (as a shield against the intrusion of the out-groupers) (Allan & Burridge, 1991, pp. 221-222).

The use of euphemisms has important implications for the practice of moral medicine. In fact, the erosion of medicine under Hitler was, at least in part, due to the way euphemisms for medicalized murder were used so effectively. The present debate about euthanasia and assisted-suicide desperately needs to be informed by this history. The language games played by the Nazi doctors have critical implications for the present debate.

In the remainder of this article, I will 1) examine some of the euphemisms used by the Nazi physicians to redefine medicalized killing, 2) compare the Nazi language games with those of contemporary proponents of medicalized killing, and 3) conclude that the consistent application of euphemisms for medicalized killing significantly weakens arguments against assisted killing.

MEDICALIZED MURDER UNDER DICTATORSHIP

Leo Alexander, a physician-consultant on duty with the Chief Counsel for War Crimes, wrote a devastating critique of "Medical Science Under Dictatorship" in the July 1949 *New England Journal of Medicine*. Alexander (1949) asserted that

"Nazi propaganda was highly effective in perverting public opinion and public conscience, in a remarkably short period of time" (p. 40). Alexander showed how the barrage of propaganda against what he called "the traditional nineteenth-century attitudes toward the chronically ill" fueled the fires of the furnaces at Dachau, Auschwitz, and the other killing centers erected under Hitler. Filmmaker John Michalczyk (1994) mentioned two silent film documentaries, *Was du erbst* (What You Inherit) and *Erb Krank* (The Hereditarily Ill), produced by the Nazi government which depicted images of the severely handicapped and mentally ill (p. 65). Later, two additional films, *Opfer der Vergangenheit* (Victims of the Past) and *Das Erbe* (The Inheritance), were shown under order of the Führer in all 5,300 German theaters. In 1939, *Dasein ohne Leben* (Existence without Life), was produced under commission of those who ran the infamous Operation T-4 euthanasia campaign. This film was "designed to reassure those involved in the euthanasia program that this was an ethical and humane procedure" (Michalczyk, 1994, p. 67). While copies of *Dasein ohne Leben* were all destroyed, a copy of the script was recovered after the war.

Commenting on the contents of the script, Michalczyk (1994) observed,

> As the professor clinically describes the masses of 400,000 German patients in mental asylums, images of the helpless wards punctuate his words . . . In a pseudo-humane tone, the lecturer uses religious language of mercy killing to help "liberate" these creatures, while simultaneously denying these individuals their humanity. How cruel it would be to maintain these spiritually dead people as "living corpses." It is a sacred demand of charity that we eliminate the suffering of these helpless individuals, the film advocates. To show how humane this process is, the lecturer concludes by confessing that if he were struck down by a crippling disease, he himself would opt for mercy killing (p. 67).

From the film:

> Isn't it the duty of those concerned to help the incapable—and that means total idiots and incurable mental patients—to their right?
> Is that not a sacred command of charity?
> Deliver those you cannot heal!
> The Director of a large mental institution asked this question of the parents of all his incurable charges.
> 73% answered "Yes."
> A mother wrote: "Don't ask, do it!" [this citation literally burned on the screen] (Burleigh, 1994, p. 199).

Finally, the film with the highest production values was made in 1941. *Ich klage an!* (I Accuse) takes up a familiar story. Hanna Heyt, the heroine of the film, shows signs of physical deterioration due to multiple sclerosis. She makes it clear that she does not wish to spend her last days in a "vegetative state." Her husband, Thomas, in consultation with her physician, gives her an overdose which kills her. A dramatic courtroom sequence follows.

> ... Thomas accuses the law of not helping in the case of his wife's suffering. The defense concludes that the law must be changed to allow mercy killing for humanitarian reasons. The film ends by putting the verdict in the hands of the audience (Burleigh, 1994, p. 69).

From the film:

> SCHÖNBRUNN Gentlemen, if you ask me, Professor Heyt must be acquitted because he is an example to every doctor. I know I am touching on a sensitive issue, but at the same time it is a very inflexible point in our current moral and social view.
>
> HUMMEL I don't know . . . if one simply allows this sort of thing—will people still go to see their doctors?
>
> SCHÖNBRUNN "Simply allows?" One must . . .
>
> ROLFS Now look, what if—and I've been drawing an invalidity pension all my life—what if I go off sick one day, then they might simply do away with me?
>
> SCHÖNBRUNN For God's sake! . . . The most important precondition would always be that the patient wished it!
>
> ROLFS Many of them will, for a moment or two.
>
> HUMMEL When one of them is mentally ill, they sometimes want it.
>
> SCHÖNBRUNN Yes: if someone is deranged, or depressed or for one reason or another has no will of his own, then the state must assume responsibility! It must establish a commission consisting of doctors and lawyers, with a proper legal character. One should no longer have to stand by watching thousands of people who in earlier times would have died a gentle death, but who nowadays have to endure the most awful suffering simply because the doctors know how to prolong their poor lives artificially (Burleigh, 1994, p. 214).

The post-war testimony of Nazi doctors confirms the impact of the film in shaping their notions of the morality of euthanasia (Lifton, 1986, p. 49). For anyone acquainted with the contemporary debate on euthanasia and assisted suicide, these are familiar word pictures and arguments. The film makes use of the euphemisms for euthanasia: "right to die," "caring," "make the poor woman's end less painful," "I delivered my wife," and others.

As we now know, the euthanasia program did not stop with the killing of the mentally disabled, the feeble, and the terminally ill. Aly (1994) recounts that "In 1941, the SD killing units active in the East reported with barbaric regularity that in addition to 'Soviet commissars,' Jews, and the mentally ill, they were shooting capital criminals, beggars, and 'trouble-makers'" (p. 59). Patients suffering from specified diseases, persons who were continually institutionalized for at least five years, the criminally insane, and those who were not German citizens or not of Aryan descent were murdered under Hitler's "Final Solution."

Interestingly, even the institutions established to evaluate prospective patients for euthanasia were euphemistically named: "Realm's Work Committee of Institutions for Cure and Care," "Realm's Committee for Scientific Approach to Severe Illness Due to Heredity and Constitution," "Charitable Foundation for Institutional Care," and "Charitable Transport Company for the Sick" (Alexander, 1949, pp. 40-41). According to Alexander (1949), this latter institution, "brought 150-250 brains at a time to a Dr. Hallervorden, a neuropathologist for the Third Reich" (p. 40). Hallervorden remarked:

> There was wonderful material among those brains, beautiful mental defectives, malformations, and early infantile diseases. I accepted those brains of course. Where they came from and how they came to me was really none of my business (Alexander, 1949, p. 40).

While examples of the ubiquitous use of euphemisms in Nazi "medicine" could go on *ad nauseam,* a few examples from Nazi diaries and journals must suffice. Christian Pross (1994) has argued persuasively that the best source for understanding the methods of Nazi medicine is not the post-war interviews with the Nazi doctors found in much of Robert J. Lifton's (1986) illuminating volume, *The Nazi Doctors: Medical Killing and the Psychology of Genocide.* Rather, says Pross, "The diaries, letters, and publications of Nazi doctors of the time . . . contain few elements of idealism or the high ethical standards of the 'physician-self,' and thus scant evidence of doubling" (p. 13). The notion of "doubling" to which Pross refers is a notion introduced by Robert Lifton to explain how the Nazi doctors could perform heinous acts while thinking themselves to be noble physicians. In brief, Lifton argues that the Nazi doctors experienced a psychological "personality split" in which the "Auschwitz-Self" and the "physician-self" existed simultaneously in the same mind.

Only a few months after the suspension of Operation T-4, legislation was introduced to legalize institutionalized euthanasia. Aly (1994) recounted that the law required the Reich Minister of the Interior to appoint a Reich Commissioner who would oversee all institutions "concerned, even in part, with the accommodation and treatment of the mentally ill, feeble-minded, epileptics, and psychopaths" (p. 165). Euthanasia was justified under the new legislation as part of "wartime economic measures" (p. 165). Beds would need to be made available for Nazi soldiers wounded in the war. Thus, something would have to be done with those who were presently occupying the beds and who were exhausting scarce medical resources. According to Aly, by the time the new law became effective the Reich Association of Mental Hospitals had already killed over 70,000 patients. Under the new law the Reich Commissioner for Mental Hospitals was subordinate to the Minister of the Interior and was authorized "to take necessary measures" to maintain the economic viability of the asylums-turned-army hospitals (p. 165). Patients were labeled as having lives which were "usable," "unusable," "worthy," and "unworthy" (Aly, 1994, p. 165).

The designation, "Life Unworthy of Living" (*lebensunwertes Leben*) was an established euphemism decades before the war. In 1920 Karl Binding and Alfred Hoche wrote what was to become a most influential tract on euthanasia, "Permitting the Destruction of Unworthy Life" (Binding & Hoche, 1992). While Binding and Hoche frequently used the term "killing" when referring to euthanasia, they were also fond of euphemisms. For instance, Binding said of killing a patient who is experiencing pain, "This is not 'an act of killing in the legal sense' but is rather the modification of an irrevocably present cause of death which can no longer be evaded. *In truth it is a purely healing act*" (p. 240, emphasis added). Interestingly, this method of referring to medicalized killing was used by some of the Nazi doctors themselves. One of the physicians who euthanized children under T-4 said, "there was no killing, strictly speaking . . . People felt this is not murder, it is a putting-to-sleep" (Lifton, 1986, p. 57).

Murderous medicine was also couched in economic euphemisms. In 1944, for instance, H. J. Becker, acting head of the Central Clearinghouse for Mental Hospitals, introduced measures to govern the so-called "practical work" of the asylums. This euphemism was, according to Aly (1994), a reference to "thousands of murders" by Nazi physicians (p. 180). Becker was an indefatigable number-cruncher. He "even calculated economic losses due to friction resulting from 'unproductive excitement' over the death of a 'useless person'" (Aly, 1994, p. 182).

> As late as February 1945, Hans Joachim Becker issued a form with which doctors were to report sick forced laborers who "would probably remain in the institution for more than four weeks, "In the final days of the Third Reich, a forced laborer who might not be able to work for more than four weeks had lost the right to live. The decision was no longer made by a physician but by the Central Clearinghouse on the basis of a few lines in a "report of findings" (Aly, 1994, p. 184).

Clearly, euphemisms for murder played a significant role in the Nazi euthanasia program. What Lifton (1986) called "detoxifying language" contributed to an ethos which allowed physicians to turn from healers to killers. Convinced that some patients and, by extension, all Jews were merely "human ballast" who had " . . . lives which have so completely lost the attribute of legal status that their continuation has permanently lost all value, both for the bearer of that life and for society" (Binding & Hoche, 1992, p. 246), Nazi physicians perpetrated undeniable atrocities in human experimentation and euthanasia.

THE CONTEMPORARY CAMPAIGN

Examples of euphemisms are ubiquitous in the contemporary debate on euthanasia and assisted-suicide. Both the popular and academic presses have inundated the book shelves with euphemistic titles. *Final Exit: The Practicalities of Self-Deliverance and Assisted Suicide for the Dying* (Humphry, 1991), *The Least Worst Death: Essays in Bioethics at the End of Life* (Battin, 1994), and *Prescription: Medicide* (Kevorkian, 1991) are just a few of the books. Such titles may be excused by acknowledging the titillating nature of marketing strategies, but a more sobering look at contemporary euphemisms and linguistic strategies is in order.

First, we have our own genre of assisted-dying films from the feature film *Who's Life is it Anyway?*, to more obscure videos such as, *Please Let Me Die,* and made-for-TV-movies such as *Last Wish. Last Wish* is an ABC-TV movie based on Betty Rollin's 1985 book about helping her mother commit suicide. The movie received mixed reactions. David Klinghoffer (1992) reviewing the film for the *Washington Times* said the movie was "a noxious concoction" which ignores "the entire body of Western moral teaching." At the same time, movie reviewer Susan Stewart (1992) of the *Detroit Free Press* said the film was so "inspiring" that "at times, you're actually able to forget you're being proselytized." In addition, there are the occasional PBS airings of documentaries which bring the Dutch euthanasia experience into our living rooms. Most recently, of course, the now infamous Dr. Kevorkian brought us face-to-face with active euthanasia on the television program *60 Minutes.*

Second, popular culture is suffused with euphemisms for euthanasia. "Mercy killing," "merciful death," "death with dignity," "painless end to suffering," "termination of life," "humane treatment," and even "comfort care" are part of the public conversation. Recently, neologisms such as "managed death" (Sulmasy, 1995, pp. 133-136) have crept into the glossary of terms for euthanasia (itself an euphemism). Former member of Congress and professor of law at Georgetown University, Robert F. Drinan (1995) published a commentary arguing that "The debate about the moral and legal issues that arise when a terminally ill patient wants to shorten the period of suffering should not be confused with suicide. Perhaps the more appropriate term is 'expedited death.'" Though unlikely to catch on, this euphemism, like the others, demonstrates how far some are willing to go to avoid the obvious.

Third, most people understand and acknowledge the need for effective euphemisms if advocacy of assisted-dying is to be successful. University of Utah professor and medical ethicist Margaret Pabst Battin (1994) takes Drinan one step further. In her challenging volume, *The Least Worst Death: Essays in Bioethics on the End of Life,* Battin argues that American medicine should learn its lesson about euthanasia and assisted suicide not from the Dutch, but from contemporary Germany.

Battin observes that Germans have at least four words for "suicide" (*Selbstmord, Selbsttötung, Suizid,* and *Freitod*). She laments the obvious poverty of the English language to equal the nuances of colloquial German. The word which possesses the preferred connotation is *Freitod* ("free death"). Says Battin, "The very concept of *Freitod*—a notion without religious, altruistic overtones and without negative moral or psychological implications, but that celebrates the voluntary choice of death as a personal expression of principled idealism— is, in short, linguistically unfamiliar to English speakers" (p. 263).

Perceptively, Battin (1994) acknowledges that some kind of language game is necessary if American culture is going to accept medicalized killing of any sort.

> Language is crucial in shaping attitudes about end-of-life practices, and because of the very different lexical resources of English and German, it is clear that English speakers cannot straightforwardly understand the very different German conception of these matters. Even in situations of terminal illness, the very concept of voluntary death resonates differently for the German speaker who conceives of it as *Freitod* than it does for the English speaker who conceives of it as *suicide* (p. 263).

Later in the chapter she admits, ". . . what we see is that we are limited by our own language, and do not have the linguistic resources for understanding the issue in the way members of another culture can" (p. 265). Clearly, then, for Battin the issue is the language we use to describe medicalized killing. This brings us full circle. Language matters.

Finally, when euphemisms find their way into public policy, clarity gives way to ambiguity. For instance, Oregon's recent narrowly passed assisted-suicide legislation makes use of at least a couple of critical euphemisms. First, the title of the legislation is, "The Oregon Death With Dignity Act." Interestingly, in §1.01, definitions are provided for a host of words found in the legislation, including definitions for "adult," "attending physician," "consulting physician," "coun-seling," "patient," and "qualified patient," among others. Yet, there is no defini-tion of "dignity" or even "death with dignity." As Paul Ramsey (1974) pointed out just over two decades ago, "death with dignity" may in fact be a gross "indignity" (pp. 47-62).

Furthermore, the "Death With Dignity Act" makes repeated reference to death in "a humane and dignified manner" without defining or distinguishing between a "humane act" and an "inhumane act." Section 4.01.1, on immunities specifies, "No person shall be subject to civil or criminal liability or professional disci-plinary action for participating in good faith with this Act. This includes being present when a qualified patient takes the prescribed medication to end his or her own life in a humane and dignified manner." Thus, the law presupposes that assisted self-murder is, within specified parameters, a "humane" act. Moreover, the language tends to imply that a physician is "inhumane" if he or she refuses to comply with the requests of a patient who wants to kill himself or herself. But what makes that the case? Unless "humane" is appropriately defined, the language of the Act remains ambiguous.

Better designed studies on attitudes toward medicalized killing have sought to rid survey language of the ambiguity of euphemisms. For instance, in a survey of 1,355 randomly selected physicians in the state of Washington, Jonathan Cohen et al. (1994), used the phrase "prescription medication [e.g., narcotics or barbiturates] or the counseling of an ill patient so he or she may use an overdose to end his or her own life" instead of "physician-assisted suicide" (pp. 89-94). Instead of "euthanasia" the survey used the phrase, "deliberate administration of an overdose of medication to an ill patient at his or her request with the primary intent to end his or her life." One must wonder what the response of voters would have been if the legislation had been titled, "The Legalized Self-Murder Act" or "The Assisted Self-Killing Act."

CONCLUSION

Euphemisms—using a less direct word or phrase for one considered offensive—are linguistic devices which are place-holders for notions or practices we would consider abhorrent if we called them what they are. Euphemisms take the sting out of practices we would otherwise disdain.

While it has not been the purpose of this article to argue that medicalized killing is wrong, it is the candid presupposition. Nevertheless, arguments can be made from "both sides of the isle" that euphemisms do not serve the purpose of perspicacious speech or informed decision-making.

I have argued that the Nazi use of euphemisms enable physicians in the Third Reich to commit horrendous atrocities and yet sleep well at night. I have argued, furthermore, that the ever-present use of euphemisms in the contemporary debate over medicalized killing contributes to ambiguity and has the effect of salving the consciences of many who embrace its tenets.

If those who oppose medicalized killing are to contribute to informed public debate on the topic, it is important that they are not accomplices in using euphemisms for murder. They must not succumb to such usage under the umbrella of being viewed as irenic debaters. In sum, we need to tell it like it is: euthanasia and assisted-suicide are really medicalized murder and complicity to self-murder respectively. The use of euphemisms significantly weakens the argument of those who find medicalized killing morally abhorrent. Such language games permit our culture to hide behind the veil of pseudo-mercy and false conceptions of the humane.

REFERENCES

Alexander, L. (1949, July 14). Medical science under dictatorship. *The New England Journal of Medicine, 241,* 39-47.

Allan, K., & Burridge, K. (1991). *Euphemism and dysphemism: Language used as a shield and weapon.* New York: Oxford University Press.

Aly, G. (1994). Medicine against the useless *and* Pure and tainted progress. In G. Aly, P. Chroust, & C. Pross (Eds.), *Cleansing the fatherland: Nazi medicine and racial hygiene* (pp. 22-98, 156-237). Baltimore, MD: Johns Hopkins University Press.

Battin, M. P. (1994). *The least worst death: Essays in bioethics on the end of life.* New York: Oxford University Press.

Binding, K., & Hoche, A. (1992, Fall). Permitting the destruction of unworthy life. *Issues in Law & Medicine, 8,* 231-265. English translation by W. E. Wright, P. G. Derr, & R. Saloman.

Burleigh, M. (1994). *Death and deliverance: "Euthanasia" in Germany 1900-1945.* New York: Cambridge University Press.

Cohen, J. S., Fihn, S. D., Boyko, E. J., Jonsen, A. R., & Wood, R. W. (1994). Attitudes toward assisted suicide and euthanasia among physicians in Washington state. *New England Journal of Medicine, 331,* 89-94.

Drinan, R. F. (1995). Commentary: Suicide the wrong term for gravely ill who want to die. *Religion News Service,* January 25, 1995.

Humphry, D. (1991). *Final exit: The practicalities of self-deliverance and assisted suicide for the dying.* Eugene, OR: The Hemlock Society.

Kevorkian, J. (1991). *Prescription: Medicide.* New York: Prometheus Books.

Klinghoffer, D. (January 12, 1992). *The Washington Times,* A-1.

Lifton, R. J. (1986). *The Nazi doctors: Medical killing and the psychology of genocide.* New York: Basic Books.

Michalczyk, J. J. (1994). Euthanasia in Nazi propaganda films: Selling murder. In J. J. Michalczyk (Ed.), *Medicine, ethics, and the Third Reich: Historical and contemporary issues* (pp. 64-70). Kansas City, MO: Sheed and Ward.

Pellegrino, E. D. (1994, November-December). Words *can* hurt you: Some reflections on the metaphors of managed care. *Journal of the American Board of Family Practitioners, 7,* 505-510.

Pross, C. (1994). Introduction. In G. Aly, P. Chroust, & C. Pross (Eds.), *Cleansing the fatherland: Nazi medicine and racial hygiene* (pp. 1-21). Baltimore, MD: Johns Hopkins University Press.

Ramsey, P. (1974, May). The indignity of "death with dignity." *Hastings Center Studies, 2,* 47-62.

Shem, S. (1978). *The house of God.* New York: Dell Publishing.

Sontag, S. (1978). *Illness as metaphor.* New York: Farrar, Straus and Giroux.

Stewart, S. (January 10, 1992). *The Detroit Free Press.*

Sulmasy, D. P. (1995). Managed care and managed death. *Archives of Internal Medicine, 155,* 133-136.

Winslow, G. R. (1994). Minding our language: Metaphors and biomedical ethics. *Update, 10,* 1, 3.

KEVORKIAN, MARTHA WICHOREK AND US:
A PERSONAL ACCOUNT*

KALMAN J. KAPLAN, PH.D.
Michael Reese Hospital and Medical Center

MARY LEONHARDI, M.S.W.
Wayne State University & Neighborhood Service Organization, Detroit

ABSTRACT

In this short article, the authors describe their attempt to do suicide-prevention with a patient that ultimately died as the result of a physician-assisted suicide. Autopsy revealed no sign of physical disease but the patient's letters indicate a preoccupation with independence as the definition of life, and conviction that people who lose independence are no longer alive.

I am not stressed, oppressed, or depressed. I don't have Alzheimer's and am not terminally ill, but I am 82 years old and I want to die.

These words were written by Martha Wichorek within a day of her death by assisted suicide at the hands of Dr. Georges Reding, a Kalamazoo, Michigan psychiatrist (who is in training for "patholysis") in the presence of Dr. Jack Kevorkian. The autopsy conducted by Dr. John Somerset of Wayne County found neither any sign of a terminal condition nor indeed any evidence of medical disease. Martha just wanted to die. This case puts into stark relief the contrast between suicide prevention and doctor assisted suicide. If a clinician encounters a person about to jump off a bridge, is it his duty to extend his hand to prevent him from jumping or to help him jump? To examine this question, let us share our involvement with Martha Wichorek.

In early December of 1996, one of us (KK), received the first of what turned out to be five unsolicited letters from Ms. Wichorek. We think that Martha wrote these letters as part of a political campaign she was personally conducting in

*An earlier version of this article appeared in *Newslink, 23* (4), 9-10, 1997.

Michigan and nationally to legalize state euthanasia clinics.[1] The first letter, like all of them, was written in impeccably neat handwriting and offered an unusual description of the stages of what she called "the life-death cycle." An excerpt of this letter follows:

> Dec. 2, 1996.
> Prof. Kaplan, Dear Friend
> In matters pertaining to the euthanasia-assisted suicide issue, we have heard and read a hundred times that "Only God gives life and only He should take it away." True, God does give life and also takes it away gradually, by way of old age, disease, drugs, etc.
> When "life" (being able to do things for yourself and others) is taken away, unless a heart attack or accident strikes first, every human being usually descends into the "miserable existence" stage (cannot do anything for yourself or others—totally helpless). This stage of that life-death cycle can last weeks, months or years and is the most dreaded of human experiences.
> We also hear and read "the sanctity of life," "concern for human life," "we must protect life," etc. Everyone agrees that it is right, moral and proper to sanctify, protect and value "life." However, when "life" is taken away and we Elderly, terminally ill, Alzheimer's, etc., descend into the "miserable existence" stage, very few officials and medical personnel acknowledge that this stage is a special stage and should receive special treatment. In fact, many just say "if the heart is beating, then the patient is alive."
> This refusal to divide the "life"—"miserable existence"—"death" cycle into distinct categories is causing most of the animosity in euthanasia discussions. Many deliberately use the word "life" when they know very well that they mean "miserable existence," hoping they can confuse listeners.

Martha went on for three full pages, speaking about the suffering of those in the "miserable existence stage" which she also called the "other death row." She called for a state approved euthanasia clinic. Among the indignities of the "miserable existence stage" she included: 1) nursing home or hospital tests and procedures, 2) living with children, 3) hospice, 4) in home and visiting nurse arrangements, 5) living wills, and 6) committing suicide without the help of a doctor. She signed the letter "a still clear thinking 81 year old human being."

Concerned, each of us (KK, ML) separately called Mrs. Wichorek. Our conversations revealed that Martha had lost her husband to cancer three years previously and had three grown daughters. She lived alone, and aside from some normal ailments associated with aging, was in reasonable health. She was not terminal, not in acute physical pain, and had a sharp mind. Yet she advocated forcefully for a state-sanctioned euthanasia clinic for "we terminally ill, elderly Alzheimer's."

---

[1] We have seen letters written back to Martha by Governor Engler and Senator Abraham of Michigan, attempting to discourage her in her endeavor.

Significantly, Martha was none of these except elderly, and by her own description "still clear thinking." Yet she insisted she wanted to die before she became incapacitated, or terminally ill. Neither of us felt, after speaking with her, that Martha Wichorek was acutely suicidal. We both were concerned, however, that her perception of her situation would lead to a more concrete death plan in the future, and also that she presented constricted thinking.

In January, 1997, Dr. Kaplan received a second letter from Martha, reiterating many of the same points. We did not contact her at this time. In March, 1997, KK received a third letter. However, this time the tone had changed—ominously. Now Martha began to write of her own death and of using the money she would save through her death to buy her grandson (who was graduating from college) a car. We both contacted her. We stressed the hostility underlying such a gift, and the ambivalent feelings that a survivor would have toward a gift brought about by her suicide. We stated that we thought her grandson would prefer a live grandmother to a car received as a result of her suicide. She told us about the death of her husband. We acknowledged her loneliness and suggested she get involved in activities or even therapy. She rejected both of these options. We then stressed Martha's capabilities and how much she had to offer in the fight for better health care for the elderly. KK invited Martha to present her views at a class he taught in suicide. Martha declined but said she enjoyed our calls. She gave KK the phone number of a speakers bureau for "problems of the elderly." Curious, KK called the number. It was the law firm of Geoffrey Feiger, the lead attorney for Jack Kevorkian! Martha's legal knowledge began to make some sense! We resolved to keep in regular contact with her.

In April, 1997, something new happened. Martha wrote KK from the hospital where she had undergone a hysterectomy after bouts with vaginal bleeding. She was doing fine and acknowledged that "she was getting stronger" but described the "torture" she endured. She specified: 1) "IVs with anesthetics, nutrients, etc.", 2) "tight rubber stockings that stretched from her toes to the crotch, and expanding and contracting legging attached to a motor for better blood circulation," 3) "tubes in my nose, for oxygen," 4) "breathing tubes to exercise my lungs," 5) "blood pressure and temperature checks every hour, an EKG, blood drawn for lab tests, etc.," and 6) she was expected to walk, one day after surgery, alone from the bathroom, holding onto the IV pole.

Martha spent three days in the hospital. Those of us who have undergone surgery recognize these "tortures" as unpleasant but temporary. For Martha, however, these tortures represented yet another reason for a state euthanasia clinic. She oddly claimed that in the absence of legalized euthanasia, she chose surgery "because the alternatives . . . such as living with children, in a nursing home, with hospice or home care arrangements were worse."

Space limitations prevent us from going on in detail with more of Martha's specific comments. She was a colorful and interesting lady whom we liked. However, we had real concerns. Among our concerns were: 1) Black and white negative thinking (she rejected all solutions to problems of the elderly and terminally ill—including her own). 2) A counterphobic stance toward dependency (rejection of all help or assistance). 3) Insistence on a non-biological definition of life (as being able to take care of oneself), 4) Use of euphemisms (she created a new life stage "miserable existence" rather than describing herself as feeling miserable), 5) Unsolicited speaking for others (she advocated for a state-sanctioned euthanasia clinic for "we terminally ill, elderly, Alzheimer's"). 6) An overly rational legal analysis of the problem of euthanasia and doctor-assisted suicide. 7) Exaggeration of annoying but relatively minor and temporary discomforts. 8) An irrational tunnel vision behind her seemingly logical arguments. 9) An apparent blurring of her personal situation with the campaign to legalize euthanasia and the eagerness to make herself a martyr for the cause. 10) Her plan to die to give her grandson a car. 11) Reluctance to accept family support (she found death preferable to living with her children). 12) Her choice to die (and be in control) rather than accept her current relatively healthy though somewhat diminished state.

This case also raised broader issues for us. 1) With legislation/permission for assisted suicide, there is more chance for abuse (both by the financially driven choices in health care, and also by families who wished their loved ones dead), 2) The extension of choice of assisted suicide to physically sound but depressed individuals, 3) The "quick" solution of death for the elderly when they feel useless (is there any relationship between the rising rates of elderly suicide and the publicity related to assisted suicide?), 4) The substitution of "dignity of death" for "meaning of life," 5) The focus of death as a right rather than a fact, and the over concern with the legal as opposed to the psychological and spiritual issues. The decriminalization of suicide in contemporary society does not mean that health care professionals should encourage it.

On a personal note, we never met Martha Wichorek but we will miss her. She was a lively intelligent person who had written three books. We suspect her death may well have represented a political act in her eyes. We don't think she had to die when she did and we wish she could have seen her value as a living person as we did. Evidently, the appeal of death as a "martyr for a cause" was too great. We wish we had been able to prevent her suicide and that she was still writing us letters.

MICHIGAN VERSUS KEVORKIAN

KALMAN J. KAPLAN, PH.D.
Wayne State University and
Michael Reese Hospital and Medical Center

M. CATHERINE MCKEON, R.N.
Wayne State University

ABSTRACT

Our personal reflections on the Michigan versus Kevorkian trial highlight the following issues: 1) the switch from physician-assisted suicide to euthanasia, 2) the television showing of the death, 3) the dropping of the prosecution of the charge of physician-assisted suicide, 4) Kevorkian serving as his own defense attorney, trying to argue that ALS was a secondary cause of Thomas Youk's death, 5) Kevorkian's attempt to employ a logical syllogism to demonstrate that euthanasia need not be murder, 6) Kevorkian's initial reference to the civil rights tradition but sudden change to the medical analogy of Nazi medicine: a *final solution,* 7) the insistence of Kevorkian on "all or nothing" sentencing, 8) the irony of Kevorkian being finally convicted by a prosector who was elected on a platform of not prosecuting Kevorkian, 9) Kevorkian hiring a lawyer after the verdict is in, and 10) Kevorkian's threat to starve himself to death if sent to prison.

It seems impossible to end the section on Kevorkian with anything other than our personal reflections gleaned attending, observing, and studying the Michigan v. Kevorkian trial (March, 1999) in which Kevorkian was prosecuted for his role in the death of Thomas Youk as shown on "60 Minutes" and discussed in a previous article in this volume (Kaplan, O'Dell, Dragovic, McKeon, Bentley, & Telmet, 1999). The experience of our research team in viewing Kevorkian's tapes from the first assisted suicide in 1991 of Janet Adkins to the first acknowledged euthanasia in 1998 of Thomas Youk has been surrealistic, to say the least. This journey has led us many times off the main highway into dimly lit alleys which seemed to be cul-de-sacs. Yet there has always been an unanticipated opening which enabled us to keep traveling on our journey which perhaps inevitably led to the Pontiac Courtroom where Jack Kevorkian was being tried and convicted for murder and the delivery of a controlled substance in the death of Thomas Youk.

A number of issues stand out for us in stark relief:

1. Kevorkian has to convince Youk to let him perform a euthanasia rather than assisted suicide, an issue which became critical as Youk seemed to be attempting to say something as he is being injected. Kevorkian ignores this sound and plunges ahead, an action disquietingly similar to his role in the death of Hugh Gale in 1993 (cf., Kaplan, 1998).

2. Kevorkian has to convince Youk's widow, Melody, and brother, Terry, to allow him to show the tape on national television, an action not in keeping with their description of Youk as a private man.

3. Kevorkian and his defense team are outmaneuvered by the prosecution who drops the assisted suicide charge, thereby excluding the issues of Thomas Youk's pain and suffering as well as the issue of Thomas Youk's consent, neither of which are relevant issues in a trial for murder. Thus the testimony of Melody and Terry Youk are not admissible in the trial, but the tape of his death is. The cleaned up tape seems to reveal a sound emerging from Youk at the point of injection as described above.

4. Kevorkian insists on being his own defense attorney, presumably because he wants to cross-examine his nemesis, Dr. L. J. Dragovic, Medical Examiner of Oakland County and offer his own closing argument. He first tries to show the logical fallacy of the death certificate by showing that ALS was also a cause of Thomas Youk's death, something that Dragovic had previously denied. Comments by members of "Not Dead Yet," an advocacy group for the disabled ubiquitous at the trial are quite telling here. Their take is that the ALS was indeed a secondary cause of death because of Kevorkian's problem with disability pushing him to poison Thomas Youk.

5. Kevorkian attempts to turn his case into a Socratic dialogue involving the legitimacy of euthanasia. Employing Dr. Dragovic's own previous statements and actions, Kevorkian plays the role of philosophy professor in writing the following logical syllogism on a blackboard: (1) Homicide is not necessarily equal to murder, (2) Euthanasia is equal to homicide, and therefore, (3) Euthanasia is not necessarily equal to murder. However, the doctor seems to have ignored the logical fallacy of the undistributed middle. In every day language, the subclass of homicide which is not equal to murder is homicide in self-defense, a category of homicide which euthanasia does not fall into. So Kevorkian is trying to use logic to try to prove the illogical, and is anything but straightforward and indeed rather dissembling in his use of language.

6. Kevorkian begins his closing argument by appealing to the tradition of civil disobedience of Rosa Parks and Martin Luther King. He says words on paper are not necessarily laws. Kevorkian tells jurors he is only doing his duty as a

dedicated physician in following Youk's wishes to end his suffering. However, Kevorkian soon deviates from this tact, as if there is not enough action in it for him. He turns on the prosecutor, John Skrzynski, for being obsessed with the words: "killing" and "murder." Kevorkian claims that he didn't kill anyone, but simply provided a medical service to Youk for the purpose of offering a *final solution* for Thomas Youk's medical problems (c.f., Mitchell, 1999). Kevorkian's public persona does not seem sufficient to contain his ever-active unconscious. How else does one explain such a loaded murderous imagery? From civil rights to Nazi medicine in one gulp should make any serious person ponder Kevorkian and what he stands for very carefully.

7. Kevorkian wants a showdown, wishing Judge Jessica Cooper to give sentencing options of only acquittal or first degree murder. This stance reminds us of Socrates' ultimately suicidal initial push to the jury in Athens to give him free meals at the senate for the rest of his life as his punishment. The prosecution wishes Judge Cooper to offer the jury the intermediary sentencing options as well of second degree murder and involuntary manslaughter. She goes along with the prosecution request. Kevorkian is convicted on the count of second degree murder after a day-and-a-half of deliberations. Members of the jury subsequently indicate that the only issue of dispute for them was whether to convict him on first degree murder (cause, intent, premeditation, and deliberation) or only second degree murder (cause and intent).

8. Ironically, Kevorkian is convicted on March 26, 1999 by the office of Oakland County Prosecutor David Gorcyca who won office against fellow Republican, incumbent and prosecutor in earlier Kevorkian trials, Richard Thompson, Gorcyca's platform: not to prosecute Kevorkian.

9. Subsequent to his conviction, Kevorkian finally decided not to act as his own attorney, turning over his appeal to Southfield lawyer Mayer Morganroth, a nationally known legal mind who had teamed in the past with Kevorkian's previous lawyer, Geoffrey Fieger, to keep Kevorkian clear of convictions in his previous trials.

10. Kevorkian continues to threaten to starve himself to death if he goes to prison, a right he does not have as a prisoner. This quixotic urge to martyrdom speaks volumes as to Kevorkian's fascination with death, whether it be another's or his own.[1]

We wish to make one point in closing. Kevorkian's imagery of a *final solution* is not an innocent slip of the tongue. For someone of Kevorkian's intelligence, this reference is no more an ideal reference than is his white out of forty-seven words in his record of Hugh Gale's death simply a correction of a typo (cf.,

---

[1] Kevorkian was sentenced to a prison term of ten to twenty-five years on April 14, 1999 on the counts of second degree murder and delivery of a controlled substance. There is no sign that Kevorkian, currently in prison, is starving himself.

Kaplan, 1998) or his calling Janet Adkins a heroine in the classical Greek sense (cf., Kaplan, Lachenmeier, Harrow, O'Dell, Uziel, Schneiderhan, & Cheyfitz, 1999-2000) some innocent historical observation. Kevorkian is engaged in a cultural war against traditional Biblical religions and their insistence on the intrinsic and indivisible value of life. Using medical sounding terminology and civil rights rhetoric, Kevorkian is raising the question of who should live and who should die. At heart he is as much a eugenicist as was his heroine, Margaret Saenger of planned parenthood renown. She always wanted people *from some groups* to practice birth control. The selective and nativistic ideas underlying this thinking were conveniently forgotten after the Nazi atrocities became public knowledge and planned parenthood groups cleaned up their act.

For both Kevorkian and Saenger, as well as for Plato (cf., Cheyfitz, 1999-2000), some lives are more worth living than others and it is the role of the physician to help implement this aesthetic. Helping people in distress seems often secondary to this process—from Janet Adkins to Thomas Youk. Belief in a patient's right to die should not blind us to this strain in the Kevorkian type of thinking. We are blinded at our peril, and ignore the possibility that a well-intentioned initiative can lead to disastrous and unintended consequences. This is what the groups of people with disabilities are warning us. If we are wise, we will listen very carefully to them in our crafting of legislation to deal with end-of-life issues.

REFERENCES

Cheyfitz, K. (1999-2000). Who decides: The connecting thread of euthanasia, eugenics and doctor-assisted suicide. *Omega, 40* (1) 5-16 (this issue).

Kaplan, K. J. (1998). The case of Dr. Kevorkian and Mr. Gale: A brief historical note. *Omega, 36,* 169-176.

Kaplan, K. J., Lachenmeier, F., Harrow, M., O'Dell, J., Uziel, O., Schneiderhan, M., & Cheyfitz, K. (1999-2000). Psychosocial versus biomedical risk factors in Kevorkian's first 47 physician-assisted deaths. *Omega, 40* (1), 109-163 (this issue).

Kaplan, K. J., O'Dell, J., Dragovic, L. J., McKeon, M.C., Bentley, E., & Telmet, K. (1999-2000). An update on the Kevorkian-Reding 93 physician-assisted deaths in Michigan: Is Kevorkian a savior, serial-killer or suicidal martyr. *Omega, 40* (1), 209-229 (this issue).

Mitchell, B. (1999-2000). Of euphemisms and euthanasia: The language games of the Nazi doctors and some implications for the modern euthanasia movement. *Omega, 40* (1) 255-265 (this issue).

PHYSICIAN, HATE THYSELF:
COMMENTS ON THE KEVORKIAN TAPES

DAVID GUTMANN
Northwestern University Medical School
Chicago, Illinois

What follows are some impressions gleaned from viewing the videotape of Dr. Kevorkian interviewing Janet Adkins, a candidate for assisted suicide, two days before he helped to put her down. Mrs. Adkins appeared with her husband, who confirmed that his wife was suffering from an early stage dementing illness, entailing some forgetfulness of tennis scores, personal belongings, etc. He was in complete accord with the planned suicide. At the outset, Mrs. Adkins seemed—in her manner, in her mood and in her alertness—to contradict the diagnosis: she appeared to be a vigorous, seemingly healthy and "together" middle-aged woman; hardly a candidate for snuffing. However, as the interview wore on, as her husband provided detailed testimony on her deterioration, and as Dr. Kevorkian eulogized her decision, Mrs. Adkins became indecisive, increasingly mute, and reliant on her husband for direction. She became, in effect, the living illustration of her diagnostic label. Almost as if there was an osmotic exchange of psychic contents, Kevorkian waxed as his "patient" faltered and waned. Once her agreement to die had been secured and registered, Kevorkian became relaxed, expansive, filled with his sense of mission: "Not since the Greeks . . . !" he declaims, has mankind been so liberated from the stigma of "therapeutic" suicide. The comments that follow are reactive to these later passages of Kevorkian's snuff tape.

For starters, Kevorkian comes through as disquietingly chipper, up-beat; he enjoys his work: there is little or no sense of a tragic personal event; instead, he escapes from the personal dimension into the depersonalized historic sphere. From this Olympian perch, the fate of one mere damaged mortal—Ms. Adkins—becomes inconsequential. Meanwhile, the doctor, as the agent of historic change, elevates himself. Nowhere does Dr. K. appear to be oppressed by the knowledge that in two days he will participate in killing a patient; instead, he is self-congratulatory about his pioneering role. As for Ms. Adkins, in his view she should also be pleased, even grateful that she has been given a bit part in this epochal event.

I am not necessarily chilled by the idea of a doctor participating in a suicide; that happens routinely, and often enough, I am sure, for good reasons. I am not against assisted suicide per se; but I am stunned and frightened when Dr. Kevorkian shows me that a doctor, with the power to kill, can take so much pleasure and derive so much self-esteem from all the activities entailed in putting a patient down.

There is some personal history behind that last statement. Incidental to my cross-cultural studies of the aging process, for a number of years I talked with Mayan Curanderos, as well as Navajo medicine men and their patients; and across these disparate societies there was a common theme: distrust of the powerful Shaman. His powers are seen as double-edged, and the healer as potentially double-faced—as a medicine man he can serve life, as a sorcerer/ witch he can bring death. The shaman is always under the suspicion that he will, as the Navajo put it, go to the "Bad Side," use his powers for personal gain, and become death's agent. Viewing these tapes, I finally grasp what they were warning against: In them, I see Kevorkian the doctor become Kevorkian the witch. He urges killing, he assists in killing—and, most important—I see him taking pleasure in killing, and in the deadly exercise of his special powers.

Again, there is nothing new about the killing per se; along with Eros, Thanatos is the great theme of human affairs. But participation in killing is usually charged with tragic emotions—terror, guilt, and remorse. Why then does Kevorkian whistle as he works? What gives him permission to combine these usually mutually exclusive categories, of murder and pleasure? I think it is because the good doctor has, in his own eyes, gained some redeeming legitimacy. His assistance in suicide is self-sanctified: He partakes of killing in the name of a higher law—in the name of LIFE itself. The superego—the internal warden against the Eros of killing—is off his back; and so he can enjoy both the participation in suicide, and the self-esteem that comes with public service: the bonus of a good conscience.

For me, the Kevorkian example sheds light on the larger issue, of assisted suicide. It teaches me at least that we should be very careful about making laws to justify killing. Kevorkian is unusual: he is a law unto himself, a law-maker rather than a law receiver. But most of us do require external sanction, usually from the system of formal laws, before we can shift the burden of conscience away from ourselves, and onto the targets for punishment that the law has designated or permitted. But once the law has accredited killing, when the superego is put on the side of killing, then sure as Hell, you are going to get lots of killing. Warfare is, of course our best example: the nation defines killing as a duty, the superego becomes the advocate rather than the antagonist of murder, and the enthusiastic slaughter begins.

As a professional class, doctors are certainly not immune from the temptations of legalized killing. Most doctors do have the vocation, the identity of "Death fighter," but a minority—small in number perhaps, but significant in their potential for harm—use the practice of medicine as a defense against the Thanatos within themselves. So as not to murder, they fight for life. It is only their professional superego that guards their patients—and themselves—against the submerged appetite for killing. But when the laws of professional practice accredit homicide, then the internal law-giver, the Superego is diminished, and a significant minority of practitioners—the enthusiastic Nazi doctors, the Tuskegee experimenters, for example—will declare themselves, front and center.

Euthanasia and assisted suicide are established but generally unacknowledged medical practices. They will go on; they should go on. But a necessary hypocrisy is required. For doctors, such extreme measures should never be routinized or legitimated by law. They should always remain measures of last resort: covert, shrouded in secrecy, guilt, doubt, and endless self-questioning. As Ingmar Bergman put it in the movie "Wild Strawberries," "The first duty of the doctor is to ask forgiveness." Physician, hate thyself. Again, the medical Superego is the patient's ultimate protection, the patient's last line of defense against the power of the physician. Weaken that, and "Que Messieurs les assassins commencent . . . !" ("Let the honorable killers begin"). It would not take much legal sanction to move far too many doctors from the status of healer to the status of witch.

LOOKING DEATH IN THE EYE:
ANOTHER CHALLENGE FROM DOCTOR KEVORKIAN

ROBERT KASTENBAUM
Arizona State University, Tempe

Scarcely a voice was raised in opposition when Herman Feifel (1959) asserted that the subject of death had become taboo in the United States and other technologically advanced nations. Once pointed out, the evidence was too pervasive to deny. This recognition, however, did not necessarily mean that society was ready to rescind the taboo—after all, it had developed for a reason and was serving a purpose. As we entered the 1960s there was little to suggest a vigorous death awareness movement. The palliative and interpersonal needs of terminally ill people were seldom addressed, nor the anxiety, sorrow, and vulnerability of family members. There were no courses on death education and counselling, few articles and books written on the subject, even fewer based upon empirical research, and no journals devoted to understanding the human encounter with death. Both peer support groups and national professional organizations were also some years away. By and large, society continued to close its eyes and look away when Death came visiting (allowing always for the robust public fascination with violent death). Still years ahead were the high profile litigations, court decisions, public debates, and media coverage of end-of-life issues.

Omega entered the picture in 1970 as the first regularly published peer-reviewed journal on dying, death, grief, suicide, and related topics—just in time to contribute to the many developments that would mark this decade. During those formative years the center of attention was the need to improve understanding and care for terminally ill people and their families, a broad-spectrum effort that included clinical, research, and educational components. Three decades later, this concern is still very much with us, but another issue has also emerged. Should physician-assisted death be accepted or rejected? On what basis should this decision be made? And who should make the decision? This issue of

Omega has been expanded to offer findings and interpretations that illuminate the physician-assisted death controversy.

This brief article, a reflection by the editor, does not attempt to add anything to the topic that has been so extensively examined throughout this issue of *Omega* as well as in many other publications. Instead, the purpose is to revisit a particular glimmering in the pre-dawn hours of the death awareness movement that was overlooked at the time and which has received little attention since. Perhaps most remarkably, this neglected contribution was made by a person who for some years now has been at the center of the physician-assisted death controversy. There is perhaps something to be learned by exhuming an article written by a pathologist then unknown to the public at a time when very few people in any of the allied health or social and behavioral science fields were addressing themselves to death-related issues.

"THE EYE IN DEATH"

None of the commonly accepted signs of death can be fully relied upon to answer the question, "Is this person really dead? (Kevorkian, 1961, p. 54).

Kevorkian begins with the reminder that physicians occasionally find themselves "assailed by uncertainty" in trying to determine whether or not a patient is dead. He offers the view that:

The border between "life" and absolute, irremediable, biological death is a hazy *area* rather than a sharp *line,* as judged by practically all clinical methods. Breathing that has apparently stopped will sustain life for some minutes. . . . In such cases, if artificial respiration or endotracheal oxygen or administration of some stimulant induces a return of respiration, it is obvious that the patient was never actually dead (p. 51).

Cessation of respiration, probably the most relied upon indice of death through the centuries, can lead to false positive conclusions. Kevorkian refers to Negovski's (1944-1945) review of the literature which found instances of people recovering from apnea as long as twenty-five minutes, as well as his own report of an asphyxiated infant reviving after two hours and forty-one minutes of apnea.

Kevorkian notes that even the introduction of electroencephalographic (EEG) and electrocardiographic (EKG) testing has not entirely resolved the question. He mentions cases in which the brain has produced electrical waves "for as long as 9 minutes after the EKG indicates cardiac arrest" (p. 51). Kevorkian also cites cases in which either EEG or EKG activity had ceased, but the other measure had continued for some time.

At this point in his article, Kevorkian is well supported by the historical record. In researching the question of live burial some years, I came across many examples of apparent false positives (i.e., a living person taken for dead). Perhaps the most compelling was an article published in *The Transylvanian Journal of Medicine* in 1835. Dr. Nathanial Shrock's uncle had suffered a temporary paralysis and events were bringing him rapidly to the coffin and grave before his plight was discovered. Shrock's article was intended to alert fellow physicians to the dangers of making hasty judgments based on a single criterion. He identified and critiqued twelve of the most common indices of death (summarized in Kastenbaum & Aisenberg, 1972). According to Shrock, physicians could and did make errors when they did not attend carefully to all the physical signs and consider alternative explanations. Years later, Dr. Charles Barker (1897) found it necessary to advise his colleagues that special conditions (e.g., hypothermia, drugs, trance) could lead to errors in certifying death. He suggested that physicians should resolve uncertainties by attempting to induce or encourage life rather than to make cursory diagnostic observations.

The socio-technical context of life-and-death determinations had changed since the writings of Shrock and Barker. Kevorkian seemed to recognize that even more change was on the way. Difficulties in determining the moment of death would become more common, therefore a more reliable form of assessment would become even more useful.

RETINAL SIGNS OF DEATH

This subheading, borrowed from Kevorkian, makes clear the approach that he favored. The physician faced with making an alive-or-dead determination in an ambiguous situation should be equipped with an ophthalmoscope, a familiar instrument that is used to examine the status of the eye. He reports on his own observations of retinal status in patients before and after their death. This report includes summary of findings from his ophthalmoscopic observations of fifty-one consecutive cases (Kevorkian, 1957) as well as presentation of two case histories.

Kevorkian's findings of eye status at death included (1) segmentation and interruption of blood circulation, (2) a haziness of the cornea, and (3) appearance of homogeneity and paleness. Cooling and the cessation of tears is also noted. Attention is given as well to the sequence of change from premortem to various periods of time after the moment of death. Kevorkian was therefore providing guidelines both for helping to determine the actual moment of death as it occurs and for estimating the time elapsed since death. He reminds physicians that retinal status, like other indices, is influenced by the general condition of the patient (e.g., age) and environmental factors (e.g., temperature).

His message to fellow physicians:

> 1. A thirty-second examination with an ophthalmoscope will provide more accurate information on the circulatory status and the exact time of irreversible biologic death, and the time since death, than can be obtained from all other criteria combined.

2. As in other fields, practice and experience are required before proficiency and confidence can be gained (p. 62).

WHAT LESSONS TO BE LEARNED?

There is something to be learned both from Kevorkian's observations and the response or nonresponse from the death awareness movement. We begin with a politically incorrect consideration of the relationship between personal characteristics of the researcher and the nature of the research.

Why is this Man Looking into the Eyes of Dead People?

It *is* politically incorrect to ask such questions. Many researchers and scholars have developed within a tradition that casts us as objective instruments of the truth. Neither individual personality nor political agenda are supposed to influence inquiry. It is unbecoming to suggest that a scientific truth-seeker is driven by a private passion: our focus should be on method and findings alone. Nevertheless, it has been known for years that observer effects occur throughout the broad spectrum of scientific and scholarly inquiry. In fact, many ethnographers insist that interpretation is inherent and must be taken into account every step of the way, from choice of topic through observational processes and conclusions. Not all investigators would go that far, but there is certainly a strong case to be made for recognition of the role of personal and situational influences in the inquiry process.

In the real world, we usually recognize that people have reasons for their significant life choices. Not everybody wants to be a physician, for example, and not every physician chooses to be a pathologist. We are not passing negative judgment on each other when we note that we have made some markedly different choices of career and lifestyle, and that these choices probably were not on a random basis. It would be a serious matter if we alleged that reports of scientific or scholarly inquiry were intentionally misrepresented in the service of a personal or political agenda. Simply having a powerful reason for conducting a study, however, does not imply lack of integrity in method and/or interpretation. Nevertheless, it is not improper to be curious about the work of people whose own curiosity has taken them into new or unusual paths of inquiry.

Why, then, did Kevorkian look into the eyes of dead people, especially during a socio-cultural frame within which few health care professionals showed much interest in dying, death, and grief? Three reasons suggest themselves:

1. Because the status of the eye at death was a biomedical question that had received relatively little attention.

2. Because the determination of the moment of death has practical consequences and can be subject to error.

3. Because . . .

Either of the first two reasons would clearly justify Kevorkian's research, and his work contributed to both the scientific and clinical side of the question. It is the less explicit reason that may be of particular interest to those who contribute to the care and understanding of terminally ill people and their families. Kevorkian has had an abiding interest in death throughout his life. He had already been given the sobriquet, "Doctor Death" by his fellow students in medical school, and largely because he had already demonstrated his interest in the moments just preceding and just following death.

From medical school days to his years of practice, Kevorkian was fascinated by the moment of death. He was not among the many oncologists who were then trying to extend the lives of suffering patients, nor was he among the few innovators of palliative care. Instead Kevorkian was right where he needed to be if he was to explore the mysterious zone between "alive" and "dead." Later he would become increasingly aware of the plight of terminally ill people who endured unrelieved pain and received little comfort from their physicians. He would then become the man known to the media, a feisty retired pathologist who reviled physicians for neglect of dying patients and offered assisted death as the solution.

Kevorkian looked into the eyes of dying and dead people for the two practical reasons already mentioned, but also because of a passion for investigating death and the dead that is uncommon in our society. The examples best known to the public are probably the "mad scientist" genre of science fantasy and horror films and books which mostly hearken back to philosophically-inspired gothic tales of the past century, notably Mary Wollstonecraft Shelley's *Frankenstein: Or the Modern Prometheus* (1974), and Bram Stoker's *Dracula* (1975). Here we begin to learn something about ourselves. Scientists who investigate the borderlands of life and death must be mad, twisted, and warped. Why should we think so? They are also frequently rendered as caricatures and parodies. What is so funny about life and death reaching out to touch each other? It is anxious-funny, is it not? Long before Kevorkian started his mid-twentieth century inquiries, our society had decided that the anxieties aroused by such inquiries must be moderated by branding the "perpetrators" as mad, and by converting a philosophical-scientific endeavor into something that should be played for laughs.

Kevorkian, then, walked right into a powerful negative stereotype that shadows him to this day. We can hardly envision what he has done and what he advocates without a shiver of—what? Revulsion? Anger? Terror? All of the above?

The specifics of Kevorkian's adventurings toward death include:

- Holding a (possibly) dead person's eyelids open and staring eye-to-eye through his hand-held optic instrument at the closest possible range.

- Transfusing cadaver blood into a living person (a consenting friend)
- Advocating the establishing of "obitorias" that would make intensive studies of the dying and newly-dead (Kevorkian, 1991).
- Creating vivid surrealistic paintings, many of which are dominated by death-related themes and piercing eyes—closer to nightmare visions than to politically correct depictions.

Additionally, Kevorkian has championed the cause of organ donations by condemned prisoners. This advocacy is not, however, as challenging to individual and societal sensibilities as his more "up close and personal" approaches to death and the dead.

The foundational "because" for Kevorkian's fascination with death and the dead most likely is based on one of the most appalling episodes in twentieth-century history: the genocidal attacks on the Armenian people by Turkish extremists during the World War I period. This horror has had enduring resonations up to this day, but insufficiently comprehended except by those who were immediately affected. Kevorkian was born about a decade after the height of the slaughter. He is a child of the Armenian genocide as others are children of The Holocaust. He is not just a child, but a partial orphan of this genocide. Many of those who would have been family to him did not survive. Where are they? Someplace else, across that distance that separates life from death, a distance that can seem as slight as a breath, but bridgeable only through the power of imagination.

Kevorkian and the Death Awareness Movement

During the last decade of the twentieth century, Kevorkian has been one of the most influential figures in the death awareness of both public and professionals in the United States, and to some extent throughout the world as well. Nevertheless, he has had little direct connection with the mainstream death awareness movement. Kevorkian does not seem to be acquainted with the contributions made by death educators, counselors, and researchers over the past four decades, nor has he entered into dialogue with them. He has demonstrated little knowledge of hospice and palliative care developments over the past quarter of a century. One cannot say that he even has any interest in what others have done. In an era of communication and teamwork, Kevorkian is notable for his self-selected apartness.

Kevorkian's disinterest in and/or rejection of the death awareness movement is scarcely endearing to those who have taken risks, labored, and persevered to improve attitudes, knowledge and human services in the sphere of terminal illness, dying, grief, and suicide. Mainstream "deathniks" (as we called ourselves for awhile) also have our own peculiarities, though. Our own research has been focusing much more on grief than the dying process, and much more on the dying process than on the moment of death and its meaning. We need not apologize for focusing on the ways in which people try to cope with dying and grieving, but it is at least *curious* that "death itself" and the final moments of life have received so little attention (Kastenbaum, 1993, in press). This is not the place to discuss the specific issues involved here, but there is cause for reflection on the limited attention that has been given to the death part of the death awareness movement. We might or might not endorse Kevorkian's approach, but we have not been doing much ourselves, with the possible exception of speculations associated with near-death experiences.

I believe Kevorkian has earned the right to be obsessed with death and the dead, a blood-right, if you like. What he has done, what he is doing, and what he advocates makes some of us very uncomfortable (myself included). However, as already noted, part of our negative response may derive from personal and societal anxieties about approaching the symbolically dangerous borderlands between life and death. Most of us have not looked death in the eye as he has done, nor have we devoted much effort to discovering other ways of doing so. If Kevorkian still has to explain why he is so interested in death, then perhaps we have a little explaining to do ourselves: why have "deathniks" found so many other things to do instead?

It does not disturb me that the person at the center of the physician-assisted death controversy is so strongly motivated, persistent, and risk-taking. It does disturb me that he has shown no inclination to expand his knowledge base and learn from others. A professional pathologist, he is not qualified as palliative care specialist, psychiatrist, psychologist, social worker, or nurse, to identify some of the types of expertise that could be called upon when people are in situations desperate enough to make death seem the solution. Dismissing this man as fanatic or criminal, however, might be to dismiss the unsettling issues he has engaged. If we are not ready to look death in the eye, perhaps we can start by looking Jack Kevorkian in the eye.

REFERENCES

Barker, C. F. (1897). On real and apparent death. *Clinical Medicine, 18*, 232-238.

Feifel, H. (Ed.) (1959). *The meaning of death.* New York: McGraw-Hill.

Kastenbaum, R. (In press). The moment of death: Is hospice making a difference? *The Hospice Journal.*

Kastenbaum, R. (1993). Last words. *The Monist, An International Journal of General Philosophical Inquiry, 76,* 270-290.

Kastenbaum, R., & Aisenberg, R. B. (1972). *The psychology of death.* (First edition). New York: Springer.

Kevorkian, J. (1957). Rapid and accurate ophthalmoscopic determination of circulatory arrest. *Journal of the American Medical Association, 164,* 1660 ff.

Kevorkian, J. (1961) The eye in death. *CIBA Clinical Symposia, 13,* 51-62.

Kevorkian, J. (1991). *Prescription: Medicide.* Buffalo, NY: Prometheus.

Negovski, V. A. (1944-1945). Agonal states and clinical death: Problems in revival of organisms. *American Review of Social Medicine, 2,* 304-316.

Shelley, M. (1974). *Frankenstein: Or, the modern Prometheus.* Indianapolis: Bobbs-Merrill.

Shrock, N. M. (1835). On the signs that distinguish real from apparent death. *Transylvanian Journal of Medicine, 13,* 210-220.

Stoker, B. (1975). *Dracula.* In L. Wolf (Ed.), *The annotated Dracula.* New York: Clarkson N. Potter.

SUMMARY

KALMAN J. KAPLAN, PH.D.
Wayne State University and
Michael Reese Hospital and Medical Center

This volume has presented a number of theoretical and empirical articles on the topic of euthanasia, physician-assisted suicide, and suicide. These articles have explored the effects of age, as in high school, college, or adult populations, and the issues of God, state, or individual control with regard to end of life decisions. We have also examined the first extended data available in America—in-depth analysis of Dr. Kevorkian's first forty-seven acknowledged suicides—in terms of biological versus psychosocial factors (Kaplan, Lachenmeier, Harrow et al., 1999). The role of gender, age, social economic status, ethnic-national-religious ancestry, and marital status have been examined in-depth through quasi-psychological autopsies conducted on these first forty-seven cases, often with very troubling implications. Important information has been obtained from secondary sources on some of the later cases of Kevorkian and his colleague, Dr. Reding as well (Canetto & Hollenshead, 1999-2000). Finally, we present an up-to-date analysis on all ninety-three publicly identified cases as of November 25, 1998 (Kaplan, O'Dell, Dragovic et al., 1999-2000). In addition, we present some preliminary work on seven cases of physician-assisted suicide in Australia (Kissane, Street, & Nitschke, 1998; Street & Kissane, 1999-2000).

Gender and age bias in particular seem to run like a thin but discernible red thread throughout these studies and also in a trio of attitude studies. Male high school students seem to be more accepting of doctor-assisted suicide for females. Female students are more tolerant of DAS for men (Kaplan & Bratman, 1999-2000). Younger people seem more accepting of doctor-assisted suicide than their elders, at least when it refers to the conceptual issue rather than the specific personal application and to others rather than for themselves. The preponderance of disability as opposed to terminality in the Kevorkian-Reding cases raises a red flag, suggesting that the fears of advocacy groups for people with disabilities may not be unfounded.

Pain seems to operate differently for men and women. In one of the most striking findings regarding the Kevorkian patients, similar proportions of men and women report pain. However, when the physiological underpinnings are examined, the two genders are radically different. Autopsies often show no anatomical basis for the pain among the pain-reporting women. What is it, then, that the women are reporting? Phantom pain, psychological misery? Finally the sheer preponderance of women in the Kevorkian patients is disquieting, resembling more the ratio of attempted suicides in America rather than completed suicides. In other words, do the women going to Kevorkian (or any health professional) want him to assist them or prevent them? This complicated question must be explored in all its ramifications.

What becomes clear is the non-uniqueness of the Kevorkian-Reding Michigan sample. Despite the flamboyant nature of Kevorkian, people going to him and Reding to seek physician-assisted suicide may not be so different from those seeking this same solution in the Netherlands, in the northern provinces of Australia, and in Oregon. The average age is over fifty, and in both Michigan and Australia, terminality is higher among men than women, and the majority of all these samples are women. This last point must be qualified with regard to the Dutch sample. Canetto and Hollenshead (1999-2000) correctly point to the greater proportion of men as opposed to women among "assisted suicide" end-of-life decisions in the Netherlands. However, the opposite trend occurs among the far more numerous "euthanasia" end-of-life decisions (van der Maas et al., 1996). The unique Dutch definitions of "physician-assisted suicide" and "euthanasia" make this difference understandable in an American context. The Dutch definition of physician-assisted suicide (i.e., the prescription or supplying of a drug to a patient to enable him to kill himself) is more like the American definition of unaided completed suicide (where males are predominant) while the Dutch definition of euthanasia (i.e., the doctor administering these drugs to the patient) is more like the Michigan definition of doctor-assisted suicides (where females seem predominant). This points to the importance of standardizing definitions in cross-cultural comparisons. In all three of the samples, more women than men opt for physician-assisted suicide, though this act is labeled euthanasia in the Netherlands. Also critical here is the emergence of "angels of death" hastened death specialists in these other venues (cf., Hendin, 1998).

Finally, the ubiquitous economic issue must be addressed. How much of the push toward legalizing doctor-assisted suicide is motivated by economic factors? Is it pure coincidence that the first state, Oregon, to legalize doctor-assisted suicide is also the first state to ration medical care to the recipients of Medicaid? Or does the mind-set in Oregon represent a lethal dialectic of the left's concern with civil liberties and the right's concern with cost-cutting, a dialectic which is ready to sacrifice the economically disadvantaged either passively (through limiting the number of medical and surgical procedures that will be paid for by society) or actively (through encouraging doctor-assisted suicide). The unholy alliance between the left and the right on this death solution eerily reflects the unanimity in 1933 Germany across the political spectrum with regard to applying the concept of racial hygiene (Franzblau, 1995; Lifton, 1986) and the ambivalent relationship between the doctor and killing (Gutmann, 1999-2000; Lifton, 1986). Licensing the patient's right for a physician-assisted death also licensed the physician's right to kill.

Mitchell (1996, 1999) shows us how insidious the metaphors regarding terms such as "quality of life" became in Nazi medicine. The road to Aushwitz was paved in the euthanasia project under the banner of liberating sick and disabled people from their suffering. Their lives were completely written off with the euphemism of "dasein ohne leiben" (existence without life). Leaving aside the analogy to Nazi euphemisms, it is worrisome that doctor-assisted death, whether passive or active, is likely to always remain within the patient's control. Consider a recent proposed policy by the Houston City Task Force on Medical Futility (Halevy & Brody, 1996). Arguing for the principle of a fundamental balance between patient autonomy and physician integrity, Halevy and Brody propose a procedure whereby doctors can choose to withdraw life support from a patient against the patient's or the family's wishes if the life support is judged futile or likely to lead to a poor "quality of life." Dinwiddie (1999-2000) points to psychodynamic issues in the doctor's response to "end of life" requests and Schneiderhan (1999-2000) stresses the problematic role of the pharmacist in this procedure. Often the pharmacist may not know for what purpose he is filling a prescription—to treat a patient or to hasten his death. Unfortunately, there is very little data on many of the above issues and a blurring of a good number of subtle issues (cf. Emanuel & Emanuel, 1992; Kaplan, Lachenmeier, Harrow et al., 1999-2000).

Clearly, not every doctor supporting physician-assisted death is an advocate of Nazi medical hygiene. However, not every patient seeking doctor-assisted suicide is terminal (indeed, most of Kevorkian's were not, especially the women) nor are all of them racked with excruciating, unbearable pain. Indeed, in six cases, no anatomical evidence of any disease emerged at autopsy. In the service of providing a theoretical framework to better discuss these issues, guide research and craft legislation, we conclude this volume by proposing a multifaceted model of doctor-assisted death focusing as a good reporter, on the six pronouns: who, what, where, when, why, and how (c.f., Wooddell & Kaplan, 1998).

Who makes the decision to end the patient's life, whether through active intervention, or passive withdrawal. Is it the patient, the family, the doctor, the institution or the government itself? What are the mechanisms for adjudication if different parties disagree? Does the patient have the final say in this? What is the process of proxy representation if the patient is not able to articulate his/her wishes?

What is the action taken? Is it simply the withdrawal of a life-supporting service or substance, or is it the introduction of a life-ending service or substance? The first procedure has traditionally been referred to as passive and the latter as active, but the difference may be more subtle than this.

Where is the action to be performed? In the patient's home, a hospital, a hospice center or a center specifically designed for this purpose? What are the implications of the particular venue in terms of pressure put on the patients?

When is the decision made in the course of a disease? When is the advanced directive obtained? Is it renewed? There is no evidence as to the time reliability of these decisions. A patient in a healthy state may feel he would want to die if some hypothetical catastrophe happened, and feel quite differently if it actually did happen. In short people adjust to their life space. The opposition of many disabled people to the idea of doctor-assisted suicide provides ample evidence of this contention.

Why is the decision made? Is the patient in physical or emotional pain/ depression, or psychological distress imposed by societal pressures. The Wooddell and Kaplan (1999-2000) and the Kaplan and Bratman (1999-2000) studies point to the extreme sensitivities of how this issue is worded. For example, wording the patient's distress as emotional pain may make physician-assisted suicide more acceptable while wording it as depression may make the alternative less acceptable. The results of these two studies suggest that the doctor's role in the patient's decision (whether discussing, accepting, or encouraging) may be more important in people's judgment than the act itself. Is the patient pressured by family, by the doctor, or institution? Also, what are the economic considerations?

How is the decision implemented? Is the doctor observing the act, assisting or performing the act itself? Is there a mechanism in place for the patient to change his/her mind and reverse the process? The case of Hugh Gale, Kevorkian's thirteenth acknowledged patient (Kaplan, 1997), raises the specter of a patient changing his mind and not being able to reverse the consequences.

We hope this set of questions provides a framework in which to consider the weighty issue of doctor aid in dying. One thing is clear. The doctor's obligation to help a patient die is not identical with the doctor's aid in helping the patient kill himself. Prematurely assisting the patient to kill oneself represents as fundamental and abandonment of the dying patient as turning one's back on his distress (Kaplan & Schwartz, 1998, 1999-2000).

REFERENCES

Canetto, S. S., & Hollenshead, J. D. (1999-2000) Gender and physician-assisted suicide: An analysis of the Kevorkian cases, 1990-1997. *Omega, 40* (1), 165-208 (this issue).

Dinwiddie, S. (1999-2000). Potential psychodynamic factors in doctor-assisted suicide. *Omega, 40* (1), 101-108 (this issue).

Emanuel, E., & Emanuel, L. (1992). Four models of the physician-patient relationship. *Journal of the American Medical Association, 267*, 2221-2226.

Franzblau, M. (1995). Ethical values in health care in 1995: Lessons from the Nazi period. *The Journal of the Medical Association of Georgia, 84*, 161-164.

Gutmann, D. (1999-2000). Physician, hate thyself—Comments on the Kevorkian tapes. *Omega, 40* (1), 275-277 (this issue).

Halevy, A. & Brody, B. A. (1996). A multi-institution collaborative policy on medical futility. *Journal of the American Medical Association, 276* (7), 571-574.

Hendin, M. C. (1998). *Seduced by death: Doctors, patients and assisted suicide* (pp. 124-127). New York: W. W. Norton and Company.

Kaplan, K. J. (1997). Dr. Kevorkian and Mr. Gale. *Omega, 36,* 169-176.

Kaplan, K. J. (1998b). *TILT: Teaching Individuals to Live Together.* London, UK: Taylor & Francis.

Kaplan, K. J., & Bratman, E. (1999-2000). Gender, pain, and doctor involvement: High school student attitudes toward doctor-assisted suicide. *Omega, 40* (1), 27-41 (this issue).

Kaplan, K. J., Lachenmeier, F., Harrow, M., O'Dell, J., Uziel, O. Schneiderhan, M., & Cheyfitz, K. (1999-2000). Psychosocial versus biomedical risk factors in Kevorkian's first 47 physician-assisted deaths. *Omega, 40* (1), 109-163 (this issue).

Kaplan, K. J., O'Dell, J., Uziel, O., Dragovic, L. J., McKeon, M. C., Bentley, E., & Telmet, K. (1999-2000). An update on the Kevorkian-Reding 93 physician-assisted deaths in Michigan: Is Kevorkian a savior, serial-killer or suicidal martyr? *Omega, 40* (1), 209-228 (this issue).

Kaplan, K. J., & Leonhardi, M. (1997). Kevorkian, Martha Wichorek and us: A personal account. *Newslink, 23,* 9-10.

Kaplan, K. J., & Schwartz, M. (1998). Watching over patient's life and death: Kevorkian, Hippocrates and Maimonides. *Ethics and Medicine, 14* (2), 49-53.

Kaplan, K. J., & Schwartz, M. B. (1999-2000). Hippocrates, Maimonides, and the doctor's responsibility. *Omega, 40* (1), 17-26 (this issue).

Kissane, D. W., Street, A., & Nitschke, P. (1998). Seven deaths in Darwin: Case studies under the Rights of the Terminally Ill Act, Northern Territory in Australia. *The Lancet, 352,* 1097-1102.

Lifton, R. J. (1986). *The Nazi doctors.* New York: Basic Books.

Mitchell, B. (1996). Nazi Germany's euphemisms. In J. F. Kilner, A. B. Miller, & E. D. Pellegrino (Eds.), *Dignity and dying: A Christian appraisal* (pp. 123-134). Grand Rapids, MI: William B. Eerdmans.

Mitchell, B. (1999-2000). Of euphemisms and euthanasia: The language games of the Nazi doctors and some implications for the modern euthanasia movement. *Omega, 40* (1) 255-265 (this issue).

Schneiderhan, M. (1999-2000). Physician-assisted suicide and euthanasia: The pharmacist's perspective. *Omega, 40* (1), 89-99 (this issue).

Street, A., & Kissane, D. (1999-2000). Dispensing death, desiring death: An exploration of medical roles and patient motivation during the period of legalized euthanasia in Australia. *Omega, 40* (1), 231-248 (this issue).

van der Maas, P., van der Wal, G., Haverkate, I., de Graaff, C. L. M., Kester, J. G. C., Onwuteaka-Philipsen, B. D., van der Heide, A., Bosma, J. M., & Willems, D. L. (1996). Euthanasia, physician-assisted suicide, and other medical practices involving the end of life in the Netherlands, 1990-1995. *New England Journal of Medicine, 335* (22), 1699-1705.

Wooddell, V., & Kaplan, K. (1998). An expanded typology of suicide, assisted suicide and euthanasia. *Omega, 36,* 219-226.

Wooddell, V., & Kaplan, K. (1999-2000). Effect of the doctor on college students' attitudes toward physician-assisted suicide. *Omega, 40* (1), 43-60 (this issue).

OMEGA—Journal of Death and Dying

Editor: KENNETH J. DOKA

Providing multidisciplinary studies and perspective on dying, death, bereavement, suicide, and other lethal behaviors for over two decades.

MANAGING EDITOR
MICHON LARTIGUE

EDITORIAL BOARD
JEAN QUINT BENOLIEL
ALBERT C. CAIN
LAWRENCE G. CALHOUN
SILVIA SARA CANETTO
MICHAEL CASERTA
CHARLES A. CORR
GEORGE DOMINO
JOSEPH A. DURLAK
NORMAN L. FARBEROW
HERMAN FEIFEL
VICTOR FLORIAN
ROBERT FULTON
EARL A. GROLLMAN
GERALD GRUMAN
KALMAN J. KAPLAN
DENNIS KLASS
RONALD KOENIG
MYRA BLUEBOND
  LANGNER
DAVID LESTER
DAN LEVITON
BRIAN L. MISHARA
RUSSELL NOYES
C.M. PARKES
VANDERLYN R. PINE
THERESE A. RANDO
RICHARD SCHULZ
BERNARD SPILKA
STEVEN STRACK
MARGARET S. STROEBE
WOLFANG STROEBE
DAVID K. SWITZER
DONALD TEMPLER
AVERY D. WEISMAN

AIMS AND SCOPE:

OMEGA: Journal of Death and Dying brings insight into terminal illness; the process of dying, bereavement, mourning, funeral customs, suicide. Fresh, lucid, responsible contributions from knowledgeable professionals in universities, hospitals, clinics, old age homes, suicide prevention centers, funeral directors and others, concerned with thanatology and the impact of death on individuals and the human community.

OMEGA is a rigorously peer-refereed journal. Drawing significant contributions from the fields of psychology, sociology, medicine, anthropology, law, education, history and literature, *OMEGA* has emerged as an internationally recognized forum on the subject of death and dying. It will serve as a reliable guide for clinicians, social workers, and health professionals who must deal with problems in crisis management, e.g., terminal illness, fatal accidents, catastrophe, suicide and bereavement.

SUBSCRIPTION INFORMATION:

Sold as a 2 volume group - 8 issues yearly.
ISSN: 0030-2228
Rates: $238.00 Institutional, $65.00 Individual
Postage & handling: $14.00 U.S. & Canada,
$25.00 elsewhere

—*Complimentary sample issue available upon request*—

Baywood Publishing Company, Inc.
26 Austin Avenue, Amityville, NY 11701 / (631) 691-1270 Fax (631) 691-1770
Orderline—**call toll-free** (800) 638-7819
e-mail: baywood@baywood.com **web site:** http://baywood.com